Advanced Personal Training

T0386488

Effective fitness instruction and training programme design require a specialist trainer to combine professional experience with strategies underpinned by scientific evidence. This book allows readers to develop their understanding of the scientific rationale behind important components of personal training, such as monitoring fitness and training programme design. Each chapter synthesizes the findings of cutting-edge scientific research to identify optimum training methods and dispel some myths that are prevalent in the fitness industry.

The chapters within this new edition have been written by internationally renowned experts from several disciplines, including strength and conditioning, physiology, psychology, and nutrition. Contributions have also been made from esteemed academics who have conducted some of the scientific studies discussed within the book. The authors have interpreted and summarised the scientific evidence and produced evidence-based recommendations, allowing readers to explore the latest concepts and research findings and apply them in practice. The book includes several new chapters, such as evidence-based practice (EBP), and designing training programmes specifically for women, older adults, and expectant mothers.

This second edition remains the essential text for fitness instructors, personal trainers, and sport and exercise students. The book provides an invaluable resource for fitness courses, exercise science degree programmes, and continued professional development for exercise professionals.

Paul Hough is a Senior Lecturer in Sport and Exercise Science at Oxford Brookes University. He began his career in the fitness industry while studying sport science and strength and conditioning. Paul is a BASES accredited Sport and Exercise Scientist, providing sport/exercise science support to professional and amateur athletes, members of the public, and various organisations. Paul has worked with elite level athletes from several sports, including athletics, tennis, and Formula One. Paul has undertaken research projects as a lead and assistant investigator and published several studies within academic journals. His current PhD research focuses on how sleep affects athletic performance.

Brad J. Schoenfeld is an associate professor of exercise science at Lehman College in the Bronx, New York, where he serves as the graduate director of the Human Performance and Fitness programme. Brad has published more than 250 peer-reviewed scientific papers on various exercise- and sports nutrition-related topics, and authored the seminal textbook, 'Science and Development of Muscle Hypertrophy'. Brad received the 2016 Dwight D. Eisenhower Fitness Award, presented by the United States Sports Academy as well as earning the 2018 National Strength and Conditioning Association Young Investigator of the Year Award. He formerly served as Sports Nutritionist for the New Jersey Devils hockey organization.

Advanced Personal Training

Science to Practice

Second Edition

**Edited by Paul Hough
and Brad J. Schoenfeld**

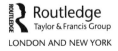

LONDON AND NEW YORK

Second edition published 2022
by Routledge
2 Park Square, Milton Park, Abingdon, Oxon, OX14 4RN

and by Routledge
605 Third Avenue, New York, NY 10158

Routledge is an imprint of the Taylor & Francis Group, an informa business

© 2022 Taylor & Francis

First edition published by Routledge 2016

Library of Congress Cataloging-in-Publication Data
A catalog record has been requested for this book

ISBN: 978-1-032-06942-5 (hbk)
ISBN: 978-0-367-90402-9 (pbk)
ISBN: 978-1-003-20465-7 (ebk)

DOI: 10.4324/9781003204657

Typeset in Baskerville
by KnowledgeWorks Global Ltd.

Contents

List of figures

List of tables

Contributors

Alan Aragon
Independent nutrition researcher and educator

Keith Baar
UC Davis Health, USA

Anoop Balachandran
University of Miami, USA

Zachery Bell
Victoria University, Australia

David Bishop
Victoria University, Australia

Martin Buchheit
Kitman Labs

Bret Contreras
Independent strength and conditioning expert

Jess Cunningham
Optima Female Performance

Marlize DeVivo
Canterbury Christ Church University, UK

Gabrielle Fundaro
Monash University, Australia & Vitamin PhD Nutrition, LLC

Jozo Grgić
Victoria University, Australia

Stuart Guppy
Edith Cowan University, Australia

G. Gregory Haff
Edith Cowan University, Australia

Cody Haun
LaGrange College, USA

Eric Helms
Auckland University of Technology, New Zealand

Paul Hough
Oxford Brookes University, UK

Alex Hutchinson
Independent endurance training expert

Mike Israetel
Renaissance Periodization & Lehman College, USA

Ian Jeffreys
Setanta College, Ireland

Ben Kirk
Australian Institute for
  Musculoskeletal Science & The
  University of Melbourne and
  Western Health, Australia

Paul Laursen
HIIT Science

Cédric Leduc
Leeds Becket University, UK

Jeremy Loenneke
The University of Mississippi, USA

Martin MacDonald
Mac-Nutrition & Mac-Nutrition Uni

Mike Matthews
Legion Athletics & Muscle for Life

Gary Mendoza
Stages of Change Ltd

Greg Nuckols
Stronger by Science

Kay Robinson
Optima Female Performance

Brad J. Schoenfeld
Lehman College, USA

Sam Spinelli
Citizen Athletics & E3 Rehab
  LLC

Neil Stanley
Independent sleep expert

Marc Surdyka
University of Southern California
  & E3 Rehab LLC

Nick Tumminello
Strength Zone Training

Sean Wilson
FitGreyStrong, Australia

Foreword

I use sports science to support what I do. Finding out about new research makes me so passionate about my work and allows me to project the importance of physical activity to the public with confidence and, most importantly, with hard evidence.

Paul is someone I take vast amounts of knowledge from, and I admire his passion for what he does. I had the opportunity to work with him on several occasions, learning about body composition, specifically reducing body fat. We have measured the body composition of my clients using the Bod Pod, which is just one example of how sports science principles, that are usually applied with athletes, can be used with personal training clients. Using detailed assessments, research, and Paul's expertise has helped me to optimise training programmes that have achieved outstanding results for my clients.

Bradley Simmonds, Personal Trainer

Acknowledgements

I would like to thank Brad and all the contributors for their hard work, professionalism, and patience during the writing and editing process. I would also like to thank Simon Penn (The Open University, UK), Will Hopkins (Victoria University, Australia), and Stu Phillips (McMaster University, Canada) for their advice. Finally, thank you to my wife, Colette, for supporting me during the many evenings and weekends I spent working on this book.

Paul Hough

1 Introduction

Paul Hough

A vast quantity of health and fitness information available on websites and social media is inaccurate because it has not been written or verified by experts. The circulation of poor-quality information seems less common in other industries, such as engineering or law, probably because fewer people have direct experience in these disciplines. More people feel confident to circulate exercise and nutrition information because they have some experience (e.g., they have tried various exercise programmes and diets). However, *experience* and *expertise* are different. Expertise involves developing a high level of knowledge or skill through training, education, and practical experience. Experience can be gained from simply doing something over time. For instance, someone who has been exercising for 20 years has extensive experience but not necessarily expertise. Inaccurate information can quickly become widespread amongst the public, which leads to numerous exercise and nutrition misconceptions. The spread of inaccurate information is problematic for fitness professionals as clients may follow advice that could be counterproductive or even unsafe.

My students and clients often learn about new health and fitness research via articles on the Internet. Unfortunately, even articles and blogs that include scientific references, published within seemingly credible publications, can be inaccurate (Kininmonth et al., 2017). Once inaccurate content is within the public domain, the misinformation can take a long time to debunk (Lewandowsky et al., 2012). As well as creating confusion amongst the public, I have found that the massive volume of freely available health, fitness, and nutrition information makes it difficult for students to determine which information is accurate and trustworthy. Therefore, the inspiration and ethos for the first edition of this book were to provide students and exercise professionals with information based on scientific evidence. The philosophy of this new edition remains the same. However, this is not just an update of the first edition; it is an entirely new book. I have commissioned esteemed experts from several disciplines, such as psychology, and nutrition, to author chapters and sub-sections of this book. The contributors to this book also include researchers who have done some of

DOI: 10.4324/9781003204657-1

the scientific studies discussed. The experts have interpreted and summarised the scientific evidence and produced evidence-based recommendations, which I hope will inform your practice.

Evidence-based practice

Evidence-based practice (EBP) broadly involves designing programmes and creating content based on your professional experience, client's preferences, *and scientific evidence.* Encouragingly, since the first edition of this book was published, it seems that more practitioners within the health and fitness industry are taking an EBP approach. However, EBP can be oversimplified as it relates to exercise and nutrition. For example, in social media discussions it is relatively common for someone to support or contend a statement with a link to a scientific study. Sharing research is a positive step, as it shows the scientific literature is being recognised and applied within the fitness community; however, EBP is more nuanced than this. One study can never prove that something works or does not work for everyone – this is not how science works. Instead, we can think of each new study as a piece in a puzzle. As the research (puzzle pieces) accumulate, we begin to get a clearer idea if/how something works. Informed conclusions can only be reached by analysing the entirety of literature related to the subject in question, which takes time and *expertise.* To explain the concept of EBP for fitness professionals, I am delighted that Dr Brad J. Schoenfeld, an internationally renowned researcher, author and evidence-based practitioner, has co-authored the new EBP chapter and edited several other chapters within this book.

Evolving as a practitioner

When I am asked a question regarding fitness, sport science or nutrition, I often begin my answer with 'it depends'. I have experienced this type of 'it depends' response in conversations with practitioners and academics, so I appreciate it can be frustrating. After all, it is human nature to seek definitive answers over ambiguous or cautionary ones (Kruglanski & Webster, 1996). Our requirement for certainty could partly explain why individuals who claim to have a panacea (silver bullet) method can prosper in the fitness industry (Guadagno & Cialdini, 2009). For example, some people sell products related to detox diets, which supposedly eliminate (unspecified) toxins and facilitate weight loss. However, there is a lack of credible evidence that detox diets and products are effective (Klein & Kiat, 2015). People who sell detox diet products unknowingly or knowingly benefit from offering clients and customers certainty.

In my experience, experts rarely have a panacea, usually provide nuanced answers, and are comfortable with uncertainty. Scientific research is always ongoing, which is why updates of textbooks like this are needed. Of course, this does not mean you can never provide your clients with straight answers. Instead, as an evidence-based practitioner, you should be mindful that there could be more than one correct answer, and your opinion might change when you become aware of further evidence. Indeed, some of the research discussed in this book might challenge your current beliefs and practices.

What does science to practice mean?

In this book, leading researchers and practitioners have interpreted the body of scientific evidence to provide evidence-based recommendations to inform your practice. However, these recommendations are not meant to dictate your practice. It is essential not to forget the 'personal' aspect of personal training. Clients will respond differently to exercise or nutrition interventions due to differences in genetics, psychology, and lifestyle factors (e.g., psychological stress and sleep). Some clients will achieve considerable improvements in a particular outcome (e.g., fat loss), whereas others may not, despite following a similar programme. This phenomenon has led some researchers to describe participants as high or low responders. Although scientific evidence enables us to develop guidelines that are likely to be effective, your clients unique physiological and psychological characteristics will influence how they will respond to exercise and nutrition strategies. Thus, a 'copy and paste' approach cannot be adopted. Instead, your advice and programmes should be individualised according to your client's capabilities, preferences, and responses. Before making decisions or offering advice it is important to consider your client's values and preferences alongside scientific evidence, and knowledge acquired from your professional experience (see Figure 1.1).

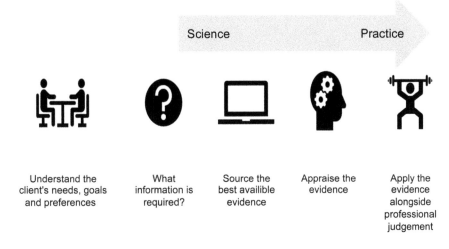

Science				Practice
Understand the client's needs, goals and preferences	What information is required?	Source the best availible evidence	Appraise the evidence	Apply the evidence alongside professional judgement

Figure 1.1 The concept of applying science to practice in personal training.

References

Guadagno, R., & Cialdini, R. (2009). Online persuasion and compliance: social influence on the internet and beyond. In *The social net* (pp. 91–113).

Kininmonth, A., Jamil, N., Almatrouk, N., et al. (2017). Quality assessment of nutrition coverage in the media: a 6-week survey of five popular UK newspapers. *BMJ Open, 7*(12), e014633.

Klein, A. V., & Kiat, H. (2015). Detox diets for toxin elimination and weight management: a critical review of the evidence. *Journal of Human Nutrition and Dietetics: The Official Journal of the British Dietetic Association, 28*(6), 675–686.

Kruglanski, A. W., & Webster, D. M. (1996). Motivated closing of the mind: 'seizing' and 'freezing'. *Psychological Review, 103*(2), 263–283.

Lewandowsky, S., Ecker, U., Seifert, C., et al. (2012). Misinformation and its correction: continued influence and successful debiasing. *Psychological Science in the Public Interest, 13*(3), 106–131.

2 Evidence-based practice in personal training

Anoop T. Balachandran and Brad J. Schoenfeld

Why is an evidence-based approach necessary?

The concept of evidence-based medicine (EBM) was developed in the early 1990s to help physicians better interpret scientific evidence to make the best clinical decisions in their everyday practice. Although the philosophical principles date back to the 19th century, modern-day EBM was introduced by Dr David Sackett, a former professor at McMaster University, Ontario (Sackett, 1997). EBM should not be confused with a new theory of knowledge; rather, it is a practical framework or heuristic to optimise the practice of health care. In light of the contributions to the field of medicine, EBM was voted the seventh most important medical milestone by the *British Medical Journal* (BMJ) (Kamerow, 2007).

Although clinical trials were required by the Food and Drug Administration (FDA) as early as the 1960s for drug approvals, medical decisions were still made based on expert opinion, unsystematic observations, and physiological/pathological mechanisms-based knowledge. EBM likely evolved because of numerous appalling medical mistakes that were made based on compelling yet flawed evidence driven by expert opinion and physiological knowledge. Below are some examples of mistakes that made an enormous impact on medical practice. These are the same reasons why an evidence-based approach should be adopted in exercise, nutrition, and other fields that require making practical decisions.

- **Sleeping babies:** Dr Benjamin Spock was one of the foremost experts in paediatrics. In the 1958 edition of his best-selling book *Baby and Child Care*, he argued that babies sleeping on their backs would be more likely to choke if they vomited. Therefore, Dr Spock advised millions of readers to encourage babies to sleep on their stomachs. Although this sounded reasonable and logical, subsequent scientific studies showed that prone sleeping increased the risk of sudden infant death syndrome. It is now apparent that Dr Spock's advice, apparently rational in theory, led to the cot deaths of tens of thousands of infants (Gilbert et al., 2005).

DOI: 10.4324/9781003204657-2

- **Heart arrhythmia and mortality:** Cardiac rhythm abnormalities are associated with an increased risk of death after a heart attack. Thus, it was theorised that if a drug would prevent these abnormalities, it might reduce the risk of early deaths. Doctors who were convinced about the efficacy of antiarrhythmic drugs prescribed them widely (Morganroth et al., 1990). To convince the minority of sceptics, the Cardiac Arrhythmia Suppression Trial (CAST) study was conducted in 1987. As expected, the antiarrhythmic drugs stopped the abnormal heart rhythms in the study; however, the drugs also stopped the heart (Cardiac Arrhythmia Suppression Trials [CAST], 1989, 1992). At the peak of their use in the late 1980s, it is estimated that the drugs may have killed as many as 70,000 people every year in the United States alone (Chalmers, 2004).

- **The ideal reepetition range for muscle hypertrophy:** Although not as impactful as the cases above, the fitness field is replete with examples where well-accepted tenets are based on flawed evidence. For instance, it was a virtually uncontested belief that training within a range of 8–12 repetitions optimised muscle growth (hypertrophy) (Schoenfeld, 2010). This was mainly based on anecdotal evidence from bodybuilders and research showing acute increases in exercise-induced anabolic hormones when training within this repetition range. However, a compelling body of evidence now shows that similar hypertrophy is achieved using lighter weights (see Chapter 13). Therefore, as claimed for decades, there are no magic hypertrophic benefits to the 8–12 repetition range.

The examples above demonstrate that an evidence-based approach evolved because relying on experts, unsystematic observations, and/or pathophysiological mechanisms, no matter how compelling and logical they may appear, can be very misleading.

What is evidence-based practice (EBP)?

The definition of EBM by Sackett (1997) is Evidence-based medicine is the conscientious, explicit, and judicious use of current best evidence in making decisions about the care of individual patients (Sackett et al., 1996). EBP involves three elements (outlined in Figure 2.1) that assume equal importance.

1 **Best available evidence:** Evidence can be obtained from a variety of sources, including well-conducted randomised controlled trials, unsystematic clinical observations, or even expert opinion. Thus, the evidence used in personal training could come from a controlled trial, a physiological mechanism, or a popular fitness guru. However, the importance or trust that is placed on the evidence differs based on

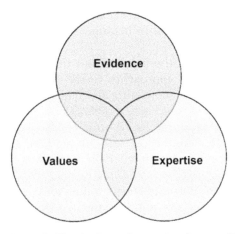

1. Best available evidence; 2. Client/patient values and preferences 3. clinical expertise

Figure 2.1 The framework of evidence-based practice.

the type of evidence. This will be discussed in the following evidence hierarchy section.

2 **Client values and preferences**: One of the guiding principles in EBP is 'evidence is not enough'. It means that decisions ultimately depend on the client's values, expectations, and preferences. Every patient or client assigns his/her values, preferences, and expectations on out-comes and choices. For example, some clients might place a high value on muscle growth, whereas others may value their general health and fitness as most important. Some clients may value the social aspect of training in a gym more than the associated muscular adaptations. The client's personal decisions have no wrong or right answer and should be heeded and respected. The job of a fitness professional is to help clients achieve whatever goals they desire, provided a given goal is not detrimental to overall health and wellness. Even if trainers have con-trasting beliefs and opinions to clients, they should not impose these on clients (see Chapter 3).

3 **Clinical expertise:** Clinical expertise is what many refer to as the 'art' of EBP. Expertise forms an integral part of EBP, and no amount of research can replace it. Likewise, no amount of clinical expertise can replace research-based evidence; the concepts are interdependent. Clinical expertise involves basic scientific knowledge, practical exper-tise, and intuition to:

- diagnose the problem (e.g., why is this client not able to squat deep; are there issues with exercise technique?)
- search for the relevant research evidence (e.g., the number of sets required to gain muscle for an advanced trainee) and critically

analyse the research evidence for methodological issues (e.g., was the study carried out in beginners? Was the outcome measured relevant?)

- understand both the benefits and the risks involved, as well as other alternative approaches to the goal (e.g., a CrossFit®-type workout might be motivating and improve general cardiovascular endurance, but could have a high risk of injury)
- alter the programme based on client feedback and results (e.g., reducing the number of sets) or modifying the exercise (e.g., range of motion) for an older client or someone with pre-existing injuries.
- Listen and understand clients' values and preferences to communicate the risk, cost, and benefits in a simple manner, and use a shared decision approach to determine the best possible plan to move forward; this is the art of an evidence-based approach.

The evidence hierarchy

An evidence hierarchy is one of the foundational concepts of EBP. It states that all evidence is not equal, and the quality of each source of evidence depends on the type of evidence. The hierarchy of evidence pyramid (see Figure 2.2) indicates that the quality of evidence and the trust practitioners can place in its conclusions increases as the pyramid is ascended. In other words, evidence higher in the pyramid is more trustworthy than that below (see Figure 2.2).

Randomised control trials (RCTs)

An RCT is regarded as the 'gold standard' study design as it is the only type of design that can infer *cause and effect*. In an RCT, participants are

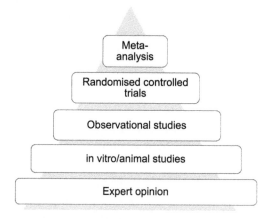

Figure 2.2 Evidence hierarchy or pyramid.

randomly assigned to groups so each person has an equal chance of falling into either of the groups. The randomisation process ensures both groups are equal in almost everything except for the intervention. For example, a study to determine the effect of strength training repetitions on muscle growth would randomise a group of participants into a low or high repetition group for a training duration of 12 weeks. Accordingly, the researchers would attempt to control all other variables as best as possible, so they have minimal influence on the outcome. After 12 weeks, the researchers could reasonably conclude that any change in muscle growth was due to the specific intervention (high or low repetitions). Differences in muscle growth could not be attributed to genetics, motivation, or diet since randomisation ensured these variables were equally distributed among both groups.

Meta-analysis

A meta-analysis is generally considered the highest form of evidence and occupies the apex of the pyramid. A meta-analysis synthesises the entire body of RCTs on a given topic and quantifies the results of all the studies using statistical techniques. The major advantage of a meta-analysis, apart from providing a single estimate of all study results, is that it looks at the totality of the evidence instead of selectively identifying (or cherry-picking) studies that fit a narrative. Meta-analyses can be important to exercise- and nutrition-related topics, as the sample sizes are often small, and thus pooling the data across studies provides greater statistical power for inference.

Observational studies

Observational studies are often conducted when an RCT is not feasible due to financial or practical constraints. For example, conducting an RCT for 5–10 years to investigate outcomes such as death, heart disease, or cancer may not be feasible. RCTs are also unethical in studies assessing harms, such as smoking. Observational studies involve observing the participants without randomising participants into groups or imposing an intervention. Study designs, such as case-control or cohort studies, are classified as 'observational studies'.

An example observational study would be investigating the effects of eating red meat on the risk of cardiovascular disease (CVD) and mortality. Since CVD or mortality from CVD takes years to develop, conducting an RCT is often not feasible. Also, it would be unethical to instruct participants to eat red meat for years to assess if they develop CVD if there is a reason to believe an association does indeed exist. Hence, an observational design allows researchers to observe people already eating red meat and compare them with people who are not. Since there is no randomisation, the groups could be different in their lifestyle, medication, habits, genetics, etc. For example, people who avoid red meat could be more health-conscious and physically active, and possibly smoke and drink less alcohol (Mihrshahi et al., 2017; Orlich et al., 2013). Therefore, it cannot be determined if an observed increase in heart disease was caused by red meat consumption or an unhealthy lifestyle. In research, these uncontrolled variables are known as confounders or covariates. Although confounders are accounted for in the statistical analysis, observational studies can only show associations and not causation. In layman's terms, 'association' means it cannot be certain if red meat played a causal role in heart disease.

In vitro/animal studies

In vitro means outside of a living organism as in a test tube or petri dish. Animal experiments use rodents and monkeys as models since there exist some similarities with humans. However, we have striking dissimilarities too. The unreliability of animal models is conveyed by the quote, "Mice lie and monkeys exaggerate". Laboratory studies and animal experiments are often utilised in drug discovery, but they are always followed by human trials, often termed as phase 1, 2, and 3 trials. In vitro/animal studies are typically used as preliminary or preclinical evidence to generate tentative hypotheses that require further confirmatory research in humans.

Expert opinion/experience

An expert's opinion or experience is often fallible, as demonstrated in the examples provided previously, and hence occupies the bottom position of the hierarchy.

There are three important points to keep in mind about the evidence hierarchy.

- First, the trustworthiness or the confidence in the study results increases towards the peak of the hierarchy, and the bias (systemic deviation from the truth) decreases. Thus, a meta-analysis or a systematic review of RCTs is the highest form of evidence with the least bias.
- Second, the hierarchy is neither set in stone nor static; depending on the quality of the study, an RCT can be downgraded in the hierarchy. Likewise, observational studies can be upgraded, too. Consequently, the methodology of a study is important.
- Third, there is always evidence. Therefore, the best evidence is what is currently available and need not necessarily come from an RCT or a meta-analysis for practitioners to act. However, recommendations will vary depending on the type of evidence and confidence in the evidence. If practitioners only have an expert opinion, they should not be confident in the evidence and acknowledge this uncertainty when providing recommendations to clients.

Critically evaluating a study

Having developed a basic understanding of the fundamentals of EBP, it is essential to develop the skills to understand and appraise a study. In our experience, most people quickly jump to conclusions before having a clear understanding of the major parts of a study. Therefore, practitioners are advised to follow the PICO framework to define and understand an RCT (Sackett, 1997).

- **Population:** Refers to the specific individuals or community being investigated (i.e., the participants' descriptive features in the study). Research is very population specific. For instance, an exercise or supplement that works in trained individuals might have no effect in untrained individuals.
- **Intervention:** Refers to the specific focus of what is being investigated. The intervention could be resistance training, supplementation, psychological therapy, etc. There is no intervention assigned in an observational study, so 'I' is replaced by 'E' (exposure). It is also important to understand the specifics of the intervention. In an exercise intervention, specific details (e.g., frequency, intensity, volume, duration) usually impact the results and conclusions. For example, a 10-week intervention could have different outcomes than a similar intervention, lasting 6 months.
- **Comparator group:** Refers to the group(s) that the intervention group is compared against. When interpreting a study, the comparator group must be considered to prevent reaching a misleading conclusion. For example, a new exercise intervention could look spectacular if compared to a control (no intervention) group of sedentary participants. However, the results might be mediocre if the comparison group performs a standard exercise protocol.
- **Outcome(s):** Refers to the primary outcome(s) or the end point(s) of the study. In exercise research, it could be maximum strength, muscle hypertrophy, or performance measures, such as a timed trial or maximum oxygen uptake (VO_{2max}). The outcome selected should be meaningful and valid.

Identifying the PICO enables the reader to develop a quick understanding of the study. The example below outlines the PICO framework for a hypothetical study.

- Population: Sedentary women aged 18–26 years with an average BMI of 22.0
- Intervention: High-intensity interval training (HIIT) 3 days/week for 12 weeks using a cycle ergometer
- Comparator Group: Sedentary control
- Outcome(s): Body fat changes (measured using skinfold calipers)

The PICO question is *Can 12 weeks of high-intensity interval training decrease body fat in young, sedentary women compared to a sedentary control group?* By stating the PICO, some of the study limitations become apparent: The population of women with a healthy BMI means the results cannot be extrapolated to either males or obese adults. Also, the study only showed changes compared to the sedentary (no training) group, and hence it is unclear if the HIIT had a causal role. To conclude that HIIT was responsible for body fat changes, the study should have used a comparator group that performed a standard moderate-intensity continuous training protocol. The outcomes assessed were body composition using skinfolds, which offers lower accuracy than other assessment measures (e.g., dual-energy x-ray absorptiometry). In summary, utilising a systematic approach, like PICO, allows the reader to gather the substance of a study quickly and reveals some of the study's strengths and limitations.

Evaluating the results of a study

When analysing the results or outcomes of a study, four primary concepts should be considered:

- **Surrogate outcomes:** Is the outcome a surrogate or substitute? Surrogate outcomes are outcomes in scientific studies that are just laboratory/physiological markers for clinically meaningful outcomes (or outcomes that people care about). For example, older adults care less about muscle mass or bench press strength but more about if they can perform everyday activities, such as climbing the stairs. Bodybuilders care about muscle size and body fat instead of EMG activity, protein synthesis, or molecular signalling pathways. Studies using surrogate outcomes usually serve as preliminary data or to generate hypotheses for proof-of-concept trials. Therefore, researchers are less confident in making practical recommendations based on surrogate outcomes.
- **Statistical significance:** Statistical significance asks the question, 'Are the study results due to chance?' Typically, in most research areas, the cut-off for the P (Probability) value is 0.05. Thus, if the P-value, usually reported in the abstract/results/figures, is less than 0.05 (5%), the result is deemed 'statistically significant'. That is, there is less than a 5% chance that the results obtained could be explained by random chance. For example, if the P-value was 0.03, the result is statistically significant. However, statistical inference is a complex topic, and numerous questions have been raised against the use of P-values at a given level of significance (Wasserstein & Lazar, 2016). We recommend using point estimates and confidence intervals to draw practical inferences (Amrhein et al., 2019), but the topic is beyond the scope of this chapter.
- **Clinical significance:** If statistical significance asks the question, 'is there a difference?', clinical significance asks, 'how big is the

difference?'. Typically, the magnitude of change in the outcome can be obtained from the tables or figures in the results section. In theory, with a large enough sample size, even a 0.5 kg reduction in body weight could be statistically significant. Thus, it is crucial to understand that statistically significant does not mean the results are practically meaningful. Hence, both statistical and practical significance must be inspected separately. In weight loss literature, a 5–7% loss of the initial body weight is considered practically meaningful. In exercise science, the research is uncertain about the practical meaningfulness of muscle gain or fat loss for performance or aesthetic goals. For example, an increase of 1 kg of muscle mass in a month for a beginner is seemingly meaningful; however, this substantial increase is almost impossible to achieve for a trained individual.

- **Adverse effects/cost/burden:** From what we have seen, people often pay less attention to the adverse effects, economic cost, and the burden or hassle of an intervention. Although the adverse effects of exercise may not be life-threatening, compared to pharmacologic/medical treatments, they could be meaningful in clinical populations, older adults, and pregnant women. The economic cost is a significant concern that is often overlooked, especially when evaluating supplements or following specific diets (e.g., recommending organic foods). In people with limited financial means, the cost is a significant concern that should be considered. The burden of the intervention should also be assessed as even seemingly small tasks, such as taking a daily pill, come with their own inconvenience. Training programmes like CrossFit®, high-frequency training, or programmes that use advanced techniques (see Chapter 13) can be highly fatiguing and burdensome. Thus, all trainers should question whether the benefits of the intervention/supplement are worth the risk, harms, burden, and cost.

Rating study quality

Critically analysing a scientific study to evaluate its quality (or trustworthiness) is a vital component of EBP. We recommend assigning three quality levels when critically appraising evidence: low, moderate, and high. Although an RCT starts at a high-quality grade, it can be downgraded to moderate or low, depending on its limitations. A downgraded RCT means there is uncertainty regarding the trustworthiness of the results. Observational studies or non-systematic observations and case series are always low-quality evidence, but observational studies can be rated up. Several issues reduce the quality of an RCT, such as lack of concealed allocation, lack of blinding, large dropouts, improper comparator group, low precision due to small sample size, indirectness of intervention/population, and surrogate outcomes.

Moving from evidence to recommendations

After critically evaluating a study, the client can be advised on what action to take. Clients expect and appreciate the guidance, so the trainer has to offer a recommendation, even when evidence is lacking, conflicting, or missing. Several formal guidelines have been developed to move from evidence to recommendation systematically and transparently. One such approach is the international Grading of Recommendations, Assessment, Development and Evaluation (GRADE) system (Guyatt et al., 2008, 2009) that is widely employed for guideline development. GRADE classifies recommendations as either strong or weak depending on the tradeoff between benefits, risk, burden/hassle, and cost:

- A *strong recommendation (for/against)* is made when the practitioner can be very certain or highly confident that the benefits outweigh the harms, cost, and burden or vice versa.
- A *weak/conditional recommendation (for/against)* is made when there is appreciable uncertainty or the benefits and risks are delicately balanced.

Strong recommendation

An example of a strong recommendation would be supplementing with creatine to increase strength in resistance training individuals. The meta-analyses, with mainly high-quality RCTs, demonstrate moderate strength

---

BOX 2.1

Common misconceptions about EBP

1 **I do not care about *why* it works. All I care about is results.**
   As shown in the examples above (sleeping babies, heart arrhythmia drugs, and ideal repetition range), EBP evolved to produce better 'results' and not simply to explain mechanisms. Hence, basic science or mechanistic studies are low in the hierarchy of evidence. Indeed, there are hundreds of life-saving treatments and drugs where the underlying mechanism(s) are still unclear or unknown.
2 **Studies report an average of the sample. There are substantial inter-individual differences.**
   The focus of many studies is the summary statistics, and individual results may vary. A promising area of research is precision medicine and artificial intelligence to individualise treatments, but they are still in infancy. A trial-and-error method always could be used, but two concerns should be acknowledged in this regard:

(*Continued*)

BOX 2.1   (Continued)

Common misconceptions about EBP

- First, if benefits with a specific programme are discovered, in many cases, it is extremely hard to identify the variable that made the difference. Was it the specific exercise, the change in diet, the placebo effect, genetics, or some unknown variable?
- Second, it may not be clear if there is a clear improvement depending on the outcome. For example, gains in muscle mass come very slowly for trained individuals. Hence, a programme could take months to produce any clear results. However, controlled research often uses measures that are highly sensitive to subtle changes in muscle mass that can be observed within weeks.

3 **There are numerous problems with scientific research, so you cannot use the results of a study to train your clients.**
One of the basic steps in EBP is to critically analyse studies to determine their quality. If the study has methodological issues, the evidence is downgraded, thereby raising the uncertainty. Consequently, the strength of recommendations becomes weak.

4 **Smoking studies are observational in nature. How can we make a strong recommendation against smoking based on low quality evidence?**
The hierarchy is neither set in stone nor static. An observational study can be rated up if it shows a large magnitude of effect and a dose-response effect. For instance, associations between smoking and lung cancer studies show a substantial effect (relative risk ranging from 5 to 25) (Ordóñez-Mena et al., 2016; Pesch et al., 2012) and a robust dose-response gradient that cannot be explained by covariates. However, most observational studies have a very small magnitude of association and hence remain as low quality. For example, a recent controversial review of red meat and adverse health outcomes showed a very small relative risk of 1.08–1.28 (Johnston et al., 2019).

5 **What are the limitations of EBP?**
Several criticisms have been raised against EBM (Greenhalgh et al., 2014; Ioannidis, 2016). Most of these (e.g., biases due to conflict of interest, poor quality studies) are valid points, but are not criticisms of EBP *per se*. Fundamentally, EBP is just a framework to make better decisions; it has no legal authority over who conducts research or how they conduct their research. Furthermore, practitioners can claim to be using EBP, but without a thorough understanding, they are likely to misinterpret and misapply EBP. Finally, and importantly, critics of EBP have not proposed an alternative approach that can overcome the limitations raised.
The critical analysis of research articles is a major limitation for personal trainers that can be a barrier in using EBP. Therefore, the resources listed at the end of this chapter are recommended to further your understanding of EBP.

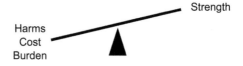

Figure 2.3 Desirable outcome outweighs the undesirable consequences for creatine supplementation.

increases (benefits) in both trained and untrained individuals across a variety of populations (Lanhers et al., 2015, 2017). Furthermore, the side effects/harms from creatine supplementation are minimal (minor gastrointestinal issues), the cost per serving is low, and supplementing carries a low burden. Therefore, practitioners can be confident, based on the high-quality evidence, that the benefits of creatine supplementation outweigh the risk/cost/burden. Still, some clients may not want to take creatine, which underlines the importance of considering the client's goals and preferences. Conversely, if only low-quality evidence were available, the certainty regarding the benefits of creatine supplementation would decrease, and a strong recommendation would be avoided.

Current physical activity guidelines for health are another excellent example of a strong recommendation in favour of the intervention (physical activity). A widely cited example of a strong recommendation against an intervention is cigarette smoking, as observational studies clearly show that the risk of smoking outweighs any benefits. Finally, strong recommendations are accompanied by phrases such as 'recommend to/recommend not to' or 'should do/should not' (Figure 2.3).

Weak recommendation

An example of a weak recommendation would be fish oil supplementation for improving physical function in older adults, as there are a few low to moderate quality RCTs showing little to no improvement in function in untrained older adults compared to a placebo (Da Boit et al., 2017; Rodacki et al., 2012). Furthermore, fish oil can be relatively expensive ($20–30/month), and there are alternatives (such as creatine) with a better risk-reward profile. Although harms are mild (gastrointestinal issues and fishy breath), it is uncertain if the small benefit outweighs the other negatives. Another example of a weak recommendation is HIIT for fat loss (see Chapter 11 and Figure 2.4).

As demonstrated in the previous examples, when the benefits, risks, cost, and burden are closely balanced, the values and preferences become more important. In other words, there is a greater role for shared decision-making when the recommendation is weak. Weak recommendations are conveyed using words such as 'suggest' and 'might' rather than words

Figure 2.4 Desirable outcome finely balanced with undesirable outcomes for interval training.

used when making strong recommendations (e.g., recommend/should). When in doubt, trainers should opt for a weak recommendation.

Decision-making is a complex process that requires considerable judgement at every step, and informed clients could disagree with the final recommendation. Hence, it is important to use a structured and transparent approach in decision-making to facilitate appraisal and to settle conflicts.

Conclusion

In closing, EBP is currently the best approach to make decisions related to health, fitness, and performance. A good evidence-based trainer should have a strong understanding of both the practical and the scientific aspects of exercise and nutrition and, more importantly, an untiring commitment and empathy to clients and their values.

Recommended resources

1. Greenhalgh T. *How to read a paper: The basics of evidence-based medicine and healthcare.* John Wiley & Sons; 2019.
2. Straus SE, Glasziou P, Richardson WS, Haynes RB. *Evidence-based medicine E-book: How to practice and teach EBM.* Elsevier Health Sciences; 2018.
3. Guyatt G, Rennie D, Meade M, Cook D. *Users' guides to the medical literature: A manual for evidence-based clinical practice.* McGraw-Hill Education; 2015.
4. Evans I, H Thornton H, Chalmers I, Glasziou P. *Testing treatments: better research for better healthcare.* Pinter & Martin; 2010.

References

Amrhein, V., Greenland, S., & McShane, B. (2019). Scientists rise up against statistical significance. *Nature, 567,* 305.

Cardiac Arrhythmia Suppression Trial (CAST) Investigators (1989). Preliminary report: effect of encainide and flecainide on mortality in a randomised trial of arrhythmia suppression after myocardial infarction. *New England Journal of Medicine, 321*(6), 406–412.

Cardiac Arrhythmia Suppression Trial II Investigators (1992). Effect of the antiarrhythmic agent moricizine on survival after myocardial infarction. *New England Journal of Medicine, 327*(4), 227–233.

Chalmers, I. (2004). In the dark: drug companies should be forced to publish all the results of clinical trials. *New Scientist, 181*(2437), 19.

Da Boit, M., Sibson, R., Sivasubramaniam, S., et al. (2017). Sex differences in the effect of fish-oil supplementation on the adaptive response to resistance exercise training in older people: a randomised controlled trial. *The American Journal of Clinical Nutrition, 105*(1), 151–158.

Gilbert, R., Salanti, G., Harden, M., et al. (2005). Infant sleeping position and the sudden infant death syndrome: systematic review of observational studies and historical review of recommendations from 1940 to 2002. *International Journal of Epidemiology, 34*(4), 874–887.

Greenhalgh, T., Howick, J., Maskrey, N., et al. (2014). Evidence based medicine: a movement in crisis? *BMJ (Clinical Research Ed.), 348,* g3725.

Guyatt, G., Oxman, A., Kunz, R., et al. (2009). GRADE: what is "quality of evidence" and why is it important to clinicians. *Chinese Journal of Evidence-Based Medicine, 9*(2), 133–137.

Guyatt, G., Oxman, A., Vist, G., et al. (2008). GRADE: an emerging consensus on rating quality of evidence and strength of recommendations. *BMJ (Clinical Research Ed.), 336*(7650), 924–926.

Ioannidis, J. (2016). Evidence-based medicine has been hijacked: a report to David Sackett. *Journal of Clinical Epidemiology, 73,* 82–86.

Johnston, B. C., Zeraatkar, D., Han, M., et al. (2019). Unprocessed red meat and processed meat consumption: dietary guideline Recommendations from the Nutritional Recommendations (NutriRECS) Consortium. *Annals of Internal Medicine, 171*(10), 756–764.

Kamerow, D. (2007). Milestones, tombstones and sex education. *BMJ (Clinical Research Ed.), 334*(7585), 126.

Lanhers, C., Pereira, B., Naughton, G., et al. (2015). Creatine supplementation and lower limb strength performance: a systematic review and meta-analyses. *Sports Medicine, 45*(9), 1285–1294.

Lanhers, C., Pereira, B., Naughton, G., et al. (2017). Creatine supplementation and upper limb strength performance: a systematic review and meta-analysis. *Sports Medicine, 47*(1), 163–173.

Mihrshahi, S., Ding, D., Gale, J., et al. (2017). Vegetarian diet and all-cause mortality: evidence from a large population-based Australian cohort – the 45 and up study. *Preventive Medicine, 97,* 1–7.

Morganroth, J., Bigger, J., & Anderson, J. (1990). Treatment of ventricular arrhythmias by United States cardiologists: a survey before the cardiac arrhythmia suppression trial results were available. *The American Journal of Cardiology, 65*(1), 40–48.

Ordóñez-Mena, J., Schöttker, B., Mons, U., et al. (2016). Quantification of the smoking-associated cancer risk with rate advancement periods: meta-analysis of individual participant data from cohorts of the CHANCES consortium. *BMC Medicine, 14*(1), 1–15.

Orlich, M., Singh, P., Sabaté, J., et al. (2013). Vegetarian dietary patterns and mortality in Adventist Health Study 2. *JAMA Internal Medicine, 173*(13), 1230–1238.

Pesch, B., Kendzia, B., Gustavsson, P., et al. (2012). Cigarette smoking and lung cancer—relative risk estimates for the major histological types from a pooled analysis of case–control studies. *International Journal of Cancer, 131*(5), 1210–1219.

Rodacki, C., Rodacki, A., Pereira, G., et al. (2012). Fish-oil supplementation enhances the effects of strength training in elderly women. *The American Journal of Clinical Nutrition, 95*(2), 428–436.

Sackett, D. (1997). Evidence-based medicine. Paper presented at the *Seminars in Perinatology, 21*(1) 3–5.

Sackett, D., Rosenberg, W., Gray, J., et al. (1996). Evidence based medicine: what it is and what it isn't. *BMJ (Clinical Research Ed.), 312*(7023), 71–72.

Schoenfeld, B. (2010). The mechanisms of muscle hypertrophy and their application to resistance training. *The Journal of Strength & Conditioning Research, 24*(10), 2857–2872.

Wasserstein, R., & Lazar, N. (2016). The ASA statement on p-values: context, process, and purpose. *The American Statistician, 32*(4), 421–423.

3 Helping clients to change

Gary Mendoza and Gabrielle Fundaro

Fitness professionals require behavioural change facilitation skills to complement their understanding of exercise prescription and nutrition (Nigg, 2016). It is well established that lifestyle factors affect physical and mental health, influencing quality of life across the lifespan (Lopez-Fontana et al., 2009). However, the Raising the Bar Report (Futurefit Training, 2018) showed that newly qualified fitness professionals often lack the required level of behaviour change facilitation skills. Therefore, the purpose of this chapter is to introduce commonly used behaviour change models and theories that are beneficial to facilitate lifestyle changes in clients.

Psychological models of behaviour change

Health psychology applies psychological theories and principles to the promotion, adoption, and maintenance of health behaviours (see Figure 3.1). The intention of motivational models is to describe underlying decisions that are related to health. The Health Belief Model (HBM) (Becker & Maiman, 1975) and Theory of Planned Behaviour (TPB) (Ajzen, 1991) fall into the category of 'motivational models' (see Figure 3.1). The HBM posits that our assessment of our perceived vulnerability to illness or injury is a major determinant of our decision to engage in virtually all health-promoting or health-harming behaviours (Gibbons et al., 1997). The TPB posits that behaviours depend on an individual's intention to perform, which arises from their attitude and perceived ability and the social norms surrounding a behaviour. The Transtheoretical Model (TTM) encompasses several theoretical concepts explaining the processes of considering, implementing, and maintaining behaviour change (Prochaska et al., 1994) (see Figure 3.1).

A point of differentiation between the TTM and TPB can be made by classifying them as a continuum model or stage model (Callaghan et al., 2002). In a continuum model, such as the TPB, an individual is placed along a continuum representing the likelihood of them taking a specified

DOI: 10.4324/9781003204657-3

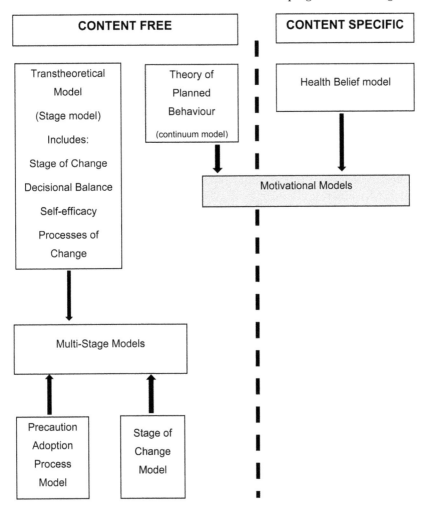

Figure 3.1 Conceptual and theoretical models.

action. This differs from the TTM stage model, where the client is classified as being in a stage of change. Because clients gradually move from one stage to the next with a degree of overlap, viewing behaviour change as a continuum is easier to visualise.

Other motivational constructs and models should not be dismissed as they will all have a degree of validity and application when considering behaviour change. Indeed, there is considerable debate within the scientific literature if stage theory is accurate and whether other behavioural models are perhaps more applicable (Weinstein et al., 1998). Behaviour change is a fast-moving field of constant learning, discovery, and new hypotheses. Therefore, it is important to keep abreast of the literature and be aware of existing and emerging behavioural models.

The Transtheoretical Model (TTM) of change

The TTM assumes that behaviour change is a multi-stage process where influences on behaviour change vary according to an individual's stage of change. The TTM was first used in tobacco dependency to explain individual differences in readiness and progression through the process of smoking cessation (Prochaska & DiClemente, 1983). It has since been applied to other health risk behaviours, weight-loss treatment, and dietary change (Kushner & Hopson, 1998). The TTM encompasses the Stages of Change Model (SCM) and the theoretical concepts of decisional balance, processes of change, and self-efficacy (SE), which can be linked to progression through the stages (Prochaska & Markus, 1994). A study on exercise behaviour in young Japanese women by Wakui et al. (2002) found a significant relationship between SE, decisional balance, and stage of change, and similar results have been reported amongst research using personal trainers (Mendoza et al., 2007). As clients progress from the pre-contemplation to the action stage, their SE increases before stabilising during maintenance, potentially indicating maximisation of their confidence in the ability to execute their desired behaviour(s). Additionally, clients' decisional balance shifts over time, with an increased proportion of reasons *favouring* change as they move from pre-contemplation to action.

Marcus et al. (1992) state that one of the strengths of the TTM is "...its focus on the dynamic nature of health behaviour change". Though the TTM is a theoretical, academic construct, it can be used as a roadmap that might indicate a client's readiness for change and the specific skills a trainer might utilise to help a client progress from only considering a lifestyle change to adopting and maintaining healthy behaviours. However, there is considerable uncertainty about how to match behaviour change techniques with theoretical constructs (Bridle et al., 2005). For example, planning is one potentially effective behaviour change technique, but its effectiveness may vary despite the client's apparent readiness for change based on the TTM.

The Stages of Change Model (SCM)

The SCM has been analysed in changing addictive behaviours, with applicability to weight management and exercise behaviours (Prochaska et al., 1992, 1994). The stages include:

- **Pre-contemplation**: The individual is not considering making any change.
- **Contemplation**: The individual seriously considers making a change in the future.

- **Preparation**: The individual who has been considering making a change over the past year(s) seriously thinks about putting this into action within the next month and prepares to make the change.
- **Action**: The individual attempts to make the changes.
- **Maintenance**: Six months after the action stage commenced, the individual attains their goal and now attempts to sustain the new behaviour.

When a client starts a programme, they may experience 'barrier underestimation' (Martin et al., 2004; Dibonaventura & Chapman, 2008) by underestimating the difficulty in overcoming a barrier. For example, underestimating the time it takes to attend the gym; this is a good point to discuss the stages of change, highlighting the client's personal journey. A client may experience a **relapse** (disruption in new habits) at any moment and may subsequently move back to an earlier stage of change (see Figure 3.2). The client should be aware that a lapse is a short-term disruption that may not result in regression to a previous stage of change; this enables a potential relapse to be perceived as 'feedback' rather than 'failure' so the client can work out how to move forward.

It is likely that most clients will be attempting to change more than one lifestyle behaviour, so the trainer must adopt a lifestyle counselling approach (Sallis, 2018). A problem that has been considered when promoting greater physical activity (PA) or changing dietary behaviour is how to identify the behaviours concerned accurately. As discussed later (self-monitoring), a behaviour that cannot be accurately identified will be difficult to match to a stage of change. Research has demonstrated that clients' progress through the change journey can be measured using psychometric

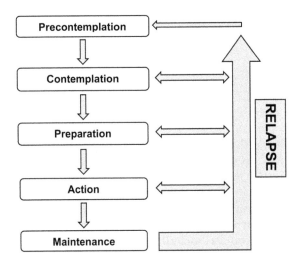

Figure 3.2 Stages of Change Model.

testing (Barasi et al., 2004). SE increases and decisional balance shifts as a client progresses through the stages, so a psychometric test can also be used to indicate when a client is starting to relapse by indicating reductions in SE or perceived benefits to maintaining a behaviour.

Self-efficacy

Self-efficacy (SE) is an individual's belief that they have the power or capacity to produce a desired effect. Bandura (1977) proposed that "...people process, weigh and integrate diverse sources of information concerning their capability, and they regulate their choice behaviour and effort expenditure accordingly". Thus, SE can be thought of as situational self-confidence. SE is measurable using psychometric testing (Mendoza et al., 2007) and can be built through education, autonomy, vicarious experience, imaginal experience, and past successes, many of which are also important for enhancing internal motivation.

Several studies have observed SE increasing as an individual progresses through the stages of the TTM (Mendoza et al., 2007). For instance, exercise SE has been shown to increase from the pre-contemplation stage to maintenance stage amongst young people (Callaghan et al., 2002; Wakui et al., 2002). In contrast, clients experiencing barrier underestimation at the onset of their lifestyle change may begin with high SE and motivation levels, but a lack of experience in facing behaviour change challenges (Wingo et al., 2013). As they initiate and attempt to integrate changes into their daily lifestyle, they may lapse or relapse in response to barriers; this perceived 'failure of self-control' may reduce SE (Duckworth et al., 2018). For example, a client who misses a gym session due to unforeseen circumstances may develop the belief that she is incapable of maintaining a consistent schedule, which could reduce her confidence in her ability to achieve her goals.

Decisional balance

Janis and Mann's (1977) decision-making model is the basis for decisional balance, or a client's perceived benefits and losses incurred by making a potential change. A balance sheet approach can be adopted by clients that involves listing the pros (items in favour) and cons (items against) of making a change. As the client progresses through stages of change, the number of pros start to outweigh the cons (O'Connell & Velicer, 1988). For example, one study indicated students in action and maintenance stages placed a stronger emphasis on the benefits of exercise (pros), whilst those in pre-contemplation and contemplation stages appeared to emphasise the negative aspects of exercise, including barriers (Callaghan et al., 2002). To facilitate movement through the stages from pre-contemplation to action and finally maintenance, it is important to first validate the client's initial lack of readiness by expressing acceptance and empathy regarding their reasons against change. Ideally, this would be followed up by facilitating their recognition of the benefits of change and progressively evoking more reasons favouring change by asking about the potential benefits or what the client might need to feel ready for the change (Schuster, 1987). In the following example, a trainer agrees with the client's statements about the difficulty in making a change and affirms positive character traits about the client, highlighting her ability to change eventually. The trainer also asks what might be necessary for the client to be willing to making change.

CLIENT: I know I should be eating more vegetables, but they're such a pain to cook. I never have time to chop them up for dinner. I buy them, and they sit in the cupboard.

TRAINER: It is quite time-consuming to prepare veggies! You are conscientious, so you have them in mind when you shop for yourself and your family, and then you're busy in the evenings when it's time to cook dinner. What would need to change for you to be able to fit more veggies into your meals?

CLIENT: Thank you! At least I have good intentions (laughing). I guess that I would need to prepare them ahead of time because I never have time after work. Now that I've thought about it, I believe that I just need to change my shopping and cooking schedule just a bit.

Self-determination theory (SDT)

Self-determination theory (SDT) is an empirically based, psychologically-focused theory of human behaviour and personality development, which differentiates types of motivation along a continuum from controlled (external) to autonomous (internal) (Ryan & Deci, 2017).

Table 3.1 shows the types of motivation on a sliding scale, from least effective (left) to most effective for long-term change.

To facilitate a client moving from external to internal motivation, the trainer must satisfy the following three basic psychological needs.

1 Competence – The client needs to feel a degree of confidence in the task and mastery.
2 Autonomy – The client needs a sense of control and be completely involved in the decision-making process.
3 Relatedness – It is important that the trainer displays empathy. The client needs to feel connected to others, be involved and cared for.

Rewards can be useful for motivation with careful presentation and application. For example, the reward of a spa day after reaching a weight loss goal would be an external motivator, and would not necessarily achieve the intended lifestyle change. The client may engage in unsafe weight-loss strategies to achieve the goal (weight loss) without the goal's desired effect (lifestyle change). Focusing entirely on the outcome goal (weight) can be

Table 3.1 Continuum of motivation

Extrinsic motivation				Intrinsic motivation
External regulation	*Introjected regulation*	*Identified regulation*	*Integrated regulation*	*Intrinsic regulation*
Client complies to gain reward or avoid punishment.	Client complies for approval from others.	Client sees value in an activity, and it endorses their goals.	The behaviour is congruent with client's sense of identity.	Client is interested and enjoys the behaviour. It also gives them inherent satisfaction.

detrimental to attainment; thus, short-term, client-developed behavioural (process) goals are preferable. For instance, doing 30 minutes of PA 5 days/week is a process goal that can be measured and rewarded (Freund & Hennecke, 2015). Adopting process goals enables the clients to be involved in the process, their autonomy is respected, and achieving the goal(s) increases their confidence (Grant, 2014). The three basic psychological needs have been met, and the motivation becomes internalised.

Habit theory

Habits are automatic responses to situational cues (Kwasnicka et al., 2016). Through developing an understanding of how habits are formed and maintained, a trainer is better placed to unravel and discover the barriers to forming a more beneficial habit. Over time, consciously controlled behaviours can become automated and habitual, and existing habitual behaviours can be overridden. The key to overriding undesirable habits is to recognise the cue or 'trigger', then disrupt the cycle by repeatedly removing the cue or responding with a new behaviour. For instance, keeping fruit on the counter (cue) to habituate daily fruit intake (behaviour) or engaging in meditation after work to reduce stress (cue) and disrupt the habit of emotional eating (behaviour). Changing habits requires skill and patience from both the trainer and the client. Unearthing the cue/trigger can often be quite complicated and establishing a new habit loop (cue-routine-reward) could take up to approximately 8 months (Lally et al., 2010).

Attitudinal aspects and soft skills: Empathy, active listening, and collaboration

The style of the trainer will be one of the biggest determinants of the client's outcomes. High-empathy counsellors and trainers seem to achieve a greater success rate (Moyers & Miller, 2013). Therefore, developing

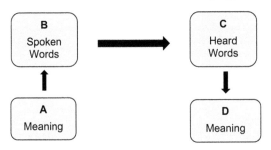

Figure 3.3 The communication process (adapted from Gordan and Edwards, 1997).

accurate empathy is a crucial skill for a trainer to master. Active listening is also an important skill to develop, as it is an integral but challenging part of the communication process (Miller & Rollnick, 2013) (see Figure 3.3).

During a conversation, the client thinks of what they want to say and then forms a sentence that has meaning to them (see Figure 3.3, box A). The client speaks those words to the trainer who hears the words and attaches his/her meaning to them (see Figure 3.3, box D). The trainer's understanding of the client's words is based upon his/her own beliefs, values, and knowledge, which can lead to a misunderstanding and a breakdown in the client/trainer relationship. Active listening involves the trainer reflecting back to the client what he/she understands the meaning of the client's words to be; this closes the loop between box D and A in Figure 3.3. Accurate reflection allows the trainer to build rapport and a more empathic relationship with the client.

Respecting the client's autonomy (right to choose), by offering choices and asking permission to give advice, may strengthen the client's degree of SE (situational self-confidence) (Amorose & Anderson-Butcher, 2007). Because persuasion seldom leads to a positive outcome, a collaborative or facilitative coaching approach (rather than a prescriptive relationship where the trainer provides answers or solutions) is more likely to achieve a long-term lifestyle change.

Navigating barriers and ambivalence

Barriers to change

Many facilitators and barriers to change have been documented, and although these vary with each client, trainers should have a broad understanding of common factors enabling and preventing change (see Table 3.2) (Kozica et al., 2015). Rather than providing solutions to barriers (known as the 'righting reflex'), trainers should facilitate collaborative discussions, enhancing the client's internal motivation and SE by

Table 3.2 Enablers and barriers to change

Enablers and barriers	Example
Motivation for participation	*Having a strong, sustainable, and predominantly internal reason for initiating the programme.*
Programme expectations	*Setting realistic expectations about the process and outcomes of the programme.*
Programme message application and utilisation	*Delivery and utility of information about the programme so that the individual can predict continued change or relapse.*
Personal knowledge, skills, and self-efficacy	*A strong educational component to enhance client self-efficacy.*
Personal achievement and programme support	*Individuals' ability to identify their personal progress throughout the programme enhances self-efficacy.*
Social and environmental barriers	*Environmental barriers included lack of child-care opportunities, geographical isolation to purchasing healthy foods, and the inability to participate in regular physical activity such as joining a local gym.*

evoking his/her capacity for change and solution-development (Resnicow & McMaster, 2012).

Motivational interviewing

In contrast to clients who seek out a trainer, clients referred to a trainer by a doctor may be ambivalent, or undecided, about making a lifestyle change. Motivational Interviewing (MI) is defined as, "…a collaborative, goal-oriented style of communication with particular attention to the language of change…designed to strengthen personal motivation for and commitment to a specific goal by eliciting and exploring the person's own reasons for change within an atmosphere of acceptance and compassion (Miller & Rollnick, 2013). MI is a collaborative, egalitarian, client-centred approach to having a conversation about change while navigating the client's ambivalence.

The treatment improvement protocol from Schuster (1987) describes MI and accounts for ambivalence:

MI is a counselling style based on the following assumptions:

- Ambivalence…is normal and constitutes an important motivational obstacle.
- Ambivalence can be resolved by working with the client's intrinsic motivations and values.
- The alliance between the trainer and client is a collaborative partnership – both bring important expertise.

- An empathic, supportive, yet directive, counselling style provides conditions where change can occur. Direct argument and aggressive confrontation may tend to increase client defensiveness and reduce the likelihood of behavioural change.

MI consists of four processes that use specific skills embodied by the 'spirit' of MI. It is beyond the scope of this chapter to explain the complete process of MI, but a range of scientific literature supports the use of MI in helping clients make behaviour changes (Frost et al., 2018; McKenzie et al. 2015; Rubak et al., 2005). The trainer's role is to facilitate the behaviour change by guiding the client in an MI-consistent manner.

The spirit and skills of motivational interviewing

Though MI is a directional conversation about change, it is *not* a technique to use 'on' a client to *persuade* them to make changes (Miller & Rollnick, 2009). A trainer embodies the spirit of MI by:

- collaborating with the client in an egalitarian way, acknowledging that the client is an expert on themselves
- expressing acceptance by meeting the client where they are and avoiding the 'righting reflex' to 'fix' the client
- showing compassion and empathy when the client expresses his/her thoughts and emotions
- evoking the client's innate capacity for change by drawing on the client's knowledge and reflecting it back with active listening skills.

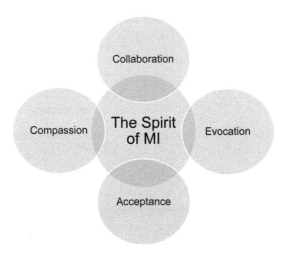

Figure 3.4 The spirit of motivational interviewing. Miller and Rollnick (2013).

Some trainers may feel expected to provide clients with answers and solutions. This form of information-giving, known as 'directing' in MI, is ineffective for evoking change. However, only listening to a client without using MI skills, known as 'following', is equally ineffective (Miller & Rollnick, 2013). The objective in MI is 'guiding' or the skilful application of active listening and information provision. However, trainers should request the client's permission before offering advice, information, and feedback; this allows the client's choice and autonomy to remain central to the process. When considering the use of MI, it is worth remembering the following rule:

- R – resist the 'righting reflex'
- U – understand the client's motivations
- L – Listen to the client (actively)
- E – Empower the client and respect his/her autonomy

Using the basic skills of OARS (see definition below), the conversation is guided in a useful and productive direction towards the client's desired outcome while using the client's knowledge and understanding to come up with solutions.

The basic skills of MI are built around OARS:

- Open-Ended Questions: Questions that require more than 'yes' or 'no' answers
- Affirmations: Statements that acknowledge a client's character strengths
- Reflections: Statements that reflect a client's words and underlying sentiments, emphasising statements in favour of a change
- Summaries: Statements that summarise a client's words to reach a mutual understanding.

Using MI skills, the counsellor/trainer moves in a general direction through the foundational steps of MI (see Figure 3.5), conceptualised by Miller and Rollnick (2013).

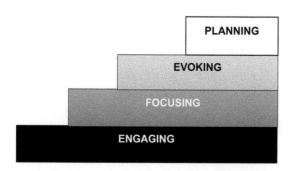

Figure 3.5 The foundational principles of MI.

Engaging

Engaging is the foundational first process of MI, during which rapport is built through mutual trust and understanding, giving rise to the effective coach-client dynamic (Miller & Rollnick, 2013). Trainers will rely heavily on all OARS skills (particularly A, R, and S) to encourage the client to continue sharing in response to the trainer's affirmation of the client's strengths, reflection of sentiments, and summaries that illustrate shared understanding. The initial engagement may also involve assessing the client's past lifestyle, history of exercise and activity, and his/her readiness to change.

Focusing

Focusing, or identifying the change a client wishes to make, can take place once engagement is established (Miller & Rollnick, 2013). The focus of a session is often apparent, but exploring all possible focal points in the initial meeting is worthwhile, as it may elicit unexpected areas of concern for the client. More open-ended questioning (O) can help guide a client who is unaware of their desired change. Focusing can be revisited as new desires for change arise.

Evoking

The evoking phase is unique and integral to MI, as it bolsters the client's readiness for change (Miller & Rollnick, 2013). During the evoking phase, OARS is used extensively (with a focus on O, R, and S) as the trainer asks about the client's reasons for change, reflects specific language in favour of change (change talk), and provides summaries of the client's positive statements about change. As the evoking stage progresses successfully, the client will provide a greater ratio of 'change talk' to 'sustain talk' (language *not* in favour of change). The specific language indicative of change and sustain talk follows the acronym DARN CATS (see definition below). DARN language indicates if a client is (or is not) ready for change. In contrast, CATS language suggests that a client has begun (or is unwilling to start) the process of change. The examples below indicate change talk, and statements opposing these examples (i.e., 'I don't want to', or 'I cannot') indicate sustain talk.

- D – Desire for change ('I want to...')
- A – Ability to change ('I can...')
- R – Reason for change ('If...then...')
- N – Need to change ('I need to...')
- C – Committed to change ('I will')
- A – Activation ('I am considering this')
- TS – Taking steps ('I have already done...')

Planning

When the amount of change talk exceeds sustain talk, the planning phase can begin. Planning, where the trainer and client collaboratively develop SMART goals (discussed later) and devise a plan for change, is the final phase of the MI process (Miller & Rollnick, 2013). The first three phases (engaging, focusing, and focusing) of MI likely occur at every session with the client, but planning may occur less frequently. A client who is ambivalent about change may spend extensive time working through each of the first three phases. Importantly, attempting to institute a plan for change *before* the client is ready can erode the trainer-client dynamics and reduce the likelihood of lifestyle change. Trainers who fail to resolve clients' ambivalence around their decision to make lifestyle changes are unlikely to achieve successful outcomes and could subsequently experience high client attrition.

Practical skills for lifestyle change programming

Scientific literature indicates there are several characteristics of successful lifestyle change programmes. A systematic review of lifestyle behaviour change factors found one of the most consistent factors associated with successful lifestyle change included the client's own beliefs (Murray et al., 2012). Thus, clients who achieve successful lifestyle-changes are able to apply strategies for dealing with setback and 'relapse' triggers, such as forward planning (with contingency plans), modifying the external environment, and making choices aligned with their identity (i.e., as a parent modelling a healthy lifestyle) (Duckworth et al., 2018; Stead et al., 2015). Research indicates that goals and goal-setting can be an important source of human motivation, and show promise in promoting diet and PA behaviour change (Brown et al., 2012). Finally, technological tools such as calorie and activity tracking apps and social media platforms have potential to promote maintenance of behaviour change by making self-monitoring easier and enhancing social support (Butryn et al., 2016; Duckworth et al., 2018).

Decisional balance sheets

Decisional balance worksheets capture client attitudes about perceived positive and negative consequences of making changes (Geller et al., 2012). Clients may use decisional balance sheets to navigate ambivalence and decide to make a change, as an increased ratio of 'pros' to 'cons' for change correlates with progression from pre-contemplation to maintenance (Di Noia & Prochaska, 2010). As clients list the potential pros and cons of making a change or not, the trainer may encourage them to think of short and long-term consequences while engaging in a discussion about possible outcomes. Additionally, with the client's permission, the discussion about the decisional

Table 3.3 The balance sheet for change

	PROS	*CONS*
Change		
No change		

balance worksheet may be an opportunity to provide education and feed-back to empower the client to make informed decisions (see Table 3.3).

Goal setting

Goal setting is an important aspect of SDT, which occurs in the planning stage of MI (Resnicow & McMaster, 2012). Well-structured goals may help clients avoid the 'intention-behaviour gap' where the intention or desire to engage in a behaviour does not always lead to action (Bailey, 2017). Trainers are advised to set short and long-term goals *with* the client in an MI-consistent manner, respecting the client's autonomy. However, the trainer should allow the client to state the initial goals, rather than suggesting goals, and reframe/refine if necessary to create SMART goals:

- Specific
- Measurable
- Achievable
- Realistic
- Time Orientated

Goals should be specific to one behaviour, observable and measurable, realistically achievable for the client, and applied to a timeline. The goals should also create coping (or contingency) plans in anticipation of potential obstacles.

Self-monitoring

Butryn et al. (2016) hypothesised that there was considerable utility in using new self-monitoring technology for the critical aspects of most dietary change and exercise/activity behaviour programmes. Indeed, self-monitoring improves the reliability of caloric intake and PA estimations and increases the potential for goal setting between the trainer and client. Reaching short-term goals can aid the success of a programme and boost intrinsic motivation as targets are achieved (Bailey, 2017). Although written food and activity diaries are useful, modern technology improves the ease and accuracy of recording several lifestyle metrics (Mendoza et al., 2007). For example, various smartphone apps enable both trainers and clients to analyse dietary intake and activity, which can improve clients' awareness of their activity level and nutrient intake (Dhurandhar et al., 2015).

Social support

During the initial engagement, trainers should inquire about the client's immediate peer support from family and friends. Lifestyle changes, especially regarding nutrition, will be easier if the peer group is supportive or even willing to adopt the changes, so it is worth exploring the level of support the client anticipates (Kwasnicka et al., 2016). Additionally, support from work colleagues is also helpful (Barasi et al., 2004). Finally, the client's trainer is clearly an important element of support. Therefore, using various communication methods (e.g., SMS messaging and e-mails), in a professional manner, may aid the client's feeling of being supported.

Summary

Personal trainers should understand and apply the basic concepts of behaviour change and refine their skills over time. The TTM is a useful construct to build an understanding of the dynamics of behaviour change. The SCM, particularly the importance of relapse, should be clearly explained to a client to manage expectations and prepare for obstacles. Assessing decisional balance and building SE will help clients identify and engage in their desired lifestyle behaviour changes. Applying principles of the Self Determination Theory enables trainers to build clients internal motivation to initiate and sustain new habits. By working in an MI consistent manner, trainers can foster a strong working relationship with clients, evoking their desires, reasons, and innate capacity for change. Finally, incorporating the key elements found in many successful behaviour change programmes enables a trainer to optimise outcomes.

References

Ajzen, I. (1991). The theory of planned behaviour. *Organisational Behaviour & Human Decision Processes, 50,* 179–211.
Amorose, A., & Anderson-Butcher, D. (2007). Autonomy-supportive coaching and self-determined motivation in high school and college athletes: a test of self-determination theory. *Psychology of Sport and Exercise, 8*(5), 654–670.
Bailey, R. (2017). Goal setting and action planning for health behavior change. *American Journal of Lifestyle Medicine, 13*(6), 615–618.
Bandura, A. (1977). Self-efficacy: toward a unifying theory of behavior change. *Psychological Review, 84,* 191–215.

Barasi, M., Mendoza, G., & Sanders, L. (2004). Weight management: a multi-dimensional approach. *Proceedings of the Nutrition Society, 63,* 79a.

Bridle, C., Riemsma, R., Pattenden, J., et al. (2005). Systematic review of the effectiveness of health behavior interventions based on the transtheoretical model. *Psychology & Health, 20*(3), 283–301.

Brown, M., Sinclair, M., Liddle, D., et al. (2012). A systematic review investigating healthy lifestyle interventions incorporating goal setting strategies for preventing excess gestational weight gain (goal setting to prevent obesity in pregnancy). *PLoS ONE, 7*(7), E39503.

Butryn, C., Arigo, D., Raggio, G., et al. (2016). Enhancing physical activity promotion in midlife women with technology-based self-monitoring and social connectivity: a pilot study. *Journal of Health Psychology, 21*(8), 1548–1555.

Callaghan, P., Eves, F., Norman, P., et al. (2002). Applying the Transtheoretical Model of Change to exercise in young Chinese people. *British Journal of Health Psychology, 7,* 267–282.

Di Noia, J., & Prochaska, J. (2010). Dietary stages of change and decisional balance: a meta-analytic review. *American Journal of Health Behavior, 34*(5), 618–632.

Dibonaventura, M., & Chapman, G. (2008). The effects of barrier underestimation on weight management and exercise change. *Psychology Health Medicine, 13,* 111–122.

Duckworth, A., Milkman, K., & Laibson, D. (2018). Beyond willpower: strategies for reducing failures of self-control. *Psychological Science in the Public Interest, 19*(3), 102–129.

Dhurandhar, N., Schoeller, D., Brown, A., et al. (2015). Energy Balance Measurement Working Group (2015). Energy Balance Measurement: when something is not better than nothing. *International Journal of Obesity, 39*(7), 1109–1113.

Freund, A., & Hennecke, M. (2015). On means and ends: the role of goal focus in successful goal pursuit. *Current Directions in Psychological Science, 24*(2), 149–153.

Frost, H., Campbell, P., Maxwell, M., et al. (2018). Effectiveness of motivational interviewing on adult behaviour change in health and social care settings: a systematic review of reviews. *PLoS ONE, 13*(10), e0204890.

Futurefit Training Ltd. (2018). Raising the bar.

Geller, K., Mendoza, I., Timbobolan, J., et al. (2012). The decisional balance sheet to promote healthy behavior among ethnically diverse older adults. *Public Health Nursing, 29*(3), 241–246.

Gibbons, F., Eggleston, T., & Benthin, A. (1997). Cognitive reactions to smoking relapse: the reciprocal relation between dissonance and self-esteem. *Journal of Personality & Social Psychology, 72,* 184–95.

Gordan, T., & Edwards, W. (1997). *Making the patient your partner: communication skills for doctors and other caregivers.* Auburn House Paperback.

Grant, A. (2014). Autonomy support, relationship satisfaction and goal focus in the coach-coachee relationship: which best predicts coaching success? *Coaching, 7*(1), 18–38.

Janis, I., & Mann, L. (1997). *Decision making: a psychological analysis of conflict, choice, and commitment.* Cassel & Collier Macmillan.

Kozica, S., Lombard, C., Teede, H., et al. (2015). Initiating and continuing behaviour change within a weight gain prevention trial: a qualitative investigation. *PLoS ONE, 10*(4), E0119773.

Kushner, R., & Hopson, S. (1998). Obesity therapy: what works – what doesn't? *Consultant, 38,* 511–516.

Kwasnicka, D., Dombrowski, S., White, M., et al. (2016). Theoretical explanations for maintenance of behaviour change: a systematic review of behaviour theories. *Health Psychology Review, 10*(3), 277–296.

Lally, P., Cornelia, H., Van Jaarsveld, H., et al. (2010). How are habits formed: modelling habit formation in the real world. *Journal of Social Psychology, 40,* 998–1009

Lopez-Fontana, I., Perrot, A., Krueger, K. et al. (2009). A global lifestyle assessment: psychometric properties of the General Lifestyle Questionnaire. *Psychologie Française,* 65, (1).

Marcus, B., Banspach, S., Lefebvre, R., et al. (1992). Using the stages of change model to increase the adoption of physical activity among community participants. *American Journal of Health promotion,* 6, 424–429.

Martin, P., Dutton, G., & Brantley, P. (2004). Self-efficacy as a predictor of weight change in African-American women. *Obesity Research, 12,* 646–651.

McKenzie, K., Pierce, D., & Gunn, J. (2015). A systematic review of motivational interviewing in healthcare: the potential of motivational interviewing to address the lifestyle factors relevant to multimorbidity. *Journal of Comorbidity,* 162–174.

Mendoza, G., et al. (2007). A multi-dimensional model for the treatment of male obesity. *Proceedings of the Nutrition Society of New Zealand, 32,* 94–100.

Miller, W., & Rollnick, S. (2009). Ten things that motivational interviewing is not. *Behavioural and Cognitive Psychotherapy, 37*(2), 129–140.

Miller, W., & Rollnick, S. (2013). *Motivational interviewing: helping people change* (3rd ed.). The Guilford Press.

Michie, S., Ashford, S., Sniehotta, F., et al. (2011). A refined taxonomy of behaviour change techniques to help people change their physical activity and healthy eating behaviours: the calorie taxonomy. *Psychology & Health, 26*(11), 1479–1498.

Moyers, T., & Miller, W. (2013). Is low therapist empathy toxic? *Psychology of Addictive Behaviors, 27*(3), 878–884.

Murray, J., Craigs, C., Hill, K., Honey, S., & House, A. (2012). A systematic review of patient reported factors associated with uptake and completion of cardiovascular lifestyle behaviour change. *BMC Cardiovascular Disorder, 12,* 120.

Nigg, J. (2016). Motivational interviewing in nutrition and fitness. *Journal of Nutrition Education and Behavior, 48*(8), 596.

O'Connell, D., & Velicer, W. (1988). A decisional balance measure and the stages of change model for weight loss. *International Journal of Addictions, 23,* 729–750.

Prochaska, J., & DiClemente, C. (1983). Stages and processes of self-change of smoking: toward an integrative model of change. *Journal of Consulting and Clinical Psychology, 51,* 390–395.

Prochaska, J., DiClemente, C., & Norcross, J. (1992). In search of how people change. *American Psychologist, 47,* 1102–1114.

Prochaska, J., Velicer, W., Rossi, J., et al. (1994). Stages of change and decisional balance for twelve problem behaviours. *Health Psychology, 13,* 39–46.

Resnicow, K., & McMaster, F. (2012). Motivational interviewing: moving from why to how with autonomy support. *International Journal of Behavioral Nutrition and Physical Activity, 9,* 19

Ryan, R., & Deci, E. (2017). *Self-determination theory.* The Guilford Press.

Rubak, S., Sandbaek, A., Lauritzen, T., et al. (2005). Motivational interviewing: a systematic review and meta-analysis. *The British journal of General Practice: the journal of the Royal College of General Practitioners, 55*(513), 305–312.

Sallis, J. (2018). Needs and challenges related to multilevel interventions: physical activity examples. *Health Education & Behavior, 45*(5), 661–67.

Stead, M., Craigie, A., Macleod, M., et al. (2015). Why are some people more successful at lifestyle change than others? Factors associated with successful weight loss in the BeWEL randomised controlled trial of adults at risk of colorectal cancer. *The International Journal of Behavioral Nutrition and Physical Activity, 12*(1), 87.

Schuster, C. (1987). Substance abuse. *JAMA: The Journal of the American Medical Association, 258*(16), 2269–2271.

Wakui, S., Shimomitsu, Y., Adagiri, S., et al. (2002). Relation of the stages of change for exercise behaviours, self-efficacy, decisional-balance, and diet related psycho-behavioural factors in young Japanese women. *The Journal of Sports Medicine and Physical Fitness, 42*, 224–232.

Weinstein, N., Rothman, A., & Sutton, S. (1998). Stage theories of health behavior: conceptual and methodological issues. *Health Psychology, 17*, 290–9.

Wingo, B., Desmond, R., Brantley, P., et al. (2013). Self-efficacy as a predictor of weight change and behavior change in the PREMIER trial. *Journal of Nutrition Education and Behavior, 45*(4), 314–321.

4 Nutrition

Alan Aragon

Scope of practice

Personal training is a dynamic, multifaceted profession with the main focus on exercise programming and instruction. However, proper nutrition is a foundational element of health and fitness. Optimal client care ideally involves a multidisciplinary team (e.g., personal trainer, dietitian/nutritionist, physiotherapist) to work with the client. However, this is not usually feasible. Thus, clients commonly rely on personal trainers for nutritional advice (Barnes et al., 2019; McKean et al., 2015). It is, therefore, essential for personal trainers to be informed and adept at providing evidence-based dietary advice and guidance within their limits of professional practice. Generally speaking, medical nutrition therapy (MNT; the nutrition-based treatment for treating or managing disease) is limited to formally credentialed nutrition professionals, such as Registered Dietitians. Licensure and registration requirements for providing nutrition care vary by country and provinces. Personal trainers should be aware of their professional limits and be ready to refer out to allied health professionals within their network.

Dietary components

Energy

Energy balance is the dynamic relationship between the energy (expressed as calories or kcal) consumed through food and beverages, versus the energy expended through basal and active physiological processes. Hypercaloric, hypocaloric, and eucaloric conditions, respectively, involve an energy surplus (weight gain), deficit (weight loss), and even balance (weight maintenance). There are several components of total daily energy expenditure (TDEE) (see Table 4.1).

Basal metabolic rate (BMR) – a term often used interchangeably with resting metabolic rate (RMR) and resting energy expenditure (REE) – is the energy expended through the body's vital physiological processes. Aside from a few exceptions (e.g., some endurance athletes), BMR is the

DOI: 10.4324/9781003204657-4

Table 4.1 Components of total daily energy expenditure (TDEE)

Component of TDEE	Per cent of TDEE	Example: 1500 kcal TDEE (kcal)	Example: 2500 kcal TDEE (kcal)	Example: 3500 kcal TDEE (kcal)
Thermic effect of food (TEF)	8–15%	120–225	200–375	280–525
Exercise activity thermogenesis (EAT)	15–30%	225–450	375–750	525–1050
Non-exercise activity thermogenesis (NEAT)	15–50%	225–750	375–1250	525–1750
Basal metabolic rate (BMR)	60–70%	900–1050	1500–1750	2100–2450

largest component of TDEE. Non-resting energy expenditure has several components. Non-exercise activity thermogenesis (NEAT) is the energy expended during basic activities of daily living, occupation activity, leisure, and fidgeting. Exercise activity thermogenesis (EAT) is the energy expended through/purposeful exercise. Unlike the relatively static BMR, NEAT and EAT vary widely across individuals. Finally, the thermic effect of food (TEF) is the energetic cost of digesting and metabolising nutrients. Protein has the highest TEF (25–30%), compared to carbohydrate (6–8%) and fat (2–3%) (Jéquier, 2002). Protein and carbohydrate contain approximately 4 kcal/g, whereas fat and alcohol contain 9 and 7 kcal/g, respectively.

There are several methods for determining total daily energy requirements. However, all methods (even highly sophisticated methods) are estimations that do not guarantee accuracy across individuals. Validated predictive equations have traditionally been used to estimate energy requirements and are systematic enough to have withstood the test of time. The first step in determining energy requirements is estimating BMR (see Table 4.2).

In most cases, the Mifflin-St. Jeor equation offers greater accuracy and reliability than other standard equations for estimating BMR (Frankenfield et al., 2005). The Katch-McArdle equation (Katch et al., 1991) is unique among the other BMR equations due to its calculation based on lean body mass. After estimating BMR, physical activity energy expenditure can be estimated by multiplying the BMR by a physical activity factor (see Table 4.3) (Tontisirin & de Haen, 2001), which produces a theoretical energy requirement to maintain body mass. If weight loss or weight gain is targeted, a caloric deficit or surplus of ~10–20%, in some cases more, can be programmed depending on how aggressively the goal is pursued. A nuanced discussion of the magnitude and composition of the energy surplus for maximising muscle hypertrophy is available in the peer-reviewed literature (see Aragon & Schoenfeld, 2020).

Table 4.2 Methods of estimating BMR

Authors	Equation
Mifflin-St. Jeor	Men: BMR = (10 × weight in kg) + (6.25 × height in cm) − (5 × age in years) + 5 Women: BMR = (10 × weight in kg) + (6.25 × height in cm) − (5 × age in years) − 161
Harris-Benedict	Men: BMR = (13.397 × weight in kg) + (4.799 × height in cm) − (5.677 × age in years) + 88.362 Women: BMR = (9.247 × weight in kg) + (3.098 × height in cm) − (4.330 × age in years) + 447.593
Katch-McArdle	BMR = (lean body mass in kg × 21.6) + 370

Protein

Dietary protein is necessary for the growth and repair of lean tissues. Protein also plays crucial roles in immunity and in the structure and function of enzymes and hormones. Protein is an essential macronutrient within the diet as the body cannot endogenously generate sufficient protein to maintain health and survival. Of the 20 amino acids that comprise proteins, nine are considered essential amino acids (EAA), and must be derived from the diet.

Table 4.3 Physical activity levels (PALs)

Category	PAL	Description
Sedentary or light activity lifestyle	1.40–1.69	• Occupations without much demand for physical effort. • Generally uses motor vehicles for transportation. • Does not exercise or participate in sports regularly. • Spends most leisure time sitting or standing (e.g., reading, talking, watching TV, using computers).
Active or moderately active lifestyle	1.70–1.99	• Occupations that are not energetically strenuous, but involve more energy expenditure than that described for sedentary lifestyles. • Sedentary occupations combined with regular moderate-to-vigorous physical activity (e.g., exercise, sports, dancing).
Vigorous or vigorously active lifestyle	2.00–2.40	• Regular engagement in strenuous work or strenuous leisure activities for several hours (e.g., prolonged, vigorous physical activities). • Occupations consisting of vigorous or strenuous physical labour (e.g., construction workers).

Proteins with higher digestibility and a greater proportion of EAA are considered higher quality (Burd et al., 2019). Protein digestibility ranking systems include the Protein Digestibility Corrected Amino Acid Score (PDCAAS), and the more recent Digestible Indispensable Amino Acid Score (DIAAS). It is important to note that digestibility ranking systems must be weighed against data on physiological and morphological outcomes (protein synthesis, muscle growth and retention, etc.) for a more holistic view of protein quality across various sources. Generally speaking, animal-derived proteins (e.g., meat, fish, poultry, dairy, egg) are higher quality than plant-derived proteins. However, a mix of animal and plant proteins can constitute a diet that provides optimal nutrition from a health standpoint.

What are the recommendations for dietary protein intake?

Daily protein requirements are population and goal-dependent but, interestingly, scientific experts consider the current 0.8 g/kg of body mass recommended daily allowance (RDA) for protein to be suboptimal (Phillips et al., 2016). For the general population, without specific athletic goals, 1.2–1.6 g/kg is appropriate for general health and preservation of lean mass, which declines with age. For athletic populations seeking to maximise training adaptations, 1.6–2.2 g/kg is appropriate (Morton et al., 2018; Schoenfeld & Aragon, 2018). Lean, resistance-trained individuals in hypocaloric conditions (dieting) can benefit from protein intakes of 2.3–3.1 g/kg of fat-free mass (Helms et al., 2014).

Is the timing and distribution of protein intake important?

Timing and distribution of protein intake are relevant to individuals aiming to maximise the hypertrophic effects of resistance training. An 'anabolic window of opportunity' has been portrayed as a narrow timeframe immediately after resistance exercise whereby rapidly digested proteins or amino acids, and highly glycaemic carbohydrate accelerate muscle recovery and growth (Aragon & Schoenfeld, 2013). However, the 'anabolic window' was challenged within the scientific literature. For example, a meta-analysis of studies comparing a protein-timed condition (feeding within an hour pre- or post-exercise) versus a non-timed condition (feeding outside of two hours pre- or post-exercise) indicated no advantage of consuming protein within an hour of training (Schoenfeld et al., 2013). Instead, greater protein intakes (~1.6 g/kg versus 1.3 g/kg) imparted the strength and hypertrophy advantages seen in the timed conditions. Subsequently, another study directly compared the effects of immediate pre- versus post-exercise protein feeding and reported no significant advantage to either protocol on resistance training adaptations (Schoenfeld et al., 2017).

The current evidence indicates that distributing daily protein intake over a minimum of three meals will support the goals of most individuals

Table 4.4 Protein requirements

Total daily amount	• General population seeking to optimise health and preservation of lean mass: 1.2–1.6 g/kg of total body mass. • Athletic populations seeking to maximise training adaptations: 1.6–2.2 g/kg of total body mass. • Lean, resistance-trained individuals in hypocaloric conditions: 2.3–3.1 g/kg of fat-free mass.
Distribution & timing throughout the day	• General population seeking to optimise health and preserve lean mass: a minimum of three relatively evenly distributed doses of protein through the day. • Athletic populations seeking to maximise training adaptations: a minimum of four protein feedings (0.4–0.55 g/kg of body mass/meal) spread relatively evenly throughout the day. • In both cases above, timing and distribution are of secondary importance to achieving the total daily protein intake.

in the general population. A minimum of four meals with protein dosed at 0.4–0.55 g/kg per meal is recommended to maximise the hypertrophic response to resistance training (Schoenfeld & Aragon, 2018). The key points regarding protein dosing and distribution are presented in Table 4.4.

Carbohydrate

In typical diets, carbohydrate is the dominant macronutrient in terms of the proportion of intake (Han et al., 2019). Like the other macronutrients, carbohydrate has multiple functions. Aside from its primary role as an inherent source of energy, carbohydrate is necessary for the efficient formation of muscle and liver glycogen to regulate blood glucose levels and fuel muscular work. Approximately 350–700 g and 100 g of glycogen is stored in skeletal muscle and the liver, respectively (Knuiman et al., 2015); however, the glycogen storage ranges vary considerably depending on lean body mass, diet composition, and training demands. Carbohydrate intake levels directly influence resting glycogen levels, which can significantly influence lean body mass since every gram of glycogen is chemically bound to 2.7–4.0 g of water (Olsson & Saltin, 1970).

Carbohydrate can broadly be classified in terms of its structure. Simple carbohydrates (monosaccharides and disaccharides) consist of single and double monosaccharide units, respectively. Complex carbohydrates (oligosaccharides, polysaccharides, and fibre) consist of short and long chains of monosaccharide units.

What are the recommendations for dietary carbohydrate intake?

Carbohydrate is often labelled as 'non-essential' since the body can biosynthesise glucose for survival by drawing upon non-carbohydrate substrates, such as lactate, glycerol, and glucogenic amino acids. While there is no

Table 4.5 Carbohydrate requirements

Total daily amount	• Clients without athletic performance concerns do not require a specific carbohydrate minimum dose. • Athletes seeking to optimally support strength/power demands and/or hypertrophy goals: 3–8 g/kg of body mass. • Athletes seeking to optimise performance in sports with endurance demands: 6–12 g/kg of body mass.
Recommended fibre intake	• 14 g/1000 kcal
Specialised tactics for endurance athletes	• Prior to competition, a loading phase with 8–12 g CHO/day for 1–3 days can maximise glycogen stores. • Within the four-hour window pre-exercise, CHO intake ranging 1–4 g/kg of body mass can benefit endurance events exceeding 90 minutes. • During exercise bouts that exceed 60 minutes, consuming 30–60 g CHO/hour within a 6–8% solution can increase endurance performance. • For maximising the rate of post-exercise glycogen resynthesis, 1.2 g CHO/kg/hour for 4–6 hours post-exercise is warranted (especially when the recovery time between bouts is eight hours or less).

minimum carbohydrate intake requirement for survival, insufficient intake can compromise athletic performance. For example, the ability to perform exercise involving high-intensity efforts can be reduced if glycogen stores are low (Hawley & Leckey, 2015). Carbohydrate dosing recommendations are presented in Table 4.5 (Kerksick et al., 2018; Slater & Phillips, 2011).

Does pre-exercise carbohydrate ingestion improve performance?

It is unclear whether ingesting carbohydrate within the hour before exercise imparts ergogenic benefits, especially if carbohydrate has been consumed during earlier feedings (e.g., a carbohydrate-rich breakfast). Consuming carbohydrate before or during exercise is unlikely to enhance performance in postprandial (fed) conditions unless the exercise exceeds 70–90 minutes. However, ingesting a combination of carbohydrate (glucose: fructose at a 1–2:1 ratio) within a 6–8% solution consumed at a rate of 30–60 g/hour is warranted during intensive exercise bouts exceeding 60 minutes.

Fat

Dietary fat is considered an essential macronutrient since the body cannot biosynthesise adequate amounts of essential fatty acids to sustain health and survival. At 9 kcal/gram, fat is a more concentrated energy source than carbohydrate and protein (which yield 4 kcal/g). The physiological roles of dietary fat include the metabolism of fat-soluble vitamins, cell membrane function, providing the structural integrity of the brain and nervous system, and hormone synthesis.

Dietary fatty acids can be broadly categorised according to their chemical structure, which determines their physical properties. At room temperature, saturated fatty acids (SFA) are solid, whereas unsaturated fatty acids (UFA) are liquid. UFA can be further stratified into polyunsaturated (PUFA) and mono-unsaturated (MUFA). SFA has historically been vilified as the 'unhealthy' type of fat due to its ability to raise low-density lipoprotein cholesterol (LDL-C), which increases cardiovascular disease risk (Borén et al., 2020); however, recent research has challenged this view (Astrup et al., 2020). Not all food sources of SFA are inherent contributors to heart disease. Evidence is mounting in support of considering the food matrix (and its diverse health-protective compounds), rather than the overly reductionist judgement of fatty acid types in isolation.

Is there an ideal ratio of omega-6 to omega-3 fatty acids?

It has been speculated that the optimal omega-6:3 ratio is somewhere between 1:1 and 4:1 (Simopoulos, 2002). However, the ratio of omega-6: omega-3 in the current Western diet is roughly 15–20:1 (Simopoulos, 2008), which may have potentially profound health implications since omega-6 FA can activate inflammatory processes, while omega-3 FA are anti-inflammatory. However, there is no inherent threat of omega-6 intake, and food source must be considered when discussing dietary fat. For example, foods such as nuts and seeds are rich sources of omega-6, yet have consistently shown favourable health outcomes (de Souza et al., 2017) and higher omega-3 intakes are associated with lower metabolic syndrome risk (Jang & Park, 2020).

Are any types of fats bad for health?

Naturally occurring trans fatty acids (TFA) in meat and dairy have shown mostly neutral effects on health. However, industrially derived TFA, from the hydrogenation of vegetable oils, increases cardiovascular risk factors and should, therefore, be avoided from the diet (Iqbal, 2014).

What are the recommendations for dietary fat intake?

The Institute of Medicine proposes that 20–35% of total energy intake should come from dietary fat (Manore, 2005). Reducing fat intake below 20% of total energy intake could have adverse health outcomes due to the role of dietary fat has in sex hormone production. For example, reductions in dietary fat from approximately 40 to 20% have resulted in significant reductions in testosterone levels (Dorgan et al., 1996; Goldin et al., 1994). Furthermore, targets below 20% may be unrealistic. Studies restricting fat calories to 20% have resulted in intakes ranging from 26 to 28% (Aragon et al., 2017). The recommended upper (35%) range of fat intake is debatable, given the substantial body of literature showing favourable effects of carbohydrate-restricted, high-fat diets (~60–80% or more) on body-weight, body composition, and various clinical outcomes (Choi et al., 2020; Hashimoto et al., 2016; Mansoor et al., 2016).

Fluid balance

Water comprises 60% of the bodyweight of healthy humans and is a vital component of all living cells, tissues, and bodily systems. Humans can survive weeks and even months without food, but insufficient fluid intake can cause death within days. Dehydration has been defined as a decrease in total body water content due to fluid loss, diminished fluid intake, or both (Shaheen et al., 2018). Dehydration by as little as 1–2% of bodyweight can impair cognition and psychomotor skills. Furthermore, exceeding a 2% decrease in bodyweight can impair athletic performance, and exceeding 8% can be lethal (Riebl & Davy, 2013). Urine colour can be used as a crude estimation of hydration status (McKenzie et al., 2015). Faint yellow indicates adequate hydration, while darker yellow and amber shades indicate progressive degrees of dehydration (Perrier et al., 2016).

Regular fluid intake/replacement is important, especially in warmer weather with physical activity and exercise. For prolonged endurance exercise, both fluid and electrolyte replacement are important. In the 2–4 hours before exercise, euhydration (adequate hydration) can be targeted by consuming fluid at 5–10 mL/kg of body mass (Thomas et al., 2016).

Is it possible to drink too much?

Excessive water intake can lead to hyponatraemia, which is a dangerous condition resulting when fluid consumption significantly exceeds sweat and urine losses. Excessive water intake can dilute plasma levels of sodium and chloride (electrolytes); thus, hyponatraemia is indicated when plasma sodium levels drop below 135 mmol/L (Thomas et al., 2016). The risk of hyponatraemia increases when a large water intake is coupled with a high sodium loss from sweating. Therefore, during exercise exceeding two hours (especially exhaustive exercise in the heat), sodium consumption of ~500–1000 mg per hour within ~0.5–1.0 L fluid per hour is recommended (Jeukendrup & Jentjens, 2005). In accordance with research data, commercial sports beverages typically contain sodium in addition to carbohydrate at a concentration of 6–8%. Post-exercise fluid intake should aim to exceed fluid loss by 25–50% (1.25–1.5 L per kg of bodyweight lost).

Vitamins and minerals

Vitamins and minerals (micronutrients) obtained from the diet are considered essential to sustain health and life as the body cannot endogenously manufacture them in adequate amounts. Vitamins are organic compounds involved in a diverse array of physiological roles including growth, homeostatic maintenance, and metabolism; they can be categorised as water-soluble or fat-soluble, based on their mode of absorption and whether or not they are stored in the body (Lykstad & Sharma, 2020). Deficiency of the water-soluble vitamins (C and the Vitamin B complex) is uncommon in North America, outside of certain at-risk populations, (e.g., alcohol use disorder and malabsorption syndromes). However, deficiencies in the fat-soluble vitamins (A, D, E, and K) are more common. The World Health Organization considers Vitamin A deficiency to be a worldwide problem in populations of low socioeconomic status (Albahrani & Greaves, 2016). Vitamin D3 deficiency is also considered to be a worldwide problem (Palacios & Gonzalez, 2014). In the USA, based on the standard of the US Endocrine Society, only 47% of Blacks and 56% of Whites have sufficient serum 25-hydroxyvitamin D (Vitamin D3) values of 30–100 ng/mL (75–250 nmol/L).

Minerals are inorganic micronutrients that are necessary for a myriad of functions, including osmotic regulation of body fluids, oxygen transport, neuromuscular transmission, and structural integrity of bones and teeth. Minerals can be categorised as macrominerals (also called major elements), which are required in amounts greater than 100 mg/ day, and microminerals (also called trace elements), required in amounts less than 100 mg/day (Morris & Mohiuddin, 2020). The macrominerals are calcium, sodium, potassium, magnesium, phosphorous, and chloride. The microminerals are iron, copper, zinc, selenium, and iodine. Worldwide anaemia prevalence is high (25%), with iron deficiency being responsible for half of the cases (Warner & Kamran, 2020). In the USA, >50% of girls aged 14–18, women aged 51–70, and both men and women older than 70 do not meet recommended calcium intakes (NIH/ODS, 2020). Furthermore, 48% of the US population consumes less than the required amount of magnesium (Rosanoff et al., 2012), and over 98% of US adults do not meet recommended intakes of potassium (Cogswell et al., 2012). Nutrients of public health concern are listed in Table 4.6 (USDHHS/USDA, 2015).

Popular supplements

Creatine

Health

Creatine is a naturally occurring compound derived from glycine and arginine by the formation of guanidinoacetate and ornithine (Persky & Brazeau, 2001) and is the most prolifically studied sports supplement. The vast majority (95%) of the endogenous creatine pool is in skeletal muscle. Creatine is found in small amounts in animal foods in the diet; omnivorous diets provide approximately 1 g/one gram per day, and vegan diets are devoid

Table 4.6 Under-consumed nutrients (and nutrients of public health concern)

Nutrient	Food sources (list is not comprehensive)
Vitamin A	Beef liver, sweet potato, spinach, pumpkin, carrots, ricotta cheese, herring, milk (fortified), cantaloupe, red peppers, mangoes, breakfast cereals (fortified)
Vitamin D	Cod liver oil, trout, mushrooms, milk (fortified), sardines, breakfast cereals (fortified)
Vitamin E	Wheat germ oil, sunflower seeds & oil, almonds & almond oil, safflower seeds & oil, hazelnuts, peanuts, peanut butter, corn oil, spinach, broccoli
Vitamin C	Red peppers, oranges, grapefruits, kiwifruit, green pepper, broccoli, strawberries, Brussels sprouts, tomato, cantaloupe, cabbage, cauliflower, potato, spinach
Choline	Beef liver, beef, eggs, soybeans, chicken, fish, potatoes
Iron	Breakfast cereals (fortified), oysters, white beans, dark chocolate. Beef liver, beef, lentils, spinach, tofu (firm), kidney beans, sardines, chickpeas, tomato paste, potatoes, cashews
Calcium	Milk, yogurt, & cheese, tofu (firm), orange juice & soy milk fortified with calcium, salmon, cottage cheese, tofu (soft), breakfast cereals (fortified)
Potassium	Beet greens, fish, chicken, beef, lentils, yam, potato, sweet potato, plantains, raisins, bananas, acorn squash, tomato, tomato paste, avocado, beans, spinach, chard, prunes, plums, apricots, oranges, carrots, milk, yogurt
Magnesium	Almonds, spinach, cashews, peanuts, soy beans (edamame), black beans, brown rice, breakfast cereals (fortified)
Fibre*	Bran cereals, various cereals, beans, peas, lentils, nuts, seeds, fruits, vegetables, most unrefined plant foods

* Fibre is the only nutrient on this list that is not considered essential, but it is beneficial to health, yet under-consumed at the population level.

of creatine (without supplementation). Supplemental creatine increases strength, power, lean mass, and sprinting performance (Kreider et al., 2017). Although several forms of creatine are commercially available, creatine monohydrate is the most stable and extensively studied form. Creatine has a consistent track record for safety, even with dosing as high as 30 g/day for five years (Kreider et al., 2017). An emerging body of research shows creatine's potential for clinical applications, such as the treatment/prevention of sarcopaenia, neurological disorders, and chronic inflammation (Riesberg et al., 2016).

Body composition

Creatine works in part through increasing cellular volume (see Figure 4.1). Due to the creatine molecule's hydrophilic nature, cellular hyperhydration occurs; thus, taking creatine is not conducive to weight loss. Indeed, a 1–2 kg increase in lean body mass is typical within 4–28 days of supplementation,

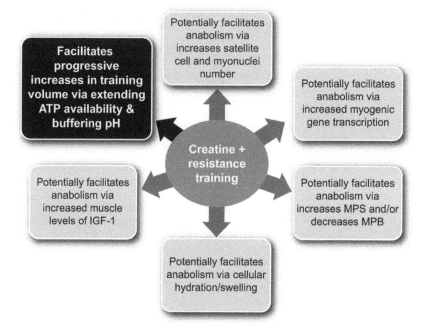

Figure 4.1 Creatine mechanism of action.

particularly when a loading phase is implemented (Persky & Brazeau, 2001).

Several creatine-loading approaches have been used in the scientific literature. The conventional week-long loading phase (20–25 g/day for 5–7 days) can be increased to two weeks with the dose halved; this approach enables muscle saturation to be achieved in two weeks and potentially avoids the gastrointestinal distress that can occur when taking 20–25 g/day. Muscle saturation can also be achieved in approximately four weeks by taking a smaller (3–5 g) daily dose. A maintenance dose of approximately 3–5 g/day is required to maintain a high level of creatine within the muscles; larger individuals may require more.

Performance

Hundreds of studies and several meta-analyses unanimously show creatine supplementation enhances performance in exercises involving intermittent, mostly anaerobic high-intensity work lasting 30–150 seconds (Cooper et al., 2012; Kreider et al., 2017). Research directly comparing pre- versus post-exercise creatine supplementation has yielded mixed results (Candow et al., 2014, 2015). Since creatine supplementation works via saturating muscle phosphocreatine levels over a shorter (1–2-week) loading period or a longer (four-week) maintenance period, the timing of dosing relative to training is unlikely to be important.

Caffeine

Health

Caffeine is a methylxanthine that naturally occurs in the leaves, seeds, and fruits of a multitude of commonly consumed plants. It is a central nervous system stimulant, and the most widely used drug in the world (Meredith et al., 2013). Caffeine acts as an adenosine receptor antagonist, thus blocking the drowsiness associated with adenosine activity. Other mechanisms include an increased shift in substrate utilisation towards fatty acids (as opposed to glycogen), and increased secretion of beta-endorphins, which can result in a decreased perception of pain or fatigue (Goldstein et al., 2010).

Potential side effects of caffeine have been reported even at low doses (250–300 mg); these include insomnia, nervousness, tremors, anxiety, nausea, gastrointestinal upset, and tachycardia (Campbell et al., 2013). Caffeine is the active ingredient in energy drinks, with doses ranging from 47–80 mg per 8 oz to 207 mg per 2 oz (Al-Shaar et al., 2017). It is, therefore, unsurprising that regular energy drink consumption has been linked with several adverse cardiovascular, metabolic, skeletal, and mental health outcomes (Al-Shaar et al., 2017). Most of these adverse effects can mainly be attributed to excessive caffeine intake.

Foods and beverages with naturally occurring caffeine such as coffee (~95 mg/cup), espresso (~64 mg/shot) tea (~27 mg/cup), and chocolate (~12 mg/oz) carry less risk than energy drinks. Indeed, there are positive findings in moderate doses. Upper safe limits of caffeine intake are 400 mg/day for healthy adults, 300 mg/day for pregnant women, and 2.5 mg/kg body weight/day for adolescents and children (Doepker et al., 2018). The acute lethal dose of caffeine is estimated to be ten grams.

Body composition

A recent systematic review and meta-analysis found that caffeine consumption reduced weight, body mass index (BMI), and body fat in a dose-dependent manner. Doubling the daily dose of caffeine resulted in 22%, 17%, and 28% greater reductions in weight, BMI, and fat, respectively, over a median duration of 12 weeks (Tabrizi et al., 2019). However, caution is necessary when using caffeine as a weight loss aid, as there is no strong evidence that caffeine-containing 'fat burner' supplements cause meaningful fat loss (>2 kg) in the long-term (Manore, 2012). Tolerance to caffeine is built over time, where its ergogenic effect diminishes (Lara et al., 2019), and by extension, its fat loss benefits could diminish as well.

Performance

Several meta-analyses demonstrate caffeine improves performance in a broad range of exercise demands across the strength-endurance continuum (Grgic et al., 2020). Performance improvements can be achieved using a dose of ~3–6 mg/kg of body mass, 30–60 minutes before exercise. Most research indicates the anhydrous form of caffeine is more effective than coffee. However, a high dose of caffeine from coffee (5 mg/kg) taken one hour before exercise was equally as effective for improving endurance performance as anhydrous caffeine (Hodgson et al., 2013). Furthermore, recent research reported that lower doses of caffeine (~3 g/kg) from coffee (the equivalent of two cups) one hour before exercise is ergogenic (Grgic et al., 2020). The interaction between genetics and caffeine can potentially explain variations in response across individuals (i.e., high and low responders). An emerging body of research has centred on two genes (CYP1A2 and ADORA2A) that can significantly impact the effectiveness of caffeine (Southward et al., 2018). The findings in this area of genotyping are equivocal, and thus do not warrant definitive conclusions for practice guidelines.

Beta-alanine

Health

Beta-alanine is a non-EAA produced endogenously and derived in small amounts from animal foods. Supplemental beta-alanine increases muscle carnosine levels, thereby acting as an intracellular pH buffering agent. Increased buffering capacity translates to greater high-intensity exercise capacity (discussed later). Doses of 4–6 g/day can increase muscle carnosine by 64% after four weeks, and 80% after ten weeks (Trexler et al., 2015). However, a side effect of beta-alanine is paresthaesia (skin tingling) in the face, neck, and hands for around 60–90 minutes. Unless the slow release form of beta-alanine is used, paresthaesia can be circumvented by breaking up the dosing into doses of 1.6 g or less.

Concerns about the safety of beta-alanine have been raised due to animal data showing its ability to decrease circulating taurine levels (García-Ayuso et al., 2019). However, this effect was not replicated in humans (Harris et al., 2006). No long-term safety data is available on beta-alanine, but as it is produced endogenously (natural occurrence within the body), it unlikely to pose any significant threat. Furthermore, a systematic risk assessment found no adverse effects of beta-alanine supplementation in healthy humans (Dolan et al., 2019).

Body composition

Most beta-alanine studies have focused on measuring intermittent and continuous high-intensity endurance performance, with little focus on changes in body composition. While an increase in lean mass and a reduction in fat mass has been reported (Smith et al., 2009), it is possible that these changes were due to the increased work output, rather than an inherent influence of beta-alanine on fuel/nutrient partitioning.

Performance

A recent and comprehensive meta-analysis found that beta-alanine improves intermittent or continuous exercise performance in events lasting 30 seconds to ten minutes (e.g., swimming, sprinting, cycling, and rowing) (Saunders et al., 2017). Furthermore, the co-ingestion of beta-alanine with sodium bicarbonate had an additive ergogenic effect beyond beta-alanine alone (Saunders et al., 2017). Despite being marketed as a supplement for weightlifters, it is unclear if beta-alanine significantly improves strength outcomes (Trexler et al., 2015). Figure 4.2 summarises sports supplements with considerable scientific support (Aragon, 2021).

Additional supplements

Sodium bicarbonate (dosed at 0.2–0.4 g/kg of body mass 1–2 hours pre-exercise) has been shown to improve performance in high-intensity exercises lasting 1–10 minutes (Carr et al., 2011; Christensen et al., 2017). However, a recent systematic review questioned the ergogenic benefit of sodium bicarbonate, citing the small sample sizes and mixed results of studies (Hadzic et al., 2019). Furthermore, the anecdotal reports of urgent gastrointestinal distress after taking sodium bicarbonate are more common than any of the

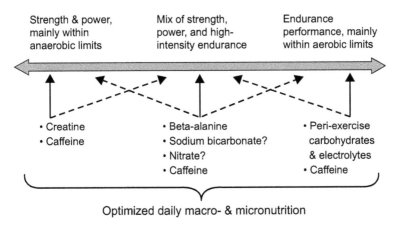

The soild lines denote stronger research evidence, the dotted lines denote weaker evidence for the compound's effectiveness in that particular region of the continuum

Figure 4.2 Supplementation along the strength-endurance continuum.

compounds listed. Nitrate, typically dosed at 10 mg/kg of body mass/day, is another well-supported compound for increasing endurance capacity (Jones, 2014). However, nitrate appears to be less effective amongst trained athletes.

Popular diets

Ketogenic diet

Health

Ketone bodies are water-soluble molecules that are produced by the liver from fatty acids. The ketogenic diet (KD) is characterised by its ability to induce *ketosis*, which is an elevation of circulating ketone bodies to ~0.5–3 mmol/L. Ketosis is objectively assessed by measuring blood levels of the ketone body beta-hydroxybutyrate (BHB) (Paoli et al., 2013). The KD typically involves restricting carbohydrate to a maximum of ~50 g or ~10% of total energy (Westman et al., 2007), while consuming a high (~60–80% or more) proportion of fat and a moderate amount (1.2–1.5 g/kg/d) of protein. Ketosis is a relatively benign state with a good track record of safety and clinically favourable outcomes, such as bodyweight reduction, decreased triacylglycerol levels, and increased high-density lipoprotein (HDL) cholesterol (Choi et al., 2020; Dashti et al., 2004).

Body composition

An abundance of research indicates KDs are superior for weight loss and fat loss compared to high-carbohydrate/low-fat controls (e.g., Choi et al., 2020). However, several studies neglected to properly control for protein and total energy intake. For example, Paoli et al. (2012) reported significant fat mass reduction and non-significant lean mass gain following a KD compared to a normal diet. However, protein intakes were substantially higher in the KD (2.9 versus 1.2 g/kg), while total energy intake was 302 kcal lower. Participants on ad libitum KDs invariably default to higher protein intakes, which can lead to greater satiety and appetite control. Therefore, Hall and Guo (2017) conducted a meta-analysis, which included only iso-caloric, protein-equated, controlled feeding studies that provided partic-ipants with all of the food intake (minimising the error of self-selected/self-reported intake). The findings showed slightly greater energy expendi-ture and fat loss in the higher carbohydrate diet, despite the carbohydrate intake ranging 1–83% and dietary fat ranging 4–84% of total energy; how-ever, the small increase in energy expenditure was not considered to be practically meaningful (Hall & Guo, 2017). Although further research is required, recent, well-controlled studies indicate, that the proportion of fat and carbohydrate in the diet can be individualised to the individual's goal, preference, and tolerance (Hall & Guo, 2017; Hall et al., 2021).

Performance

It has been postulated that a state of 'keto-adaptation', which is a physiological shift towards increased fat oxidation and decreased glycogen utilisation (Burke, 2015), can improve exercise performance. Fat yields significantly more (9 kcal/g) energy compared to carbohydrate and protein (~4 kcal/g). However, ATP can be generated approximately 2–5 times faster from glucose oxidation compared to fat oxidation (Spriet, 2002; Spriet & Watt, 2003); thus, glucose oxidation increases concurrently with exercise intensity, which has implications for carbohydrate dosing to optimise performance (Hawley & Leckey, 2015). As exercise intensity increases above ~60% of maximal oxygen consumption, the primary fuels in circulation oxidised to produce ATP are blood glucose and muscle glycogen due to progressively greater recruitment of fast-twitch motor units (Murray & Rosenbloom, 2018). Therefore, clients considering adopting a KD should proceed with caution if they perform regular high-intensity (>75% VO_{2max}) exercise, as restricting carbohydrate could impede performance (Burke et al., 2017, 2020).

Intermittent fasting

Health

Intermittent fasting (IF) can be categorised as alternate-day fasting (ADF), whole-day fasting (WDF), and time-restricted feeding (TRF) (Tinsley & Bounty, 2015). Alongside the publication of several systematic reviews and meta-analyses on the health effects of the different IF variants, IF has experienced growing popularity in recent years. To the surprise (and sometimes chagrin) of those holding on to conventional wisdom promoting a 'grazing' pattern of smaller, more frequent meals, the overall picture is favourable for IF in terms of fat loss and lean mass preservation. However, IF has not outperformed daily caloric restriction for improving cardiometabolic health parameters, including blood glucose control and lipid profile (Cioffi et al., 2018; Harris et al., 2018; Meng et al., 2020; Seimon et al., 2015). As the evidence stands, claims of IF being superior to conventional, linear caloric restriction from a health standpoint is unfounded. The advantages of IF on glucose metabolism and insulin sensitivity seen in earlier research on rodents have thus far not been replicated in humans – particularly when the control group undergoes an equivalent caloric deficit.

Body composition

Studies that compared IF and daily caloric restriction reported that intermittent energy restriction and continuous energy restriction are similarly effective for improving body composition and weight loss (Cioffi et al.,

2018; Harris et al., 2018; Headland et al., 2016; Meng et al., 2020; Seimon et al., 2015). A more significant reduction in fat mass was reported in a TRF versus a normal diet control group (Moro et al., 2016). Conversely, no significant changes in body composition (measured via DXA) were observed between participants adopting TRF compared to a regular eating pattern (Tinsley et al., 2017). TRF may not be ideal for clients training for muscle hypertrophy as one study reported participants on a control diet gained more (2.3 kg) lean mass compared to a TRF group who lost 0.2 kg; although, this difference was not statistically significant (Tinsley et al., 2017). Furthermore, the TRF group consumed less protein, which prevents firm conclusions from being drawn.

The lack of difference between IF and conventional calorie-restricted diets for reducing body fat means that clients and practitioners have the flexibility to individualise diets focused on decreasing body fat based on the client's preference and tolerance (i.e., no dietary pattern is superior for fat loss). Emerging research on TRF combined with resistance training has shown mostly equivalent effectiveness of an eight-hour feeding window versus a 12-hour window in terms of body composition improvements under hypocaloric conditions (Moro et al., 2016; Stratton et al., 2020; Tinsley et al., 2017, 2019).

Performance

The longer time periods without fuel provision during IF would, intuitively, seem to have a negative effect on performance. However, current research indicates there is no significant difference in training performance outcomes (maximal strength and muscular endurance) between IF and linear dieting (Moro et al., 2016; Stratton et al., 2020; Tinsley et al., 2017, 2019).

Veganism

Health

There are several variants of vegetarianism according to which animal foods are allowed; however, Veganism strictly excludes all animal-derived foods (even honey). Veganism is commonly adopted for ideological reasons, but this discussion will focus on health, body composition, and performance. Although observational data are not capable of demonstrating causation (see Chapter 1), there is considerable evidence showing health benefits of vegan diets, such as a reduced risk of cancer, and protection against obesity, hypertension, type-2 diabetes, and cardiovascular disease (Dinu et al., 2017; Le & Sabaté, 2014). Vegan diets have also outperformed non-vegan control diets in controlled interventions for lowering plasma lipids, reducing bodyweight, and improving glycaemic control in people with type-2 diabetes (Barnard et al., 2009; Mishra et al., 2013; Wang et al., 2015). Whether the favourable results from vegan studies are a testament to the superiority of vegan diets or merely the suboptimality of the control diets is unclear.

Humans are omnivorous in their capability to survive and thrive on a diet containing foods of both plant and animal origin. However, complete avoidance of animal foods from the diet presents nutritional deficiency risks. Supplementation or fortification of foods is, therefore, necessary to render vegan diets nutritionally complete (Rogerson, 2017). However, the extent of supplementation depends on individual goals and circumstances. The most commonly cited population-wide nutritional shortcomings among vegans are omega-3 fatty acids (EPA/DHA), vitamin B12, vitamin D, calcium, iodine, iron, and zinc (Dinu et al., 2017; Rogerson, 2017; Schüpbach et al., 2017). Additional important nutrients that are lacking or missing in vegan diets are creatine, carnosine, taurine, anserine, and 4-hydroxyproline (Wu, 2020).

Body composition

Animal-based proteins are generally of higher quality than plant-based proteins by virtue of their greater proportion of EAAs. Among the EAAs is a higher branched-chain amino acid (BCAA) content, with leucine playing a key role in driving muscle protein synthesis (MPS) (Tang et al., 2009). However, whether the short-term anabolic response indicated by MPS affects muscle hypertrophy requires corroboration by longitudinal studies. Recent evidence suggests that in response to resistance training, soy protein supplementation causes similar strength and lean mass gains as whey protein (Lynch et al., 2020; Messina et al., 2018). Additionally, pea protein supplementation has been shown to perform similarly to whey for increasing muscle thickness and force production (Banaszek et al., 2019). However, these recent plant protein studies only compared single doses of protein per day, not entirely vegan versus non-vegan diets.

A recent 12-week resistance training study compared changes in lower-body strength and muscle size between untrained vegans and omnivores who consumed a protein-matched diet (1.6g/kg/day). Both groups experienced the same gains in muscle size and strength, suggesting that protein source does not affect adaptations from resistance training (Hevia-Larraín et al., 2021). However, further research is required amongst trained individuals.

Performance

A recent narrative review proposed that vegan diets are beneficial for endurance performance based on the following benefits: reducing bodyweight, higher carbohydrate content to fuel muscular work, improvement of tissue oxygenation via improved arterial flexibility, lower oxidative stress, and inflammation via the antioxidant/anti-inflammatory foods in the diet (Barnard et al., 2019). However, the same benefits from a vegan diet suggested by Barnard et al. (2019) can be accomplished with the inclusion of animal foods while maintaining an abundance of plant foods. At present, there is a lack of compelling scientific evidence that indicates veganism is superior for athletic performance.

Summary

Nutrition is extremely complex, and numerous grey areas require scientific investigation. When dwelling on the maze of details, it is important to maintain a 'big-picture' perspective of nutrition (see Figure 4.3) (Aragon, 2021). Nutritional claims reported anecdotally and within mass/social media often lack scientific validation; however, the claims can impact clients' perspectives and behaviours. Thus, the scope of practice of the personal trainer has evolved and requires trainers to develop scientific literacy to evaluate the evidence behind nutritional claims. The fundamentals of energy balance, macronutrient and fluid intake, and supplementation for various goals along the strength-endurance continuum are rapidly developing knowledge bases. Application is a matter of weighing the research with field observations, and individualising recommendations to suit the goals, preferences, and tolerances of clients. Due to space/word limits, this chapter only covers a fraction of each topic. If you have any unanswered questions, feel free to contact me (alaneats@gmail.com), and I will do my best to answer them or point you in the right direction.

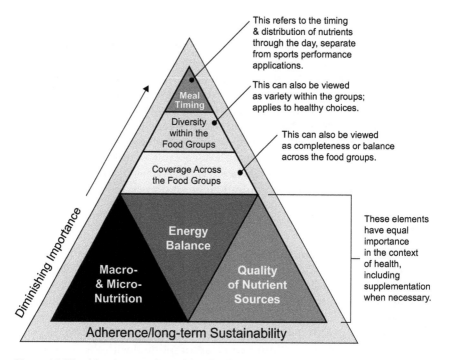

Figure 4.3 The big picture of nutrition for health.

References

Albahrani, A., & Greaves, R. (2016). Fat-soluble vitamins: clinical indications and current challenges for chromatographic measurement. *The Clinical Biochemist. Reviews, 37*(1), 27–47.

Al-Shaar, L., Vercammen, K., Lu, C., et al. (2017). Health effects and public health concerns of energy drink consumption in the United States: a mini-review. *Frontiers in Public Health, 5,* 225.

Aragon, A., & Schoenfeld, B. (2013). Nutrient timing revisited: is there a post-exercise anabolic window? *Journal of International Society of Sports Nutrition, 10*(1), 5.

Aragon, A., Schoenfeld, B., Wildman, R., et al. (2017). International society of sports nutrition position stand: diets and body composition. *Journal of the International Society of Sports Nutrition, 14,* 16.

Aragon, A., & Schoenfeld, B. (2020). Magnitude and composition of the energy surplus for maximizing muscle hypertrophy: implications for bodybuilding and physique athletes. *Strength and Conditioning Journal.* Published online ahead of print.

Aragon, A. (2021). *Advanced personal training: science to practice (2nd ed.).* Routledge.

Astrup, A., Magkos, F., Bier, D., et al. (2020). Saturated fats and health: a reassessment and proposal for food-based recommendations: JACC State-of-the-Art Review. *American College of Cardiology.* Published online ahead of print.

Banaszek, A., Townsend, J., Bender, D., et al. (2019). The effects of whey vs. pea protein on physical adaptations following 8-weeks of high-intensity functional training (HIFT): a pilot study. *Sports (Basel, Switzerland), 7*(1), 12.

Barnard, N., Cohen, J., Jenkins, D., et al. (2009). A low-fat vegan diet and a conventional diabetes diet in the treatment of type 2 diabetes: a randomized, controlled, 74-wk clinical trial. *The American Journal of Clinical Nutrition, 89*(5), 1588S–1596S.

Barnard, N., Goldman, D., Loomis, J., et al. (2019). Plant-based diets for cardiovascular safety and performance in endurance sports. *Nutrients, 11*(1), 130.

Barnes, K., Beach, B., Ball, L., et al. (2019). Clients expect nutrition care to be provided by personal trainers in Australia. *Nutrition & dietetics, 76*(4), 421–427.

Borén, J., Chapman, M., Krauss, R., et al. (2020). Low-density lipoproteins cause atherosclerotic cardiovascular disease: pathophysiological, genetic, and therapeutic insights: a consensus statement from the European Atherosclerosis Society Consensus Panel. *European Heart Journal, 41*(24), 2313–2330.

Burd, N., McKenna, C., Salvador, A., et al. (2019). Dietary protein quantity, quality, and exercise are key to healthy living: a muscle-centric perspective across the lifespan. *Frontiers in Nutrition, 6,* 83.

Burke, L. (2015). Re-examining High-fat diets for sports performance: did we call the 'Nail in the Coffin' too soon? *Sports Medicine, 4*(1), S33–S49.

Burke, L., Ross, M., Garvican-Lewis, L., et al. (2017). Low carbohydrate, high fat diet impairs exercise economy and negates the performance benefit from intensified training in elite race walkers. *The Journal of Physiology, 595*(9), 2785–2807.

Burke, L., Sharma, A., Heikura, I., et al. (2020). Crisis of confidence averted: Impairment of exercise economy and performance in elite race walkers by ketogenic low carbohydrate, high fat (LCHF) diet is reproducible. *PloS one, 15*(6), e0234027.

Campbell, B., Wilborn, C., Bounty, L. P., et al. (2013). International Society of Sports Nutrition position stand: energy drinks. *Journal of the International Society of Sports Nutrition, 10*(1), 1.

Candow, D., Vogt, E., Johannsmeyer, S., et al. (2015). Strategic creatine supplementation and resistance training in healthy older adults. *Applied Physiology, Nutrition, and Metabolism, 40*(7), 689–694.

Candow, D., Zello, G., Ling, B., et al. (2014). Comparison of creatine supplementation before versus after supervised resistance training in healthy older adults. *Research in Sports Medicine, 22*(1), 61–74.

Carr, A., Hopkins, W., & Gore, C. (2011). Effects of acute alkalosis and acidosis on performance: a meta-analysis. *Sports Medicine, 41*(10), 801–814.

Choi, Y., Jeon, S., & Shin, S. (2020). Impact of a ketogenic diet on metabolic parameters in patients with obesity or overweight and with or without type 2 diabetes: a meta-analysis. *Nutrients, 12*(7), E2005.

Christensen, P., Shirai, Y., Ritz, C., et al. (2017). Caffeine and bicarbonate for speed. A meta-analysis of legal supplements potential for improving intense endurance exercise performance. *Frontiers in Physiology, 8*, 240.

Cioffi, I., Evangelista, A., Ponzo, V., et al. (2018). Intermittent versus continuous energy restriction on weight loss and cardiometabolic outcomes: a systematic review and meta-analysis of randomized controlled trials. *Journal of Translational Medicine, 16*(1), 371.

Cogswell, M., Zhang, Z., Carriquiry, A., et al. (2012). Sodium and potassium intakes among US adults: NHANES 2003–2008. *The American Journal of Clinical Nutrition, 96*(3), 647–657.

Cooper, R., Naclerio, F., Allgrove, J., et al. (2012). Creatine supplementation with specific view to exercise/sports performance: an update. *Journal of the International Society of Sports Nutrition, 9*(1), 33.

Dashti, H., Mathew, T., Hussein, T., et al. (2004). Long-term effects of a ketogenic diet in obese patients. *Experimental & Clinical Cardiology, 9*(3), 200–205.

de Souza, R., Schincaglia, R., Pimentel, G., et al. (2017). Nuts and human health outcomes: a systematic review. *Nutrients, 9*(12), 1311.

Dinu, M., Abbate, R., Gensini, G., et al. (2017). Vegetarian, vegan diets and multiple health outcomes: a systematic review with meta-analysis of observational studies. *Critical Reviews in Food Science & Nutrition, 57*(17), 3640–3649.

Doepker, C., Franke, K., Myers, E., et al. (2018). Key findings and implications of a recent systematic review of the potential adverse effects of caffeine consumption in healthy adults. *Nutrients, 10*(10), 1536.

Dolan, E., Swinton, P., Painelli, V., et al. (2019). A systematic risk assessment and meta-analysis on the use of oral β-alanine supplementation. *Advances in Nutrition, 10*(3), 452–463.

Dorgan, J., Judd, J., Longcope, C., et al. (1996). Effects of dietary fat and fiber on plasma and urine androgens and estrogens in men: a controlled feeding study. *American Journal of Clinical Nutrition, 64*(6), 850–855.

Frankenfield, D., Roth-Yousey, L., & Compher, C. (2005). Comparison of predictive equations for resting metabolic rate in healthy nonobese and obese adults: a systematic review. *Journal of the American Dietetic Association, 105*(5), 775–789.

García-Ayuso, D., Di Pierdomenico, J., Valiente-Soriano, F., et al. (2019). β-alanine supplementation induces taurine depletion and causes alterations of the retinal nerve fiber layer and axonal transport by retinal ganglion cells. *Experimental Eye Research, 188*, 107781.

Goldin, B., Woods, M., Spiegelman, D., et al. (1994). The effect of dietary fat and fiber on serum estrogen concentrations in premenopausal women under controlled dietary conditions. *Cancer, 74*(3), 1125–1131.

Goldstein, E., Ziegenfuss, T., Kalman, D., et al. (2010). International society of sports nutrition position stand: caffeine and performance. *Journal of the International Society of Sports Nutrition, 7*(1), 5.

Grgic, J., Grgic, I., Pickering, C., et al. (2020). Wake up and smell the coffee: caffeine supplementation and exercise performance-an umbrella review of 21 published meta-analyses. *British Journal of Sports Medicine, 54*(11), 681–688.

Hadzic, M., Eckstein, M., & Schugardt, M. (2019). The impact of sodium bicarbonate on performance in response to exercise duration in athletes: a systematic review. *Journal of Sports Science & Medicine, 18*(2), 271–281.

Hall, K., & Guo, J. (2017). Obesity energetics: body weight regulation and the effects of diet composition. *Gastroenterology, 152*(7), 1718–1727.

Hall, K., Guo, J., Courville, A., et al. (2021). Effect of a plant-based, low-fat diet versus an animal-based, ketogenic diet on ad libitum energy intake. *Nature medicine, 27*(2), 344–353.

Han, S., Wu, L., Wang, W., et al. (2019). Trends in dietary nutrients by demographic characteristics and BMI among US Adults, 2003–2016. *Nutrients, 11*(11), 2617.

Harris, L., Hamilton, S., Azevedo, L., et al. (2018). Intermittent fasting interventions for treatment of overweight and obesity in adults: a systematic review and meta-analysis. *JBI Database of Systematic Reviews and Implementation Reports, 16*(2), 507–547.

Harris, R., Tallon, M., Dunnett, M., et al. (2006). The absorption of orally supplied beta-alanine and its effect on muscle carnosine synthesis in human vastus lateralis. *Amino Acids, 30*(3), 279–289.

Hashimoto, Y., Fukuda, T., Oyabu, C., et al. (2016). Impact of low-carbohydrate diet on body composition: meta-analysis of randomized controlled studies. *Obesity Reviews, 17*(6), 499–509.

Hawley, J., & Leckey, J. (2015). Carbohydrate dependence during prolonged, intense endurance exercise. *Sports Medicine, 45*(1), S5–S12.

Headland, M., Clifton, P., Carter, S., et al. (2016). Weight-loss outcomes: a systematic review and meta-analysis of intermittent energy restriction trials lasting a minimum of 6 months. *Nutrients, 8*(6), 354.

Helms, E., Zinn, C., Rowlands, D., et al. (2014). A systematic review of dietary protein during caloric restriction in resistance trained lean athletes: a case for higher intakes. *International Journal of Sport Nutrition & Exercise Metabolism, 24*(2), 127–138.

Hevia-Larraín, V., Gualano, B., Longobardi, I., et al. (2021). High-protein plant-based diet versus a protein-matched omnivorous diet to support resistance training adaptations: a comparison between habitual vegans and omnivores. *Sports Medicine, 51*(6), 1317–1330.

Hodgson, A., Randell, R., & Jeukendrup, A. (2013). The metabolic and performance effects of caffeine compared to coffee during endurance exercise. *PLoS One, 8*(4), e59561.

Iqbal, M. (2014). Trans fatty acids – a risk factor for cardiovascular disease. *Pakistan Journal of Medical Sciences, 30*(1), 194–197.

Jang, H., & Park, K. (2020). Omega-3 and omega-6 polyunsaturated fatty acids and metabolic syndrome: A systematic review and meta-analysis. *Clinical Nutrition, 39*(3), 765–773.

Jéquier, E. (2002). Pathways to obesity. *International Journal of Obesity & Related Metabolic Disorders, 26*(2), S12–S17.

Jeukendrup, A., Jentjens, R., & Moseley, L. (2005). Nutritional considerations in triathlon. *Sports Medicine, 35*(2), 163–181.

Jones, A. (2014). Dietary nitrate supplementation and exercise performance. *Sports Medicine, 44*(1), S35–S45.

Kerksick, C., Wilborn, C., Roberts, M., et al. (2018). ISSN exercise & sports nutrition review update: research & recommendations. *Journal of the International Society of Sports Nutrition, 15*(1), 38.

Knuiman, P., Hopman, M., & Mensink, M. (2015). Glycogen availability and skeletal muscle adaptations with endurance and resistance exercise. *Nutrition & Metabolism, 12*, 59.

Kreider, R., Kalman, D., Antonio, J., et al. (2017). International Society of Sports Nutrition position stand: safety and efficacy of creatine supplementation in exercise, sport, and medicine. *Journal of the International Society of Sports Nutrition, 14*, 18.

Lara, B., Ruiz-Moreno, C., Salinero, J., et al. (2019). Time course of tolerance to the performance benefits of caffeine. *PLoS One, 14*(1), e0210275.

Le, L., & Sabaté, J. (2014). Beyond meatless, the health effects of vegan diets: findings from the Adventist cohorts. *Nutrients, 6*(6), 2131–2147.

Lykstad, J., Sharma, S. (updated 2020 January). Biochemistry, water soluble vitamins. In *StatPearls* [Internet]. Treasure Island (FL): StatPearls Publishing. Available from https://www.ncbi.nlm.nih.gov/books/NBK538510/.

Lynch, H., Buman, M., Dickinson, J., et al. (2020). No significant differences in muscle growth and strength development when consuming soy and whey protein supplements matched for leucine following a 12 week resistance training program in men and women: a randomized trial. *International Journal of Environmental Research & Public Health, 17*(11), 3871.

Manore, M. (2005). Exercise and the Institute of Medicine recommendations for nutrition. *Current Sports Medicine Reports, 4*(4), 193–198.

Manore, M. (2012). Dietary supplements for improving body composition and reducing body weight: where is the evidence? *International Journal of Sport Nutrition & Exercise Metabolism, 22*(2), 139–154.

Mansoor, N., Vinknes, K., Veierød, M., et al. (2016). Effects of low-carbohydrate diets v. low-fat diets on body weight and cardiovascular risk factors: a meta-analysis of randomised controlled trials. *The British Journal of Nutrition, 115*(3), 466–479.

McArdle, W., Katch, F., & Katch, V. (1991). *Exercise physiology* (3rd ed.) Lippincott Williams & Wilkins.

McKean, M., Slater, G., Oprescu, F., & Burkett, B. (2015). Do the nutrition qualifications and professional practices of registered exercise professionals align? *International Journal of Sport Nutrition & Exercise Metabolism, 25*(2), 154–162.

McKenzie, A., Muñoz, C., & Armstrong, L. (2015). Accuracy of urine color to detect equal to or Greater than 2% body mass loss in men. *Journal of Athletic Training, 50*(12), 1306–1309.

Meng, H., Zhu, L., Kord-Varkaneh, H., et al. (2020). Effects of intermittent fasting and energy-restricted diets on lipid profile: a systematic review and meta-analysis. *Nutrition, 77,* 110801.

Meredith, S., Juliano, L., Hughes, J., et al. (2013). Caffeine use disorder: a comprehensive review and research agenda. *Journal of Caffeine Research, 3*(3), 114–130.

Messina, M., Lynch, H., Dickinson, J., et al. (2018). No difference between the effects of supplementing with soy protein versus animal protein on gains in muscle mass and strength in response to resistance exercise. *International Journal of Sport Nutrition & Exercise Metabolism, 28*(6), 674–685.

Mishra, S., Xu, J., Agarwal, U., et al. (2013). A multicenter randomized controlled trial of a plant-based nutrition program to reduce body weight and cardiovascular risk in the corporate setting: the GEICO study. *European Journal of Clinical Nutrition, 67*(7), 718–724.

Moro, T., Tinsley, G., Bianco, A., et al. (2016). Effects of eight weeks of time-restricted feeding (16/8) on basal metabolism, maximal strength, body composition, inflammation, and cardiovascular risk factors in resistance-trained males. *Journal of Translational Medicine, 14*(1), 290.

Morris, A., & Mohiuddin, S. (updated 2020 February). Biochemistry, nutrients. In *StatPearls* [Internet]. Treasure Island (FL): StatPearls Publishing; 2020 January. Available from https://www.ncbi.nlm.nih.gov/books/NBK554545/.

Morton, R., Murphy, K., McKellar, S., et al. (2018). A systematic review, meta-analysis and meta-regression of the effect of protein supplementation on resistance training-induced gains in muscle mass and strength in healthy adults. *British Journal of Sports Medicine, 52*(6), 376–384.

Murray, B., & Rosenbloom, C. (2018). Fundamentals of glycogen metabolism for coaches and athletes. *Nutrition Reviews, 76*(4), 243–259.

National Institutes of Health, Office of Dietary Supplements. (updated 2020 March). *Calcium fact sheet for health professionals* [Internet]. Available from https://ods.od.nih.gov/factsheets/Calcium-HealthProfessional/.

Olsson, K., & Saltin, B. (1970). Variation in total body water with muscle glycogen changes in man. *Acta Physiologica Scandinavica, 80*(1), 11–18.

Palacios, C., & Gonzalez, L. (2014). Is vitamin D deficiency a major global public health problem? *The Journal of Steroid Biochemistry & Molecular Biology, 144*(Pt A), 138–145.

Paoli, A., Grimaldi, K., D'Agostino, D., et al. (2012). Ketogenic diet does not affect strength performance in elite artistic gymnasts. *Journal of the International Society of Sports Nutrition, 9*(1), 34.

Paoli, A., Rubini, A., Volek, J., et al. (2013). Beyond weight loss: a review of the therapeutic uses of very-low-carbohydrate (ketogenic) diets. *European Journal of Clinical Nutrition, 67*(8), 789–796.

Perrier, E., Johnson, E., McKenzie, A., et al. (2016). Urine colour change as an indicator of change in daily water intake: a quantitative analysis. *European Journal of Nutrition, 55*(5), 1943–1949.

Persky, A., & Brazeau, G. (2001). Clinical pharmacology of the dietary supplement creatine monohydrate. *Pharmacological Reviews, 53*(2), 161–176.

Phillips, S., Chevalier, S., & Leidy, H. (2016). Protein "requirements" beyond the RDA: implications for optimizing health. *Applied Physiology, Nutrition, & Metabolism, 41*(5), 565–572.

Riebl, S., & Davy, B. (2013). The hydration equation: update on water balance and cognitive performance. *ACSM's health & Fitness Journal, 17*(6), 21–28.

Riesberg, L., Weed, S., McDonald, T., et al. (2016). Beyond muscles: the untapped potential of creatine. *International Immunopharmacology, 37*, 31–42.

Rogerson, D. (2017). Vegan diets: practical advice for athletes and exercisers. *Journal of the International Society of Sports Nutrition, 14*, 36.

Rosanoff, A., Weaver, C., & Rude, R. (2012). Suboptimal magnesium status in the United States: are the health consequences underestimated? *Nutrition Reviews, 70*(3), 153–164.

Saunders, B., Elliott-Sale, K., Artioli, G., et al. (2017). β-alanine supplementation to improve exercise capacity and performance: a systematic review and meta-analysis. *British Journal of Sports Medicine, 51*(8), 658–669.

Schoenfeld, B., Aragon, A., Wilborn, C., et al. (2017). Pre- versus post-exercise protein intake has similar effects on muscular adaptations. *PeerJ, 5*, e2825.

Schoenfeld, B., & Aragon, A. (2018). How much protein can the body use in a single meal for muscle-building? Implications for daily protein distribution. *Journal of the International Society of Sports Nutrition, 15*, 10.

Schoenfeld, B., Aragon, A., & Krieger, J. (2013). The effect of protein timing on muscle strength and hypertrophy: a meta-analysis. *Journal of the International Society of Sports Nutrition, 10*(1), 53.

Schüpbach, R., Wegmüller, R., Berguerand, C., et al. (2017). Micronutrient status and intake in omnivores, vegetarians and vegans in Switzerland. *European Journal of Nutrition, 56*(1), 283–293.

Seimon, R., Roekenes, J., Zibellini, J., et al. (2015). Do intermittent diets provide physiological benefits over continuous diets for weight loss? A systematic review of clinical trials. *Molecular & Cellular Endocrinology, 418*(2), 153–172.

Shaheen, N., Alqahtani, A., Assiri, H., et al. (2018). Public knowledge of dehydration and fluid intake practices: variation by participants' characteristics. *BMC Public Health, 18*(1), 1346.

Simopoulos, A. (2002). The importance of the ratio of omega-6/omega-3 essential fatty acids. *Biomedicine Pharmacotherapy, 56*(8), 365–379.

Simopoulos, A. (2008). The omega-6/omega-3 fatty acid ratio, genetic variation, and cardiovascular disease. *Asia Pacific Journal of Clinical Nutrition, 17*(1), 131–134.

Slater, G., & Phillips, S. (2011). Nutrition guidelines for strength sports: sprinting, weightlifting, throwing events, and bodybuilding. *Journal of Sports Sciences, 29*(1), S67–S77.

Smith, A., Walter, A., Graef, J., et al. (2009). Effects of beta-alanine supplementation and high-intensity interval training on endurance performance and body composition in men; A double-blind trial. *Journal of the International Society of Sports Nutrition, 6*, 5.

Southward, K., Rutherfurd-Markwick, K., Badenhorst, C., et al. (2018). The role of genetics in moderating the inter-individual differences in the ergogenicity of caffeine. *Nutrients, 10*(10), 1352.

Spriet, L., & Watt, M. (2003). Regulatory mechanisms in the interaction between carbohydrate and lipid oxidation during exercise. *Acta Physiologica Scandanavia, 178*(4), 443–452.

Spriet, L. (2002). Regulation of skeletal muscle fat oxidation during exercise in humans. *Medicine and Science in Sports and Exercise, 34*(9), 1477–1484.

Stratton, M., Tinsley, G., Alesi, M., et al. (2020). Four weeks of time-restricted feeding combined with resistance training does not differentially influence measures of body composition, muscle performance, resting energy expenditure, and blood biomarkers. *Nutrients, 12*(4), 1126.

Tabrizi, R., Saneei, P., Lankarani, K., et al. (2019). The effects of caffeine intake on weight loss: a systematic review and dose-response meta-analysis of randomized controlled trials. *Critical Reviews in Food Science & Nutrition, 59*(16), 2688–2696.

Tang, J., Moore, D., Kujbida, G., et al. (2009). Ingestion of whey hydrolysate, casein, or soy protein isolate: effects on mixed muscle protein synthesis at rest and following resistance exercise in young men. *Journal of Applied Physiology, 107*(3), 987–992.

Thomas, D., Erdman, K., & Burke, L. (2016). Position of the Academy of Nutrition and Dietetics, Dietitians of Canada, and the American College of Sports Medicine: nutrition and athletic performance. *Journal of the Academy of Nutrition & Dietetics, 116*(3), 501–528.

Tinsley, G., & Bounty, L. (2015). Effects of intermittent fasting on body composition and clinical health markers in humans. *Nutrition Reviews, 73*(10), 661–674.

Tinsley, G., Forsse, J., Butler, N., et al. (2017). Time-restricted feeding in young men performing resistance training: a randomized controlled trial. *European Journal of Sport Science, 17*(2), 200–207.

Tinsley, G., Moore, M., Graybeal, A., et al. (2019). Time-restricted feeding plus resistance training in active females: a randomized trial. *The American Journal of Clinical Nutrition, 110*(3), 628–640.

Tontisirin, K., & de Haen, H. (2001). Human energy requirements: report of a Joint FAO/WHO/UNU Expert Consultation.

Trexler, E., Smith-Ryan, A., Stout, J., et al. (2015). International society of sports nutrition position stand: beta-alanine. *Journal of the International Society of Sports Nutrition, 12*, 30.

U.S. Department of Health and Human Services and U.S. Department of Agriculture (2015). 2015–2020 Dietary Guidelines for Americans (8th ed.). December 2015.

Wang, F., Zheng, J., Yang, B., et al. (2015). Effects of vegetarian diets on blood lipids: a systematic review and meta-analysis of randomized controlled trials. *Journal of the American Heart Association, 4*(10), e002408.

Warner, M., & Kamran, M. (updated 2020 August). *StatPearls* [Internet]. Treasure Island (FL): StatPearls Publishing. Available from https://www.ncbi.nlm.nih.gov/books/NBK448065/.

Westman, E., Feinman, R., Mavropoulos, J., et al. (2007). Low-carbohydrate nutrition and metabolism. *The American Journal of Clinical Nutrition, 86*(2), 276–284.

Wu, G. (2020). Important roles of dietary taurine, creatine, carnosine, anserine and 4-hydroxyproline in human nutrition and health. *Amino Acids, 52*(3), 329–360.

5 Health and fitness assessment

Paul Hough, Cody Haun, Neil Stanley,
and Nick Tumminello

The regular collection of clients' health and fitness data enables trainers to establish strengths and weaknesses, monitor progress, and identify training needs. Various health and fitness assessment tools, techniques, and technologies (TTTs) enable the trainer and client to evaluate progress and set goals. Fitness assessments are usually performed several times per year to evaluate changes in components of fitness (e.g., strength) and body composition. Alongside periodic fitness assessments, certain data can be collected and monitored daily or weekly, which enables training and nutrition programmes to be refined based on the client's recent physical/psychological status and lifestyle. Collecting data regularly to inform programme design is known as 'monitoring'. Clients can collect data without the trainer (i.e., self-monitoring) using a simple logbook or technologies, such as smartphone apps. Self-monitoring could improve long-term outcomes by promoting a collaborative relationship between the trainer and client, cultivating adherence, and maintaining intrinsic motivation (see Chapter 3).

The first part of this chapter outlines a process for selecting health and fitness TTTs. Part two of the chapter includes some practical examples of monitoring methods that can be used daily, and assessments that can be done periodically.

Selecting health and fitness tools, techniques, and technologies (TTTs)

Components of health and fitness can be measured using direct or indirect measurements. Direct measurements avoid assumptions or estimates, are usually recorded in a laboratory setting, and typically require specialist TTTs and technical expertise. Laboratory-based TTTs offer the highest validity and reliability (discussed later); however, laboratory assessments are often impractical to conduct regularly due to time, logistical, and financial limitations. Therefore, most personal trainers use indirect assessment methods in a gym or field setting. For example, a direct measure of maximal oxygen uptake (VO_{2max}) requires the exerciser to breathe into a mask connected to a gas analyser during incremental exercise on an

DOI: 10.4324/9781003204657-5

ergometer. Alternatively, indirect approaches, such as measuring the heart rate (HR) response during sub-maximal exercise, can be used to predict VO_{2max} (see Table 5.3).

Numerous health and fitness TTTs, such as body fat measurement scales and activity monitors (discussed later), are available for trainers to use with clients. The abundance of TTTs can make it challenging to identify which ones to apply. The first step in deciding which TTT to select is ensuring the TTT is practically and financially viable for the trainer and client. The second step is to evaluate the TTT regarding its specificity, validity, and reliability.

Specificity

Health and fitness assessments should be specific to the client's needs and goals and inform the subsequent training and nutrition interventions. For example, clients seeking to improve maximal strength should perform periodic strength tests (see Chapter 13). Similarly, clients seeking to reduce body fat or increase muscle size should have their body composition measured using appropriate methods, such as dual x-ray absorptiometry (DXA) or anthropometry (skinfolds and limb girths). Subjective assessments can also be used alongside objective ones. For example, changes in body composition can be monitored based on appearance, alongside skinfolds (see page 72).

Reliability and validity

Trainers should select TTTs that produce measures that are as precise as possible, which requires a basic understanding of the principles of validity and reliability. Validity refers to how well the measure reflects the true value. Reliability refers to the reproducibility of the measurement. Reliability and validity are related, as a test cannot be valid if it is not reliable. However, a test can be reliable but invalid (see Figure 5.1). For instance, incorrectly

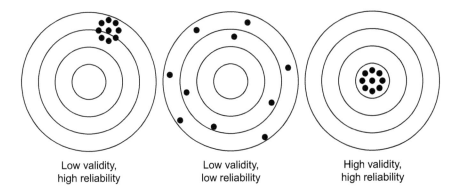

Low validity,   Low validity,   High validity,
high reliability   low reliability   high reliability

Figure 5.1 Validity and reliability.

calibrated weighing scales that consistently read 1.5 kg heavier would produce a reliable but inaccurate reflection of the user's true body mass.

Various TTTs have been studied with respect to their validity and reliability. It is a good idea to source these studies to understand if the TTT being considered offers an acceptable level of precision. Trainers should attempt to establish the validity and reliability of a TTT before using the data to inform decisions. The following section provides a brief introduction to the principles of validity and reliability.

Validity

Establishing if there is agreement between a measurement and its true value is known as concurrent validity. Concurrent validity is quantified by comparing a particular measurement against values obtained from the most accurate method of measurement, known as the criterion or 'gold standard'. For example, an electrocardiogram (ECG) is considered the most accurate (gold standard) method to measure HR. Therefore, the validity of some commercially available HR monitors has been established by comparing the HR data from the devices against an ECG (Pasadyn et al., 2019).

Two common statistical measures of validity are the standard or typical error of estimate (TEE) and validity correlation coefficient. The TEE represents the typical amount by which the measure is incorrect versus the criterion measure when an individual is assessed. For example, the TEE for the YMCA cycle ergometer test (an indirect assessment of VO_{2max}) is ±9.8 mL/kg/min compared to a direct measurement of VO_{2max} (Beekley et al., 2004). In this example, if the direct (criterion) VO_{2max} was 51 mL/kg/min, the result of the indirect method (YMCA test) could typically be 9.8 mL/kg/min above or below the true VO_{2max} in any given individual from the population for which the validity measures were derived. A reduced TEE is associated with increased validity (Heyward & Gibson, 2014).

A validity coefficient provides an indication of the strength of the relationship between a measure and the criterion measure. For example, during a 12-minute Cooper run, the distance covered showed a correlation of 0.93 with directly measured VO_{2max} during a laboratory test (Bandyopadhyay, 2015). A validity correlation (r value) closer to 1.0 indicates the relationship between the measure and the criterion measure is strong. In contrast, an r value closer to 0.0 indicates there is a weak relationship between the measurements (Cohen, 1988).

Reliability

Reliability refers to the consistency of a measure that is repeated on two or more occasions. Health and fitness metrics usually fluctuate daily. For example, the client's daily body mass shown in Table 5.1 is variable. This variation between repeated measures is known as the random error or

Table 5.1 Repeated measures of body mass and sum of skinfolds

	Body mass (kg)	*Σ 7 Skinfolds*
Monday	73.5	65
Tuesday	73.1	60
Wednesday	73.9	70
Thursday	73.6	68
Friday	74.1	
Saturday	73.4	
Average	**73.6**	**65.8**
SD = TEM	**0.4**	**4.3**

TEM = Typical error of measurement.

'noise', which can arise from the equipment (e.g., weighing scales), the operator (trainer), and the client being tested.

If there is no existing reliability data for a measure, trainers can determine reliability by repeating the measure with the same client (i.e., retest reliability) when no true change is expected (e.g., measuring a client's body mass and skinfolds on 3–4 consecutive days). Following repeated measures, the random error within the data can be accounted for by calculating the standard deviation (see Table 5.1), which represents the dispersion (spread) of a dataset relative to its mean. The data in Table 5.1 have been collected from the same client, so the SD represents the typical error of measurement (TEM). Measures with a smaller TEM offer better reliability than those with a higher TEM.

Understanding the TEM is practically useful for trainers to determine if a real change has likely occurred (i.e., deciding if the change is meaningful). Moreover, a basic appreciation of TEM can be useful for clients. For example, if the client who was weighed (see Table 5.1) understood that his body mass fluctuates daily by about 0.5 kg, mainly due to changes in body fluid stores, he would only start to be concerned about a body mass change in the region of ≥1 kg.

Inspecting future changes in a measure alongside the TEM provides a basic method for judging if a change in measurement is meaningful. More comprehensive data analysis approaches, such as considering the smallest important change from a clinical or performance perspective, offer an even better interpretation of change in an individual. For further information on data analysis approaches, refer to *resources for assessing individuals* at the sport science website: sportsci.org.

How can the precision of measurements be improved?

If a published validation study is not available, the reliability of measurement can be established by following the process outlined above. Health and fitness assessments must be suitable for the age and physical capacity of the client. Moreover, assessments should only be implemented if suitable equipment is available and the testing environment is appropriate (Burnstein et al., 2011). The following considerations must be accounted for to ensure the data collected is as precise as possible.

Pre-test guidelines: Several factors, such as dietary intake and when the client last exercised, can influence the results of assessments. Therefore, clear, standardised guidelines should be provided for clients to follow beforehand.

Environment/attire: Assessments should be conducted in similar conditions. Changes in climate (e.g., temperature), training surface, and type of clothing and footwear can influence performance.

Test familiarisation: A client's performance can often improve from having done the test before, which known as a learning effect. Generally, clients should perform 2–3 familiarisation trials to ensure an accurate measurement has been recorded.

Test protocol: Measurement techniques, equipment, and procedures should all be standardised. Where applicable, equipment should be regularly calibrated. Tests should be repeated at the same time of day and rest periods between tests kept the same. Additionally, the same instructions and motivational statements should be provided – a standardised script can be useful in this regard.

Health and fitness assessments do not need to be complex or complicated. Indeed, simple assessments are easier to standardise and often produce more reliable data than complex assessments. By following the guidelines above, bespoke assessments can be designed and modified based on the client's goals and circumstances.

Summary

Various methods are available to assess the health and fitness status of clients. Regular assessment and monitoring of appropriate metrics enable the client's progress to be evaluated and the training programme to be adapted. Alongside periodic assessments, trainers and clients can monitor certain data daily or weekly, enabling training and nutrition programmes to be frequently refined. Assessments do not need to be complex, but they should be relevant to the client's goals, and physical capacity. Several procedures should be followed to improve validity and reliability, including providing the client with clear instructions and performing assessments under standardised conditions.

Part 2: Examples of assessment and monitoring methods

Components of fitness and body composition that take weeks or months to modify (e.g., cardiorespiratory fitness and body fat) do not need to be measured on a daily or weekly basis. However, factors that can fluctuate daily, such as sleep and nutrition, influence training responses and are suited to a

Table 5.2 Examples of health and fitness assessments

Component	Parameter	Methods/instruments	Monitoring (daily or weekly)	Assessment. (monthly or quarterly)
General health	Resting heart rate	Palpation; HR monitor; mobile apps	✓	✓
	Blood pressure (BP)	BP monitor	✓	✓
	Sleep	Diary; actigraphy; mobile apps	✓	
	Dietary habits	Food diary; mobile apps	✓	
		FFQ	✓	✓
Body composition	Body mass	Body mass scales	✓	✓
	Fat mas & FFM	Circumferences (waist, hip, limb)	✓	✓
		Skinfolds, Bod Pod, DXA		✓
		BIA	✓	✓
		Photos (see page 73)		✓
				✓
Cardiorespiratory fitness		See page 77		✓
Strength	Maximal strength	RM or 1RM (see Chapter 7)		✓
	Strength symmetry	See page 72		✓
	Strength endurance	AMRAP on a body weight exercise or an exercise with a prescribed load		✓
Power	Lower body power	Vertical and broad jumps; 5–30 second sprint performance (e.g., 20-m sprint, Wingate test)		✓
	Upper body power	Medicine ball throw		✓

AMRAP = As many repetitions as possible; BIA = Bioelectrical impedance analysis; DXA = Dual-energy x-ray absorptiometry; FFM = Fat free mass; FFQ = Food frequency questionnaire; RM = Repetition maximum.

monitoring approach rather than periodic assessments (see Table 5.2). In this section, experts in sleep, exercise physiology, and strength and conditioning outline some monitoring (sleep and HR) and assessment (body composition, strength, and cardiorespiratory fitness) methods listed in Table 5.2.

Monitoring sleep
Dr Neil Stanley

Over the last decade, two developments have increased interest in sleep tracking within the sports/fitness science community. Firstly, there has been an increased appreciation of the importance of sleep to physical, mental and emotional health, athletic performance, and recovery from exercise (Erlacher et al., 2011; Roberts et al., 2019; Skein et al., 2011). Secondly, the increased commercial availability of inexpensive activity monitors that measure sleep has enabled users to objectively monitor their sleep.

Most wearable activity monitors record sleep quantity and quality by measuring the wrist movements of the sleeper, which is known as wrist actigraphy. Since the first solid-state wrist-worn actigraph that was described in the 1970s (Colburn et al., 1976), advances in technology improved the sophistication and usability of the monitoring devices, and several actigraphy devices became commercially available (Kripke et al., 1978; Redmond & Hegge, 1985). While there are variances in how different actigraphy devices work, essentially, the device's motion sensor generates a signal voltage each time it moves. The number of movements above a certain count or threshold in a set period (usually 30–60 seconds) equates to 'wake', and movements below that threshold equate to 'sleep'.

During the 1980s and 1990s, several automatic sleep/wake detection algorithms were developed to correlate with sophisticated sleep measurements recorded in sleep laboratories (Stanley, 2003). The advancement in algorithms lead to several studies reporting a significant correlation between actigraphy and electrical activity in the brain, which is used, alongside other measures, to measure total sleep time (TST), sleep efficiency (SE%), and sleep onset latency (SOL), in normal healthy participants (Cole et al., 1992; Sadeh et al., 1994). Therefore, several wearable activity monitors have been developed, which provide a reasonable estimate of TST, SE%, and SOL (de Zambotti et al., 2020).

It is not always easy to judge the accuracy of commercially available wearable activity monitors as few have been independently validated, and the algorithms are not usually published (de Zambotti et al., 2020; Evenson et al., 2015). Therefore, it is recommended that a wearable device is used in conjunction with a sleep diary (Vallières & Morin, 2003). Moreover, using a sleep diary helps to identify quiet wakefulness (e.g., before sleep onset), which activity monitors may inaccurately record as sleep. Some wearable devices claim to differentiate between sleep stages (e.g., light and deep sleep) (Roberts et al., 2020), which is not possible using movement data alone. Devices that combine movement data with heart rate (HR) data tend to offer better accuracy; however, sleep stages still cannot be reliably identified using actigraphy and HR data (Grander & Rosenberger, 2019).

Wearable activity monitors are a useful technique to measure sleep and provide a reasonable estimate of TST, SE%, and SOL. However, to improve confidence in the data, they should be used in conjunction with a sleep diary.

Monitoring heart rate
Dr Cody Haun

The autonomic nervous system (ANS) controls functions of the body that are completely or mostly independent of voluntary control. The ANS consists of a sympathetic and parasympathetic branch. The sympathetic branch promotes a so called 'fight or flight response' by increasing certain physiological parameters, such as HR and blood pressure. The parasympathetic branch dominates during periods of rest and digestion (e.g., during sleep). Monitoring resting heart rate (RHR) and/or HR variability (HRV) (defined below) may provide insight into a client's recovery from previous training and potentially indicate if the client is prepared to complete challenging training (i.e., readiness to train). Additionally, a consistently high RHR is associated with an elevated risk of cardiovascular disease (Jensen et al., 2013).

The RHR can be measured using the manual palpation method, where the base of the thumb is applied to the radial artery and the number of pulses in 15 seconds is counted and multiplied by four to calculate the RHR in beats per minute (b/min). However, for accuracy, RHR should be measured using a validated HR monitor in standardised conditions (e.g., quiet, no distractions, comfortable temperature) at the same time of day.

HRV is the variation in time between heartbeats over a specific sampling period. The ANS regulates HR and HRV; thus, changes in these variables can reflect alterations in the activity of the sympathetic or parasympathetic branches of the ANS (Acharya et al., 2006). Atypical elevations in RHR, or decreases in HRV, *may* suggest that body systems are still recovering from a prior training bout or a lower readiness to complete a challenging training session (Thamm et al., 2019). The accurate measurement of HRV requires using a validated device (e.g., chest strap) and specialised software. Several commercially available mobile applications and devices can measure HRV. However, a detailed discussion of the available HRV products is beyond this section's scope. Practitioners are encouraged to research the most appropriate research-validated technologies.

Abnormal elevations in RHR, or decreases in resting HRV, may reflect increased sympathetic nervous system activity at rest; this *may* indicate more time should be allowed for recovery, or that training load should be reduced for that day. Conversely, a normal or slightly below average RHR coupled with a normal or slightly elevated HRV, indicates lower SNS activity and a more recovered state. Some evidence suggests HRV can help guide training prescription for better training outcomes (Flatt et al., 2017). For example, HRV tended to be higher in collegiate swimmers when perceived sleep quality, fatigue, stress, and mood were better than average (Flatt et al., 2017).

Considering HRV is relatively simple to measure, it is worth considering alongside other monitoring techniques. However, scientific evidence that HR variables are reliable enough to guide training prescription, or predict readiness to train, is still needed. Some studies have shown no significant relationship between HRV measurements and adaptive outcomes (De Oliveira et al., 2019; Thamm et al., 2019). For example, Thamm et al. (2019) observed no associations between changes in HRV and other common markers of recovery (e.g., force production, creatine kinase, and subjective well-being). Researchers have concluded that several recovery markers should be used, as HRV alone may not be sensitive enough to determine the individual's recovery and readiness to train (Flatt et al., 2017; Thamm et al., 2019). Consequently, trainers should not use HR or HRV to dictate the training programme.

Subjective assessment of body composition
Dr Cody Haun

Standardised photos can be taken to compare changes in body appearance over time. The images should be recorded with the date and, where possible, body composition data (e.g., body mass and body fat %). Taking photos is not always appropriate and should only be suggested if a client is comfortable and provides consent. The practitioner must consider the client's goals and personality before suggesting photos. There are cases where photos are contraindicated (e.g., clients with a known history or susceptibility to body dysmorphic disorder). Furthermore, the appearance of a client's physique is only one subjective indicator of progress and not every client has aesthetic goals. Several positive outcomes can be achieved from regular training that photos cannot detect (e.g., improvements in cardiorespiratory fitness and strength).

Photos can be taken every 2–4 weeks in a standardised setting with consistent lighting, posing, and camera angle. Three (front, side, and rear-facing) full-body photos provide a relatively complete assessment (see Figure 5.2). Recurrent photos should be taken at a similar time of day in the same clothing. Wearing tight clothing, such as compression shorts, minimises shadows and allows body contours to be more clearly defined.

Assessing lower body strength symmetry
Nick Tumminello

An *assessment* is a process-oriented procedure used to create internally defined goals. An *evaluation* is a product-oriented procedure based on externally imposed standards. For example, in the back-squat exercise, an assessment would involve determining the client's needs to modify her

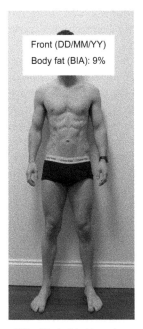
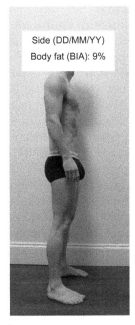
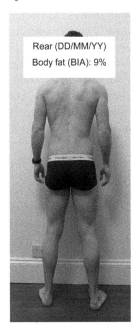

BIA = Bioelectrical impedance analysis

Figure 5.2 Example progress photos.

stance to suit her skeletal framework, injury history, and current ability. An evaluation of the back-squat would involve determining if the client is strong or weak, based on her back-squat strength relative to her body weight. Assessments and evaluations can help the fitness professional develop a safe and individualised training programme for clients and athletes.

Muscle strength and power asymmetry describes the differences in strength and power between limbs for a specific joint action. Knowledge of lower extremity asymmetry may provide insights into injury risk, rehabilitation, and performance (Croisier et al., 2002; Newton et al., 2006). For example, single-leg exercises can be used to detect deficits in unilateral strength and power (Myer et al., 2012). Indeed, several studies analysing males and females, with a variety of sporting backgrounds, have demonstrated that strength asymmetries greater than 15% between the right and left leg may be an indicator of increased injury risk (Impellizzeri et al., 2007; Knapik et al., 1991; Rohman et al., 2015). However, a certain amount of strength asymmetry is expected, especially when confounding factors, such as side dominance and injury history, are considered (Paterno et al., 2007, 2011). It is important to note that the purpose of asymmetry assessment is not to offset physical biases, developed from playing certain sports, or making naturally asymmetrical bodies move or become perfectly symmetrical. Strength asymmetries are expected, normal and allowed within a less than 15% differential. However, well-designed training interventions that reduce significant sporting asymmetries could potentially improve performance (Bishop et al., 2021).

From a performance perspective, a clear link between asymmetry and athletic performance has yet to be determined, as there is a lack of consistency between studies (Maloney, 2019). Several studies that have investigated the relationship between muscle function, performance, injury, and left to right leg asymmetry have reported no association between asymmetry and impaired performance or injury risk referring (Mertz et al., 2019; Lockie et al., 2014, 2017). However, these reports typically refer to asymmetries below 15%, which is the suggested limit where an asymmetry becomes an issue. Therefore, between-leg strength differences of less than 15% are generally not considered to be functionally significant (Knapik et al., 1991; Lockie et al., 2017) and should not have a negative impact on performance, such as running speed (Lockie et al., 2014).

Clients with a between limb strength asymmetry above 15% (see above) would likely benefit from an exercise intervention to reduce the imbalance, as this could potentially improve performance and decrease injury risk (Myer et al., 2012). Performing a lower body strength asymmetry evaluation can facilitate the programme design process by enabling more accurate prescription of exercises and volume, based on the client's individual needs. The following example is an evaluation of lower body strength symmetry.

The trainer is looking for a difference in strength above 15% between left and right sides, using one of the two unilateral lower body exercise evaluations provided at the end of this section. If there is a greater (>15%) strength difference between left and right sides, the trainer can programme to reduce the existing strength asymmetry (to <15%) using unilateral exercises as follows:

- Perform one or two more sets on the weaker side
- Start each set with the weaker side
- Use the same load on both sides, but limit the repetitions on the stronger side to match the repetitions achieved on the weaker side.

An equal volume (i.e., sets and repetitions) on unilateral lower body exercises can be resumed when strength asymmetry is within the baseline cutoff of 15% (or less).

Evaluation rules

- The trainer only counts the repetition when it is performed in the full range of motion described below.

- The set ends when the client cannot successfully perform a full range of motion repetition.
- Perform all repetitions on the same side before switching sides.
- Rest 5–6 minutes between sides to ensure fatigue is not a limiting factor.
- The client can regain his/her balance as many times as needed; this does not count against him/her.
- Choose a weight that allows the client to complete at least 8–30 repetitions per leg (30 maximum).
- The evaluations require the client to perform as many repetitions as possible, therefore, it is not recommended for beginners who have not acquired exercise familiarity, and at least six weeks of recent resistance training experience.

1a. Single-Leg Knee Tap Squat
If the client is unable to balance on a single leg, use the Bulgarian Split-Squat as an alternative exercise (see Figure 5.4). Perform all repetitions on one side before switching to the other leg. Instruct the client to keep the weight on the front foot throughout the exercise.

Action and coaching tips
- Stand in front of a pad (2–3 inches thick), a small stack of weight plates with a mat on top, or a workout step.
- Shift weight onto the left leg and lift the right foot off the floor, with the knee bent and slightly behind the left leg (see Figure 5.3a).
- Keep the hands outstretched in front of the torso at roughly shoulder level.
- Stronger clients can perform the exercise while holding a dumbbell at each shoulder.
- Slowly lower oneself towards the floor by bending the weight-bearing knee and sitting back at the hips until the back knee lightly taps on the object (see Figure 5.3b).

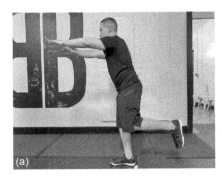 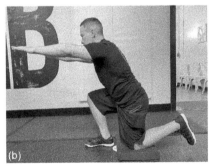

Figure 5.3 Single-leg knee tap squat.

- Do not allow the rear (non-weight-bearing) foot to touch the floor unless catching one's balance.
- Reverse the motion (stand up) to complete one repetition.

1b. Bulgarian Split-Squat
Place the rear foot on top of a stable platform that is roughly at knee height.

Action and coaching tips
- Stand tall while holding a dumbbell in each hand at the sides.
- Place the left foot on the platform behind.
- The right leg should be far enough in front of the platform so the shin can stay close to vertical as the body is lowered on each repetition (see Figure 5.4a).
- This exercise can also be performed without any load. The hands can be placed behind the head (see Figure 5.4a) or at the side of the body.
- A slight forward lean of the torso is normal and acceptable. Lower the body towards the floor, allowing the rear knee to lightly tap the floor without resting on the floor (see Figure 5.4b).
- Drive the front foot into the ground to raise the body to the starting position.
- Keep the front foot flat on the floor throughout.

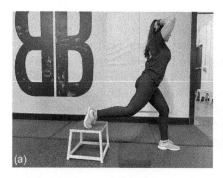 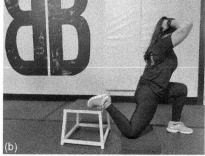

Figure 5.4 Bulgarian split-squat.

Assessing cardiorespiratory fitness

Several validated cardiorespiratory fitness (endurance) assessments have been developed for different populations (Heyward & Gibson, 2014). The direct measurement of cardiorespiratory fitness (i.e., VO_{2max}) is not usually practical, and trainers more commonly perform indirect assessments. Indirect endurance assessments can be sub-maximal or maximal. Most sub-maximal assessments involve measuring the client's heart rate (HR) throughout and ending the test before the client reaches his/her maximum HR (generally between 80 and 85% of HR_{max}). The HR data are then

Table 5.3 Example indirect cardiorespiratory fitness assessments

	Assessment	*Type*
Running/walking (continuous)	Åstrand treadmill test*	Maximal
	Balke treadmill test*	Maximal
	Balke 15-minute run*	Maximal
	Cooper 12-minute run*	Maximal
	Rockport 1-mile walk test*	Maximal
	2.4 km (1.5 mile) run*	Maximal
	5 km run (3.1 mile) run	Maximal
	6-Minute Walk Test (6MWT)	Sub-maximal**
Running (intermittent)	Multistage Fitness Test (MSFT)*	Maximal
	The Yo-Yo test battery*	Maximal
	30–15 Intermittent Fitness Test (30–15 IFT)*	Maximal
Stepping	Chester Step Test*	Sub-maximal
	Harvard Step Test*	Sub-maximal
Cycling	YMCA cycle ergometer test*	Sub-maximal
	Åstrand-Rhyming cycle ergometer test*	Sub-maximal
	Watt Bike™ assessments	Maximal
	Maximal Ramp Test	
	20-minute Functional Threshold Power	
	3-Minute Test	
Rowing	2 km rowing ergometer test	Maximal

* VO_{2max} prediction equation available.

** Some clients may reach maximal exertion before test completion.

applied to a population-specific (e.g., age, sex, activity status) equation to predict VO_{2max}.

Maximal cardiorespiratory fitness tests involve (1) exercising until exhaustion (e.g., the Multistage Fitness Test), (2) covering as much distance as possible over a set time (e.g., the Cooper 12-minute run) or (3) completing a set distance as quickly as possible (e.g., 5 km run). As with sub-maximal assessments, VO_{2max} prediction equations have been developed based on performance data (Ramsbottom et al., 1988), although the validity of some prediction equations has been questioned (e.g., Cooper et al., 2005). However, estimating VO_{2max} is not always necessary, as the ability to sustain a high-speed or power output during endurance exercise lasting ~6–15 minutes is indicative of a high VO_{2max}. Thus, an improvement in a performance metric, such as running a set distance in less time (e.g., a 5km race), can be used to infer that cardiorespiratory fitness has improved. Examples of cardiorespiratory fitness assessments are presented in Table 5.3.

References

Acharya, R., Joseph, P., Kannathal, N., et al. (2006). Heart rate variability: a review. *Medical & Biological Engineering & Computing, 44*(12), 1031–1051.

Bandyopadhyay A. (2015). Validity of Cooper's 12-minute run test for estimation of maximum oxygen uptake in male university students. *Biology of sport, 32*(1), 59–63.

Beekley, M., Brechue, W., Dehoyos, D., et al. (2004). Cross-validation of the YMCA submaximal cycle ergometer test to predict VO_{2max}. *Research Quarterly for Exercise and Sport, 75*(3), 337–342.

Bishop, C., Lake, J., Loturco, I., et al. (2021). Interlimb Asymmetries: The Need for an Individual Approach to Data Analysis. *Journal of Strength and Conditioning Research, 35*(3), 695–701.

Burnstein, B., Steele, R., & Shrier, I. (2011). Reliability of fitness tests using methods and time periods common in sport and occupational management. *Journal of Athletic Training, 46*(5), 505–513.

Cohen, J. (1988). Set Correlation and Contingency Tables. *Applied Psychological Measurement, 12*(4), 425–434.

Colburn, T., Smith, B., Guarini, J., et al. (1976). An ambulatory activity monitor with solid state memory. *Biomedical Sciences Instrumentation, 12*, 117–122.

Cole, R., Kripke, D., Gruen, W., et al. (1992). Automatic sleep/wake identification from wrist activity. *Sleep, 15*(5), 461–469.

Cooper, S., Baker, J., Tong, R., et al. (2005). The repeatability and criterion related validity of the 20 m multistage fitness test as a predictor of maximal oxygen uptake in active young men. *British Journal of Sports Medicine, 39*(4), e19.

Croisier, J., Forthomme, B., Namurois, M., et al. (2002). Hamstring muscle strain recurrence and strength performance disorders. *The American Journal of Sports Medicine, 30*(2), 199–203.

De Oliveira, R., Ugrinowitsch, C., Kingsley, J., et al. (2019). Effect of individualised resistance training prescription with heart rate variability on individual muscle hypertrophy and strength responses. *European Journal of Sport Science, 19*(8), 1092–1100.

de Zambotti, M., Cellini, N., Menghini, L., et al. (2020). Sensors capabilities, performance, and use of consumer sleep technology. *Sleep Medicine Clinics, 15*(1), 1–30.

Erlacher, D., Ehrlenspiel, F., Adegbesan, O., et al. (2011). Sleep habits in German athletes before important competitions or games. *Journal of Sports Sciences, 29*(8), 859–866.

Evenson, K., Goto, M., Furberg, R., et al. (2015). Systematic review of the validity and reliability of consumer-wearable activity trackers. *The International Journal of Behavioral Nutrition and Physical Activity, 12*, 159.

Flatt, A., Hornikel, B., & Esco, M. R. (2017). Heart rate variability and psychometric responses to overload and tapering in collegiate sprint-swimmers. *Journal of Science and Medicine in Sport, 20*(6), 606–610.

Grander, M., & Rosenberger, M. (2019). Actigraphic sleep tracking and wearables: historical context, scientific applications and guidelines, limitations, and considerations for commercial sleep devices. In *Sleep and health* (pp. 147–157). Academic Press.

Heyward, A., & Gibson, A. (2014). *Advanced fitness assessment and exercise prescription* (7th ed.). Human Kinetics.

Impellizzeri, F., Rampinini, E., Maffiuletti, N., et al. (2007). A vertical jump force test for assessing bilateral strength asymmetry in athletes. *Medicine and Science in Sports and Exercise, 39*(11), 2044–2050.

Jensen, M., Suadicani, P., Hein, H., et al. (2013). Elevated resting heart rate, physical fitness and all-cause mortality: a 16-year follow-up in the Copenhagen Male Study. *Heart, 99*(12), 882–887.

Kripke, D., Mullaney, D., Messin, S., et al. (1978). Wrist actigraphic measures of sleep and rhythms. *Electroencephalography and Clinical Neurophysiology, 44*(5), 674–676.

Knapik, J., Bauman, C., Jones, B., et al. (1991). Preseason strength and flexibility imbalances associated with athletic injuries in female collegiate athletes. *The American Journal of Sports Medicine, 19*(1), 76–81.

Lockie, R., Callaghan, S., Berry, S., et al. (2014). Relationship between unilateral jumping ability and asymmetry on multidirectional speed in team-sport athletes. *Journal of Strength and Conditioning Research, 28*(12), 3557–3566.

Lockie, R., Risso, F., Lazar, A., et al. (2017). Between-leg mechanical differences as measured by the Bulgarian Split-Squat: exploring Asymmetries and relationships with sprint acceleration. *Sports (Basel, Switzerland), 5*(3), 65.

Maloney, S. (2019). The Relationship Between Asymmetry and Athletic Performance: A Critical Review. *Journal of Strength and Conditioning Research, 33*(9), 2579–2593.

Mertz, K., Reitelseder, S., Jensen, M., et al. (2019). Influence of between-limb asymmetry in muscle mass, strength, and power on functional capacity in healthy older adults. *Scandinavian Journal of Medicine & Science in Sports, 29*(12), 1901–1908.

Myer, G., Martin, L., Jr, Ford, K., et al. (2012). No association of time from surgery with functional deficits in athletes after anterior cruciate ligament reconstruction: evidence for objective return-to-sport criteria. *The American Journal of Sports Medicine, 40*(10), 2256–2263.

Newton, R., Gerber, A., Nimphius, S., et al. (2006). Determination of functional strength imbalance of the lower extremities. *Journal of Strength and Conditioning Research, 20*(4), 971–977.

Pasadyn, S. R., Soudan, M., Gillinov, M., et al. (2019). Accuracy of commercially available heart rate monitors in athletes: a prospective study. *Cardiovascular Diagnosis and Therapy, 9*(4), 379–385.

Paterno, M., Ford, K., Myer, G., et al. (2007). Limb asymmetries in landing and jumping 2 years following anterior cruciate ligament reconstruction. *Clinical Journal of Sport Medicine, 17*(4), 258–262.

Ramsbottom, R., Brewer, J., & Williams, C. (1988). A progressive shuttle run test to estimate maximal oxygen uptake. *British Journal of Sports Medicine, 22*(4), 141–144.

Redmond, D., & Hegge, F. (1985). Observations on the design and specification of a wrist-worn human activity monitoring system. *Behavior Research Methods, Instruments, & Computers, 17*(6), 659–669.

Roberts, D., Schade, M., Mathew, G., et al. (2020). Detecting sleep using heart rate and motion data from multisensor consumer-grade wearables, relative to wrist actigraphy and polysomnography. *Sleep, 43*(7).

Roberts, S., Teo, W., Aisbett, B., et al. (2019). Extended sleep maintains endurance performance better than normal or restricted sleep. *Medicine and Science in Sports and Exercise, 51*(12), 2516–2523.

Rohman, E., Steubs, J., & Tompkins, M. (2015). Changes in involved and uninvolved limb function during rehabilitation after anterior cruciate ligament reconstruction: implications for Limb Symmetry Index measures. *The American Journal of Sports Medicine, 43*(6), 1391–1398.

Sadeh, A., Sharkey, K., & Carskadon, M. (1994). Activity-based sleep-wake identification: an empirical test of methodological issues. *Sleep, 17*(3), 201–207.

Skein, M., Duffield, R., Edge, J., et al. (2011). Intermittent-sprint performance and muscle glycogen after 30 h of sleep deprivation: *Medicine & Science in Sports & Exercise, 43*(7), 1301–1311.

Stanley, N. (2003). Actigraphy in human psychopharmacology: a review. *Human Psychopharmacology, 18*(1), 39–49. https://doi.org/10.1002/hup.471.

Thamm, A., Freitag, N., Figueiredo, P., et al. (2019). Can heart rate variability determine recovery following distinct strength loadings? A randomised cross-over trial. *International Journal of Environmental Research and Public Health, 16*(22), 1–16.

Vallières, A., & Morin, C. (2003). Actigraphy in the assessment of insomnia. *Sleep, 26*(7), 902–906.

6 Principles of training

Eric Helms

In this information age there are copious training programmes available that claim to be the 'best' because scientific or pseudo-scientific claims are used to support them. However, trainers who do not have the knowledge to evaluate such claims are left to follow trends, which often produces inconsistent and unsatisfactory results. Developing knowledge of sport and exercise science gives fitness professionals *the potential* to improve their practice through evaluating programmes using scientific evidence alongside professional experience. However, a sound understanding of the principles of training must be developed before science can be effectively incorporated into one's practice.

Adaptation

The purpose of any training programme is to induce adaptations. An adaptation is a change in a structural, physiological, or behavioural characteristic that enables a living organism to survive. In humans, biological adaptations occur within the body to meet the demands that are placed upon it. In the context of exercise, a biological system (e.g., cardiorespiratory) must be subjected to a stress (exercise) to stimulate adaptation. Therefore, training can be regarded as physical exercises designed to stimulate biological adaptations in order to improve health and/or performance outcomes.

Adaptations can be classified as acute (short-term) or chronic (long-term). For example, when a muscle is required to produce force to overcome a load (resistance training), there is an immediate increase in muscle activation and blood flow. Following the exercise, the muscles' ability to produce force is typically reduced due to fatigue. These acute changes diminish shortly after exercise. However, repeated exposure to the exercise provides a consistent stimulus to the muscle, causing it to adapt (i.e., become stronger). This process of adaptation is known as the *General Adaptation Syndrome* (GAS) (Selye, 1950). In the context of exercise, GAS states that exercise stresses biological systems, which initiates

DOI: 10.4324/9781003204657-6

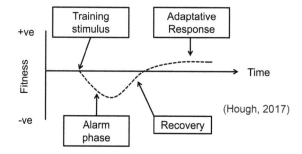

Figure 6.1 Schematic of the adaptive response following a suitable training stimulus and recovery period.

an 'alarm phase' where there is a temporary decrease in performance/ physical capacity. The alarm phase initiates a compensation effect termed the 'resistance phase', causing the system's physical capacity to return to or exceed the initial capacity. The resistance phase manifests as improvements in fitness following exposure to repeated training stress (exercise). Provided the training stimulus continues to provide a sufficient overload (see below), each training session initiates acute physiological changes that induce a cycle of stress and adaptation. Repeating this cycle of stress and recovery (i.e., consistent training) induces chronic adaptations. The final phase of GAS is the 'exhaustion phase', describing when a stressor is beyond the adaptive capacity of the biological system. The parallel to the exhaustion phase in an exercise setting is exposing a client to an excessive magnitude and/or rate of overload beyond which they can adapt to chronically (Figure 6.1).

Fitness and fatigue

To better understand how GAS plays out in the context of exercise, the interaction between the two outputs of training, fitness and fatigue, must be considered (Banister et al., 1975). The cycle of adaptation is not as simple as being the outcome of wholly separate inputs and outputs. While a stressor (i.e., exercise) can be easily quantified based on its variables (load, sets, reps, duration, intensity), the stressor of training simultaneously produces both fitness and fatigue. The chronic adaptations from training and the ability to express those adaptations (e.g., improvements in performance) depend on the dynamic and continuous interaction of fitness and fatigue. The fitness produced from training is acutely suppressed by fatigue; thus, it can be unclear whether gains in fitness occurred following a training programme when fatigue is present. However, fitness fades slowly with detraining (see below) or from training that is too easy, but fatigue fades more quickly. Thus, improving fitness and performance requires balancing the magnitude of the training stimulus and recovery from the stress

CASE STUDY 6.1

'Go hard or go home'

Terry has rekindled his passion for resistance training (RT) following a 3-year break. He has started to train with his friend who adopts the mantra 'go hard or go home' for every session. This involves using advanced RT methods and training to failure on every exercise (see Chapter 13). After three sessions Terry has started to experience severe muscle soreness and joint pain, and he is unable to train again for 3 days. Terry is significantly exceeding his adaptation threshold, which is not enabling him to recover adequately between sessions. Terry needs to reduce his training volume/intensity and avoid training to failure until his body has adapted to an introductory period of RT.

that training causes; programmes that achieve this balance enable fitness to improve without injury or burn out (Chiu & Barnes, 2003).

Recovery

Clients can often overlook the importance of post-exercise recovery, but it is fundamental to the adaptation process (see Chapter 18). Without adequate recovery, fitness can stagnate or even decline due to an accumulation of fatigue. An accumulation of fatigue can have negative physical outcomes (e.g., excess muscle soreness and joint pain) and adverse psychological outcomes, such as mood disturbances (Piacentini et al., 2016). Therefore, improving fitness can be perceived as a 'balancing act', whereby optimal adaptation takes place when the training provides an appropriate stimulus (the adaptation threshold, see below) and a suitable amount of recovery time is provided.

Biopsychosocial factors and individualisation

The fitness fatigue model clarifies the original GAS model and provides a more comprehensive picture of the biological response to training. However, further nuance is required to apply training principles in the real world. While useful conceptually, the GAS and Fitness-Fatigue models do not provide sufficient accuracy to reliably predict changes in performance, possibly because they cannot fully account for the individual response to training (Borresen & Lambert, 2009).

Our understanding of stress and the individual response to it has evolved, and subsequently, our understanding of training theory must advance as well (Kiely, 2018). For example, the magnitude and proportion of stimulus and fatigue that two individuals experience from the same training programme can differ tremendously. Further, the stimulus and fatigue responses to training also change within an individual as they age, adapt to prior training, and experience changes in their life circumstances (Kiely, 2012). Broadly, one's genetic make-up, prior training experience, injury history, nutrition, sleep, motivation, cumulative life stress, and arousal level during exercise (and more) can all impact the stimulus of a programme and the fatigue it induces. Consequently, a programme must be designed based on the client's health/fitness status, training background, and health/fitness goals.

All clients will have different needs, meaning there is no such thing as a 'one size fits all' training programme. For example, if two clients (A and B) were performing a similar resistance training programme and the intensity was increased by 10%, client A might barely notice the overload. In contrast, client B might feel more fatigued and require a longer recovery period. Programme variable guidelines must be refined based on the individual client's response to the training and the trainer's professional judgment; hence, successful training programme design can be seen as an art as well as a science.

The fitness and fatigue responses to exercise, which differ between and within individuals, are also affected by less quantifiable emotional responses to environmental and social factors (Kiely, 2012). For example, negative perceived life stress can reduce the magnitude of strength development following resistance training (Bartholomew et al., 2008). In essence, the fitness and fatigue responses to training and the necessary recovery are highly individual and also modified by the ever-present and highly influential backdrop of clients' lives, experiences, beliefs, and emotions. Thus, to successfully elicit positive adaptations, training programmes need to be flexible and adaptable so that they remain appropriate given the current state of the client.

The health-performance continuum

Each client will be at a different point on the health-performance continuum (see Figure 6.2). This model presents a framework of how exercise can be prescribed to clients with different levels of fitness and health/fitness goals (Hough, 2017). In the context of cardiorespiratory fitness, a sedentary client would be at the health end of the continuum and advanced training methods, such as HIIT, may not be required. Conversely, a keen amateur runner would be towards the performance end of the continuum, meaning their exercise goals are performance related (i.e., faster race times) and require a greater volume and intensity of exercise.

Progressive overload

Progressive overload is required in order to keep adapting to training and improving fitness. Typically, progressive overload is viewed as a proactive process of applying systematic increases in the physical demands placed

	Health	Fitness	Performance
Example client profile	Sedentary, limited exercise experience. Not meeting minimum PA guidelines	Regularly active (2-3 training sessions p/w)	Experienced exerciser (>2 years regular running, 4 training sessions p/w)
Objectives	• Achieve minimum PA guidelines • Avoidance of disease • Achieve the health benefits of regular PA	• Improve cardiorespiratory fitness • Further health improvements	• Improve 10 km race personal best time
Example exercise programme	Intensity: moderate Weekly volume: 150 minutes moderate or 75 minutes vigorous Example week: 5 x 30 minute walks	Intensity: Moderate – severe Weekly volume: 3-4 hours Example week: 3 x 5k runs	Intensity: Moderate – maximal Weekly volume: 5+ hours Example week: x 1 long run, x 2 tempo runs, x 1 interval session, x 2 resistance training

(Hough, 2017)

Figure 6.2 The health-performance training continuum.

upon the body. For example, by systematically manipulating acute training programme variables:

• Volume (quantity of work)
• Intensity (rate of work or magnitude of load)
• Frequency (number of training sessions within a set period)
• Exercise selection
• Order of exercises
• Rest periods

As discussed, the rate and magnitude of adaptation to exercise varies significantly between individuals. Therefore, an appropriate progressive stimulus for one client could be under- or overtraining for another. Thus, instead of viewing progressive overload as an active process where it is the trainer's role to *progress the overload*, it may be more practical to view progress as the consequence of sufficient overload (i.e., increasing the stimulus to correspond with improvements in the client's fitness).

The adaptation threshold

The goal of all training programmes is to consistently meet the client's adaptation threshold (i.e., provide an appropriate training stimulus to induce gains in fitness). Following the description of progressive overload above, it should be clear that the adaptation threshold increases over time as a client's fitness improves. For example, an 8-minute mile running pace or a set of 10 repetitions with 60 kg at the beginning of a programme may be perceived as similarly challenging as a 7-minute mile pace or a set of 10 repetitions with 65 kg near its end. Thus, while the objective training load increased, the subjective training difficulty is the same due to increases in fitness.

The adaptation threshold is dependent on several individual factors (e.g., training status, recovery from the previous exercise, and psychological stress levels). Therefore, the adaptation threshold is different between individual clients. As a client's fitness improves, the exercises must provide an adequate overload to meet the client's adaptation threshold. If this threshold is not met, fitness will not significantly improve. Conversely, significantly exceeding the adaptation threshold will induce a high degree of fatigue, decrease physical capacity and increase the duration of the necessary recovery period (see Figure 6.3).

Clients adapt at different rates and magnitudes and have different time courses of recovery and recuperative abilities. Further, these qualities change over time as the client's fitness progresses. Therefore, proactive increases in certain training variables to achieve progressive overload are not always ideal. The intensity at a given volume is often used to measure fitness; for example, a 5-repetition maximum for a single set or a 1-mile time trial. The trainer can always increase volume, adding distance or sets, as a way of inducing overload. Indeed, at certain stages, clients with a high level of fitness will need to use volume progression to reach their adaptation threshold, to be able to demonstrate high intensities. However, once these clients have achieved a very high level of fitness, they are simply unable to

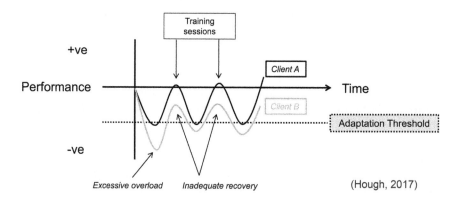

(Hough, 2017)

Client A performs training sessions which meet their adaptation threshold and there is sufficient recovery time following training. Client B is subjected to an excessive overload and inadequate period of recovery, resulting in reduced performance.

Figure 6.3 The adaptation threshold.

CASE STUDY 6.2

Diminishing returns

Colette is a gym enthusiast who has been training regularly for 2 years. She enjoys running and runs 5 km three times per week. Her strategy has been to improve her best 5 km time by 5–10 seconds every week (i.e., increasing average speed). However, her best time is no longer improving. Colette is focusing on one programme variable (intensity). Although adaptation requires a progressive overload, it is important that a variety of programme variables are modified over time (variation) rather than focusing on one. If one variable is increased while others remain constant, the client will reach a point where the training yields progressively smaller improvements in fitness, this is known as *the law of diminishing returns*. Therefore, Colette should systematically change other programme variables, such as volume (distance).

For clients who progress slowly and accumulate fatigue quickly, an increase in volume might not be needed on a session-to-session or even a weekly basis (see Chapter 7). If fitness is steadily increasing (e.g., the client can increase intensity) with a stable volume, while the client experiences noticeable but manageable fatigue, it is unnecessary and potentially counterproductive to increase training stress via volume progression. If the adaptation threshold is consistently exceeded without adequate recovery, the client's fitness will actually decrease due to an accumulation of fatigue (see Case Study 6.1).

increase intensity regularly due to a slower rate of adaptation and a higher level of fatigue from the training it took to get there. For these 'advanced clients', manipulating volume and intensity over time is especially important to facilitate further improvements in fitness (see Chapter 8).

Accommodation

If the adaptation threshold is not met (i.e., there is insufficient overload) the body is not forced to adapt and will accommodate to the training stress, resulting in no further improvements in physical fitness (i.e., a training plateau). However, fitness can also plateau if the adaptation threshold is far surpassed by excessive training, as fatigue prevents subsequent training from being effective due to inadequate recovery. A tool that can be applied to provide progressive overload and help manage fatigue is training variation.

Variation

Variation is the systematic process of varying one or more programme variables over time to ensure the training stimulus remains challenging and accommodation is avoided. Variation can be applied through implementing a long-term training programme design process known as periodisation (see Chapter 8).

Specificity

The principle of specificity dictates that training adaptations are specific to the exercise stimulus applied. Components of fitness can be improved using general programmes, but general programmes will not achieve specific outcomes. For example, the load and volume used within a RT programme have specific effects on the performance and physiological adaptations. Training with a heavier (8–12 RM) load produces superior increases in strength, compared to a lighter load (25–35 RM); whereas lifting a lighter load for many repetitions produces a more significant improvement in muscular endurance, compared to lifting a heavier load for fewer repetitions (Schoenfeld et al., 2015).

The physiological adaptations achieved following a period of training are influenced by the acute programme variables as well as specific factors related to each individual exercise, such as the speed at which the exercise is performed and the range of movement that is used (Verkhoshansky, 1977). For example, a client who usually performs her squats to a knee flexion angle of 90° will improve strength within this range of motion. However, she will find the exercise more challenging if she is asked to squat to a greater depth (80° knee flexion) as this is outside of the ROM where the strength has been developed.

Trainability

As discussed in relation to advanced clients, trainability refers to the magnitude of adaptations that have been achieved through exercise and the theoretical capacity a client has for improvement. In general, the more fitness a client has attained (generally seen in clients with a longer training

CASE STUDY 6.3

Fitness cross-over effect

John plays football three times per week (two training, one match). He plays in midfield and scored the highest result when his team performed the Multistage Fitness Test, which measures cardiorespiratory fitness. John recently entered a 20-minute cycling fitness challenge at his gym; however, he was beaten by three of his team mates. This demonstrates that fitness is specific to the mode of exercise performed. Although John has a superior level of cardiorespiratory fitness when running, this does not directly cross-over to cycling due to the different nature of the exercise. Thus, the principle of specificity must be considered when selecting training exercises and fitness assessments.

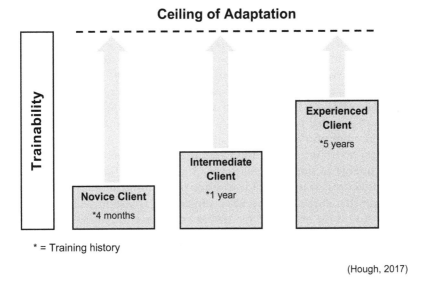

Ceiling of Adaptation

* = Training history

(Hough, 2017)

Figure 6.4 Trainability.

history), the less trainability they have. This is because physiological adaptations occur rapidly at the onset of a training programme, but the rate of improvement declines as the body becomes more adapted. For example, following a 21-week resistance training programme, untrained individuals have been demonstrated to experience a twofold greater increase in relative isometric strength compared to trained individuals (Ahtiainen et al., 2003).

As a client becomes more trained, they reach a level of fitness closer to their ceiling of adaptation (see Figure 6.4). This ceiling represents a theoretical point where no further adaptation takes place (i.e., a genetic limit). In reality this point is rarely reached, as it is not actually a point, but rather an asymptote. Even world class athletes experience small improvements in fitness during their careers, and it is difficult to determine whether their eventual inability to progress further (or decline) is related to age, accumulated injury, or truly reaching their ceiling. Nevertheless, as a client accrues more fitness they come closer to their ceiling of adaptation. Therefore, they require a greater training load to make further improvements. However, if the balance of training and recovery is incorrect the client may experience no improvement or even a decline in fitness and/ or injury. This demonstrates why trained clients require a very different approach to training programme design than novice clients.

Detraining

When exercise training is ceased for extended periods the diminished physiological demand on the body causes a decline in the physiological adaptations achieved through previous training – this is also known as 'reversibility'. The magnitude of detraining is dependent on the training status of the client, specific fitness component, and the length of time training has been ceased or reduced. For example, a study on trained endurance athletes reported a 7% reduction in maximal oxygen uptake, a measure of cardiorespiratory fitness, after 12 days without training (Coyle et al., 1984). Training status also has a large effect on the magnitude of detraining, whereby the fitness of clients with a long training history declines at a slower rate compared to novice clients (Mujika & Padilla, 2000). The magnitude of detraining during periods of reduced training can be decreased by maintaining training intensity where possible. Clients who are unable to perform their typical exercise routine can use a technique called cross-training. This involves performing an alternative mode of training that stimulates the same physiological system. For example, a runner could train on a cycle or rowing ergometer to help reduce or prevent a decline in cardiorespiratory fitness.

Does 'muscle memory' exist?

Emerging data suggests that there are physiological mechanisms of fitness 'memory'. Specifically, skeletal muscle adaptations can be regained at a faster rate upon a return to training following detraining in individuals with a long training history who have developed such a 'memory' (Snijders et al., 2020). Thus, clients who experience short periods of time off from training due to changes in life circumstances or injury will likely experience a fast return to their prior fitness levels upon returning to training.

Summary

Trainers can apply numerous training methods and techniques to achieve the same health, fitness, and performance outcomes. However, for a programme to be successful and ensure that clients get the maximum benefits from their training, the fundamental principles of training have to be applied. Having a clear understanding of the principles of training enables the trainer to create, implement and evaluate a range of training programmes based on the individual needs of their clients.

References

Ahtiainen, J., Pakarinen, A., Alen, M., et al. (2003). Muscle hypertrophy, hormonal adaptations and strength development during strength training in strength-trained and untrained men. *European Journal of Applied Physiology, 89*(6), 555–563.

Banister, E., Calvert, T., Savage, M., et al. (1975). System model of training for athletic performance. *Australian Journal of Sports Medicine, 7*, 170–176.

Bartholomew, J., Stults-Kolehmainen, M., Elrod, C., et al. (2008). Strength gains after resistance training: the effect of stressful, negative life events. *Journal of Strength and Conditioning Research, 22*(4), 1215–1221.

Borresen, J., & Lambert, M. (2009). The quantification of training load, the training response and the effect on performance. *Sports Medicine (Auckland, N.Z.)*, *39*(9), 779–795.

Chiu, L., & Barnes, J. (2003). The fitness-fatigue model revisited: implications for planning short- and long-term training. *Strength & Conditioning Journal*, *25*(6), 42–51.

Coyle, E., Martin, W., Sinacore, D., et al. (1984). Time course of loss of adaptations after stopping prolonged intense endurance training. *Journal of Applied Physiology: Respiratory, Environmental Exercise Physiology. 57*(6), 1857–1864.

Hough, P. (2017). Fundamental principles of training. In P. Hough, P., & S. Penn (Eds.). *Advanced Personal Training: science to practice* (pp. 59–82). Routledge.

Kiely, J. (2012). Periodization paradigms in the 21st century: evidence-led or tradition-driven? *International Journal of Sports Physiology and Performance*, *7*(3), 242–250.

Kiely, J. (2018). Periodization theory: confronting an inconvenient truth. *Sports Medicine*, *48*(4), 753–764.

Mujika, I., & Padilla, S. (2000). Detraining: loss of training-induced physiological and performance adaptations. Part II: Long term insufficient training stimulus. *Sports Medicine*, *30*(3), 145–154.

Piacentini, M., Witard, O., Tonoli, C., et al. (2016). Effect of intensive training on mood with no effect on brain-derived neurotrophic factor. *International Journal of Sports Physiology and Performance*, *11*(6), 824–830.

Schoenfeld, B., Peterson, M., Ogborn, D., et al. (2015). Effects of low- vs. high-load resistance training on muscle strength and hypertrophy in well-trained men. *Journal of Strength and Conditioning Research*, *29*(10), 2954–2963.

Selye, H. (1950). Stress and the General adaptation syndrome. *British Medical Journal*, *1*(4667), 1383–1392.

Snijders, T., Aussieker, T., Holwerda, A., et al. (2020). The concept of skeletal muscle memory: evidence from animal and human studies. *Acta Physiologica (Oxford, England)*, *229*(3), e13465.

Verkhoshansky, Y. (1977). *Fundamentals of Special strength-training in sport*. Moscow: Fuzkultura I Spovt.

7 Training session design

Paul Hough and Cody Haun

Training should become more challenging over time to induce anatomical and physiological adaptations and improve fitness. If a long-term training programme does not include some form of progressive overload, adaptations will plateau or stagnate. Conversely, an inappropriate overload could cause excessive fatigue and possibly lead to injury. The application of progressive overload is not as simple as making each training session more challenging than the last. Training that maintains fitness must be differentiated from training that stimulates improvements in fitness, as this will influence session design. Overload training must be balanced with recovery so that training is difficult enough to elicit adaptations, but not so difficult that it induces excessive fatigue.

This chapter will explore how fundamental training programme variables (e.g., volume, intensity, and frequency) can be measured and modified to achieve various training goals. Volume and intensity will be discussed separately; however, both short and long-term training responses are dependent on an interaction between volume and intensity. Therefore, volume and intensity must be considered together when designing, monitoring, and evaluating training sessions.

Structuring a training session

Depending on the client's goals, time demands, and level of fitness, a training session may incorporate several forms of exercise within a single session, such as endurance, resistance, and flexibility training. Alternatively, the session may just focus on one component. Regardless of the type of training, each session should begin with a warm-up (see Chapter 9). Following the warm-up, the acute training programme variables (see Chapter 6) must be considered to ensure the exercises stress the relevant physiological systems and induce the required adaptations. Therefore, the goal of each training session must be clear.

DOI: 10.4324/9781003204657-7

Training goals

The goals that have been agreed upon by the client and trainer form the foundation of the short and long-term training programme design and dictate the training methods that will be implemented. For example, if the client's primary goal is to improve cardiorespiratory fitness (endurance), then the principle of specificity dictates that the training programme must incorporate exercises that stress the cardiorespiratory system. Occasionally, a client's goals or reasons for exercising may be ambiguous and not align with a specific training modality. Therefore, trainers must be able to interpret the client's goals and make appropriate recommendations (see Case Study 7.1).

CASE STUDY 7.1

'Toning-up'

Aaron is a 40-year-old office worker who has not exercised regularly for three years. He states that he wants to 'tone-up' his arms and waist. Before designing Aaron's programme, it is important to clarify his goal. Muscle tone (aka tonus) is the normal state of tension developed within the muscle that is maintained continuously, even when a muscle is at rest. Although there are certain pathologies that can decrease muscle tone, clients who report a lack of muscle tone are usually referring to the subcutaneous fat tissue that surrounds the muscles, which can make muscle groups appear and feel soft. Therefore, in most cases, when a client cites a goal to 'tone-up', this can be interpreted as a decrease in subcutaneous fat and an increase in muscle density or size (hypertrophy) – designing a programme to achieve these body composition goals is discussed in Chapter 14.

Concurrent training
Keith Baar

To optimise overall fitness, a client's training should focus on both endurance and strength. This type of concurrent training (CT) is optimal for health-oriented programmes and forms the basis for elite performance in many sports. CT can improve cardiorespiratory fitness, strength and power in untrained individuals (Kazior et al., 2016). However, in trained clients improvements in muscle mass and strength can be negatively affected when training simultaneously to improve endurance (Hickson, 1980; Kraemer et al., 1995; Wilson et al., 2012). The compromised improvement in muscle mass and strength as a result of CT is known as the 'interference effect'.

Several theories have been presented to explain the interference effect. The scientific basis for these theories is that endurance and strength training use different molecular mechanisms to drive adaptation. Therefore, when an individual performs a high volume of endurance and strength training (>10 sessions per week), the molecular endurance signals make it harder to produce strength adaptations (Baar, 2014).

Simple strategies can be implemented to reduce or avoid the interference effect when working with trained clients. First, and most importantly, it is essential to increase the protein content of a post workout snack or supplement to 0.4 g/kg body weight (Areta et al., 2014) or more if completing a full-body workout. This is because one of the molecular changes required for endurance adaptation increases Sestrin, which is a protein that senses the amount of leucine in the diet and limits muscle growth (Kim et al., 2020). Performing regular endurance exercise can induce an energy deficit, which is another source of interference. Therefore, a second strategy is to separate endurance and resistance training (RT) sessions. Ideally, endurance training would be performed in the morning followed (within an hour) by recovery nutrition to replenish nutritional stores and counterbalance the energy expended. Strength training would then be performed in the late afternoon, prior to dinner (Baar, 2014). Individuals that cannot separate training sessions should prioritise the primary training goal. If improving strength is the priority, strength work should be completed first and the intensity and volume of the endurance sessions reduced. Clients who prioritise endurance can perform strength training immediately after endurance training (Wang et al., 2011).

Designing an endurance training session
Paul Hough

Exercise selection

Continuous and rhythmic exercises that involve major muscle groups should be selected to stress the cardiorespiratory system. Low skill exercises, such as walking and cycling, are recommended for novices. Technical exercises, such as rowing, often produce more peripheral fatigue and the risk of injury increases if the client's technique deteriorates. Furthermore, exercises involving the upper and lower body musculature increase the oxygen demand and impose greater stress on the cardiorespiratory system, which could be inappropriate for deconditioned clients. The specificity principle, discussed in Chapter 6, is particularly important for clients who want to improve cardiorespiratory fitness (CRF) for a specific activity. For instance, a client who wants to improve CRF for playing football should perform running as the primary endurance exercise mode.

Can resistance training improve cardiorespiratory fitness?

Performing a series of RT exercises (i.e., circuit training) can improve CRF and muscular strength, with less time commitment compared to separate endurance and RT sessions (Myers et al., 2015; Schmidt et al., 2016). Therefore, circuit training is a viable option for clients wishing to improve CRF and strength in a short period. However, circuit training may not provide an effective training stimulus to improve CRF for clients with a history of endurance training, such as runners and cyclists.

Calculating and monitoring endurance training intensity

Endurance training (ET) intensity can be defined and prescribed using several objective metrics, including heart rate (HR), oxygen consumption, power and metabolic equivalents (METs). Objective measures are usually calculated relative to the individual's maximum capacity; for example, as a percentage of HR maximum ($\%HR_{max}$) or maximum oxygen uptake ($\%VO_{2max}$). Prescribing training using relative intensity metrics is effective for improving CRF (Garber et al., 2011). However, objective metrics (e.g., $\%HR_{max}$ or $\%VO_{2max}$) do not always correspond to the client's subjective intensity of effort (i.e., the rating of perceived exertion [RPE]). Therefore, objective intensity metrics should be used in conjunction with subjective metrics, such as RPE (see Figure 7.1) and the Talk Test.

Heart rate

HR is commonly used to quantify ET intensity as there is a linear relationship between intensity and HR during continuous endurance exercise (i.e., HR increases as intensity increases). The maximum HR (HR_{max}) can be interpreted as the upper limit of central cardiorespiratory function; thus, a client's training intensity can be programmed relative to his/her HR_{max}.

Calculating heart rate maximum (HR_{max})

A valid method to establish a client's HR_{max} is to perform an incremental exercise test to exhaustion. However, maximal exercise testing is not always practical so HR_{max} is often estimated using an equation. There is a gradual decline in HR_{max} throughout adulthood; thus, HR_{max} equations factor in age (Christou & Seals, 2008). A commonly applied HR_{max} prediction equation is 220 – age (Fox et al., 1971). However, the (220 – age) equation has a large (~20 B/min) error of estimate and can overestimate the HR_{max} of young people and underestimate HR_{max} in older people (Nes et al., 2013). Therefore, Tanaka et al. (2001) used a meta-analysis, cross-validated by a study of 514 participants, to formulate a more accurate HR_{max} equation (208 – 0.7 × age). Research indicates that Tanaka's equation offers better accuracy than the 220 – age equation (Gellish et al., 2007).

6	No exertion at all
7	Extremely light
8	
9	Very light
10	
11	Light
12	
13	Somewhat hard
14	
15	Hard (heavy)
16	
17	Very hard
18	
19	Extremely hard
20	Maximal exertion

Figure 7.1 The Borg Rating of Perceived Exertion Scale.

Reproduced with permission from Borg (1998). Borg's Perceived Exertion and Pain Scales. Campaign, IL: Human Kinetics.

Equations that estimate HR_{max} should only be used as a broad guideline as they can still have a large (~11 B/min) error of estimate (Arena et al., 2016; Nes et al., 2013). Also, it is important to recognise the limitations of using HR to prescribe and monitor intensity. Certain medications can affect HR (e.g., ß-blockers) and factors not directly related to the exercise intensity can influence the HR response. For example:

- Psychology: emotional factors such as stress and anxiety can elevate HR
- Environment (i.e., temperature and humidity)
- Time of day – HR is typically lower in the morning
- Pregnancy
- Clinical conditions (e.g., arrhythmia)

Heart rate training zones

After measuring or estimating HR_{max} it is possible to formulate HR training zones using a fixed percentage of HR_{max} (%HR_{max}) where training zones are calculated based on HR_{max}. HR zones can also be calculated as a percentage of HR reserve (HRR), also known as *The Karvonen method*. Unlike the HR_{max} method, the HRR equation includes resting HR as follows: $HRR = HR_{max}$ – Resting HR (Karvonen et al., 1957). It is preferable to calculate HR training zones using the HRR method with trained clients because regular endurance training increases the volume of blood pumped by the heart in one contraction (stroke volume). Therefore, endurance-trained individuals tend to have a lower resting HR (bradycardia) and a broader HRR (Spina, 1999). An example of %HR_{max} and %HRR zones are presented in Table 7.1. These training zones have been calculated for a male client (age 31) using the exercise intensity zones described by the American College of Sports Medicine (Garber et al., 2011).

Rating of perceived exertion (RPE)

A RPE scale is a psychophysiological scale that is used to rate an individual's perception of effort during physical work. The scale measures feelings of effort and/or fatigue experienced using an incremental, numerical scale. Unlike objective measures (e.g., HR or oxygen consumption), RPE is subjective and relies on individuals evaluating their level of exertion based on several intrinsic physiological factors (e.g., HR, oxygen uptake, respiration rate) and psychological factors, such as mood and motivation (Borg, 1982, 1998). A widely adopted RPE scale is the 15 point (6–20) 'Borg RPE Scale®' developed by a professor of perception and psychophysics named Gunnar Borg in the 1970s (see Figure 7.1). The scale assumes that as the exercise intensity increases, physiological and perceptual strain increase together. The Borg scale begins at six as it was formulated to correlate approximately with HR within the range of 60–200 B/min (Borg, 1982, 1998). Borg also developed the CR10 scale, a general intensity category scale with ratio properties (0–10) for symptoms, such as dyspnoea, angina, and fatigue. The CR10 scale is conceptually different from the 15-point Borg scale and requires careful administration using the proper guidelines (refer to http://www.borgperception.se/).

Subjective RPE is strongly associated with cardiorespiratory, metabolic, and neuromuscular measures of internal exercise intensity during endurance exercises (Chen et al., 2002). However, in some cases, an RPE scale can produce an unreliable measure of intensity due to several factors, including how the scale is explained and whether the scale is visible (Abadie, 1996). Misinterpretation of the RPE scale can lead a client to provide an inappropriate rating, such as a very low RPE during vigorous exercise. Therefore, the RPE scale should be carefully explained to the client using a standardised script (see Borg, 1998). For instance, '*I would like you to rate how heavy and strenuous this exercise feels to you on this scale (show visual scale) from 6–20. A rating of 6 corresponds to no exertion, i.e., not doing anything, and 20 represents your maximal exertion*'. By anchoring feelings to the numerical values, the client can contextualise the scale and provide an appropriate RPE. Additionally, to improve accuracy and avoid confusion, it is important to use the same scale, which should be visible to the client.

Table 7.1 Heart rate training zones for a male age 31 years

Method	HR_max training zones*	Calculations	HR (B/min)	RPE* (6–20)
Heart rate maximum (HR$_{max}$)	Light (57–63%)	63%: 186 × 0.63 = 117	106–117	9–11
208 – 0.7(31) = 186 B/min	Moderate (64–76%)	76%: 186 × 0.76 = 141	118–141	12–13
	Heavy (77–95%)	95%: 186 × 0.95 = 177	143–177	14–17
	Severe (≥96%)		≥178	≥18

Method	HRR Training Zones*	Calculations	HR (B/min)	RPE* (6–20)
Heart rate reserve (HRR)	Light (30–39%)	39%: (126 × 0.39) + 60 = 109	98–109	9–11
HR$_{max}$: 208 – 0.7(31) = 186 B/min	Moderate (40–59%)	59%: (126 × 0.59) + 60 = 134	110–134	12–13
Resting HR: 60 B/min	Heavy (60–89%)	89%: (126 × 0.89) + 60 = 172	135–172	14–17
HRR: 186 – 60 = 126 B/min	Severe (≥90%)		≥173	≥18

B/min = Beats per minute; RPE = Rating of perceived exertion.

*American College of Sports Medicine (Garber et al., 2011).

The Talk Test

The Talk Test is a simple method where the trainer speaks with the client during an endurance training (ET)exercise to gauge intensity (Persinger et al., 2004). In general, the client can hold a conversation with infrequent pauses during light-moderate exercise (see Table 7.2). During vigorous-intensity exercise, the client cannot maintain a conversation and frequently pauses for breaths; this inability to talk provides a reasonable estimation that the client is exercising within the heavy to severe intensity domain, discussed in Chapter 10 (Foster et al., 2008). Finally, being unable to speak is indicative of maximal intensity exercise.

Table 7.2 Using the Talk Test during endurance exercise

Client's response to questions	*Approximate exercise intensity*
Can hold a conversation without frequent pauses	Light
Infrequent pauses	Moderate
Unable to talk without regular pauses (2–3 words between breathes)	Heavy-severe
Unable to talk	Extreme (maximal)

Metabolic equivalents (METs)

The MET metric is often displayed on cardiovascular training equipment. A MET is the amount of oxygen consumed during seated rest. One MET is equal to consuming approximately 3.5 mL O_2/kg/min or an energy expenditure corresponding to ~1 kcal/kg/hour. For example, an activity performed at 6 METs expends roughly six times more energy than seated rest. Therefore, a higher MET value corresponds to an increase in intensity. Although the MET value of an exercise or activity can be estimated using published activity tables (e.g., Ainsworth et al., 2011); calculating METs for activities outside the gym can be time-consuming and is associated with limitations, such as inaccurate reporting. Consequently, HR and RPE methods are more practical to prescribe and monitor ET intensity.

Calculating and monitoring endurance training load

Epidemiologic and clinical studies have used energy expenditure measures, such as kilocalories/minute/week, to quantify physical activity volume (Jetté et al., 1990; Melanson & Freedson, 1996). The volume of ET can also be expressed as a distance (e.g., running 60 miles/week) but this does not consider the intensity and, therefore, the physiological demand of the training. For example, the physiological stress of running at a relatively easy pace for a long distance is different than running a shorter distance at a fast pace (Nuuttila et al., 2020). Therefore, simply calculating and comparing training volume in units of time or distance can be misleading. Instead, volume and intensity (the training load) should be considered when prescribing, monitoring and evaluating ET.

Combining volume and intensity enables the training load or training impulse (TRIMP) to be calculated, which can be used to plan and monitor training. Technologies, such as GPS watches, calculate the TRIMP by combining external load (e.g., speed and distance) and internal load (e.g., HR) metrics using proprietary algorithms. However, measures of external training load (e.g., distance) do always reflect the true psychophysiological stress (i.e., the internal load) of training. Other factors, such as recovery from previous training (see Chapter 18) or the training environment can influence the TRIMP. Therefore, the client's RPE should also be considered.

The TRIMP rating of perceived exertion method

The simplest method to quantify the TRIMP involves the client rating the difficulty of a session using a 0–10 RPE scale (see Figure 7.2). The perceived exertion score is selected 30 minutes after the training session and is multiplied by the training session's duration to produce a TRIMP score (Foster et al., 1998, 2001). For example, if a client performed a 20-minute circuit training session and selected a session perceived exertion rating of 7, the TRIMP would be calculated as 20 × 7 = 140 TRIMP units. As with

Perceived Rating	Descriptor
0	Rest
1	Very, very easy
2	Easy
3	Moderate
4	Somewhat Hard
5	Hard
6	
7	Very Hard
8	
9	
10	Maximal

Figure 7.2 Training session perceived exertion scale.

all TRIMP calculations, the RPE method has limitations. For example, the training duration becomes the primary determinant of the TRIMP for clients who consistently train for a set-duration (e.g., one hour).

Heart rate and exercise duration TRIMP

The TRIMP can also be calculated using training time and average HR recorded during the session. A simple equation (training time [minutes] × average HR [B/min]) is applied to calculate the TRIMP. For example, 30 minutes cycling at an average HR of 160 B/min = 4800 TRIMP units (30 × 160). However, this method does not account for the increased physiological load associated with training at high (≥80% HR_{max}) intensities (Stagno et al., 2007). For example, cycling for 45 minutes at an average HR of 130 B/min produces a TRIMP score of 5850. However, cycling for 30 minutes at an average HR of 175 B/min produces a lower (5250) TRIMP score. The shorter session, performed at a higher intensity, involves greater physiological stress (Nuuttila et al., 2020), but this is not reflected in the TRIMP scores. Consequently, the five-zone TRIMP method is recommended when ET is performed at different intensities (see Case Study 7.2).

Five zone TRIMP method

The five-zone method, first described in the 1990s, applies a weighting factor to each HR zone (time in HR zone × weighting factor), with higher HR zones corresponding to a higher weighting score (Bannister, 1991; Foster et al., 2001). Variations of the five-zone method include an exponential weighting scale to recognise that as HR increases, the imposed physiological stress increases exponentially rather than linearly (See Table 7.3). For example, exercising for 30 minutes at 87% of HR_{max} (108 TRIMP units) is considerably more demanding than exercising at 65% of HR_{max} for the same duration (38 TRIMP units).

Table 7.3 Training zones based upon a percentage of maximum heart rate (Stagno et al., 2007)

Zone	% Maximum heart rate	Weighting factor
5	93–100	5.16
4	86–92	3.61
3	79–85	2.54
2	72–78	1.71
1	65–71	1.25

Training impulse limitations

Calculating a training load or TRIMP using HR and RPE provides a simple means of estimating the client's psychological (RPE) and physiological (HR) responses to the training load, which can be used to adjust the current training programme and plan future training sessions. However, there are limitations of TRIMP calculation methods that depend on RPE and HR. For example, non-exercise factors, such as psychology (e.g., motivation and anxiety), nutrition (e.g., caffeine ingestion) and environment (e.g., temperature and spectators) can increase HR and skew the physiological demand of a training session. Although weighting factors improve the accuracy of TRIMP calculations (Manzi et al., 2009; Stagno et al., 2007), using HR still has limitations during exercise involving short bouts of maximal exercise (e.g., football and resistance training). Short-duration, high-intensity efforts impose a high neuromuscular load but do not necessarily produce a large increase in HR. For example, a rugby player who performs 40 sprints and experiences 25 collisions in a match will be subjected to a high neuromuscular load. However, if the player performs frequent bouts of walking or jogging, his (80 minute) average HR will be reduced. Consequently, the TRIMP score would not accurately reflect the high neuromuscular load he experienced.

CASE STUDY 7.2

Marathon training

Simon is training for a marathon, and his trainer has asked him to record HR and time during his runs to calculate the TRIMP. Although Simon performed a greater volume of training on Wednesday (see Table 7.4), the shorter (higher intensity) run produced a slightly higher TRIMP. Simon does not use the five-zone TRIMP calculation method during high-intensity exercises, such as sprint interval or resistance training, for reasons discussed above. Instead, Simon's TRIMP score is quantified using the session RPE method.

Table 7.4 Example training impulse calculation using percentage of maximum heart rate

Day	Training	Duration (min)	Average HR (B/min)	% HRmax	Zone & (weighting factor)*	TRIMP
Monday	Run	45	155	86	4 (3.61)	162
Wednesday	Run	90	130	72	1 (1.71)	154

*Weighting factor applied from Table 7.3.

Designing a resistance training session
Cody Haun and Paul Hough

The following section provides an overview of important considerations when designing a resistance training (RT) session, including RT exercise selection systems and methods of prescribing/calculating volume and intensity. The proceeding sections will provide guidelines for designing a RT session to increase muscle size (hypertrophy) and improve maximum strength. A detailed discussion of RT considerations for health, hypertrophy, and strength follows in Chapter 13.

Session structure

Four common RT exercise sequencing methods are (1) the muscle group method; (2) the push-pull method; (3) full-body, and (4). upper-lower split. The sequencing method should be selected based on the session goal, the client's ability, and time available. For example, a client who can only train 2 days/week would likely benefit from the full-body approach. In contrast, a bodybuilder, training daily, would usually adopt the muscle group or upper-lower split method to manage fatigue and ensure a sufficient balance of exercises between training sessions.

Muscle group method

The muscle group method, also known as a 'body-part split', involves dedicating each training session to specific muscle groups, ensuring all the major muscle groups are targeted within a training week. When adopting this method, the target muscle groups will dictate the selected exercises (e.g., deltoids: shoulder press, lateral raise, etc.).

Push-pull method

In the push-pull method, exercises are selected based on their actions: pushing (moving away from the body) or pulling (moving towards the body). Selecting a balance of exercise actions usually ensures that agonists and antagonists are trained equally. For example, horizontal pushing exercises involve anterior muscles (e.g., pectorals, anterior deltoids) and horizontal pulling exercises involve posterior muscles (e.g., trapezius, rhomboids). The push-pull method works effectively for the upper body but can be problematic with the lower body, as the same muscle groups are often worked during pushing and pulling exercises. For example, the lying leg curl (pulling) and squat (pushing) both work posterior muscles (e.g., hamstrings and gluteals); to solve this issue, lower body exercises can be classified as knee or hip dominant (see Table 7.5). Hip dominant exercises involve flexion/extension around the hip joint (e.g., deadlift), with less movement around the knee joint than knee dominant exercises (e.g., squats).

Table 7.5 Resistance training exercise selection methods

Muscle group method		Push-pull method		Upper-lower body method	
Session	Example exercises	Session	Example exercises	Session	Example exercises
Chest & back	Bench press Bent-over row	Horizontal push Horizontal pull	Bench press Bent over row	Upper-body	Bench press Bent over row
Biceps & triceps	DB curls Triceps pushdown	Vertical push Vertical pull	DB shoulder press Pull-up		DB shoulder press DB curls
Shoulders & abdominals	DB shoulder press Plank	Knee dominant	BB Lunges Leg press		Triceps pushdown Plank
Hamstrings & quadriceps	Romanian Deadlift Front squat	Hip dominant	Deadlift Good mornings	Lower-body	Back squat BB hip thrust
Glutes & calves	BB hip thrust DB calf raise	Trunk	Plank Bird-Dog		Leg curls Leg extensions

DB = Dumbbell; BB = Barbell.

Upper-lower body and full-body training

Upper-lower body training splits involve training the upper and lower body on separate days (see Table 7.5). Full-body training sessions include exercises for the upper and lower body in the same session (e.g., bench press, squat, bench row, and lunges).

Exercise order

Exercises should be selected based on the client's individual characteristics, exercises completed in recent sessions, exercises planned for later in the week, and equipment availability. Exercises should also be adapted to accommodate the client's biomechanics, anthropometry, and skill. The order of exercises in a session should depend on the client's goal(s) and the objective of the training plan. Performing a compound (multiple-joint) exercise towards the end of a session, compared to the start of the session, usually reduces the number of repetitions that can be completed (Simão et al., 2012; Spineti et al., 2010). Over several weeks, exercises performed earlier in a training session often exhibit larger improvements in strength compared to doing the exercises later (Nunes et al., 2020). Therefore, to improve strength in a specific exercise, it is logical to perform the exercise earlier in a training session. However, the ordering of exercises (e.g., isolation to compound or vice versa) appears to be less important for hypertrophy after multiple weeks of training (Nunes et al., 2020).

Calculating and monitoring resistance training intensity

Repetition maximum methods

The intensity of a RT exercise is traditionally expressed as a percentage of the one-repetition maximum (%1RM), which is the maximal load that can be lifted for one repetition. The %1RM method allows the intensity to be calculated relative to the client's maximum strength. Training with a higher (e.g., ≥80%) percentage of 1RM tends to result in greater improvements in dynamic strength; therefore, the %1RM approach is often used to prescribe load in RT programmes focused on improving maximum strength (Rhea et al., 2003).

The repetition maximum (RM) corresponds to the maximum load lifted for a specified number of repetitions. Training using a RM approach generally involves working up to the heaviest load that can be lifted for a certain number of repetitions or completing multiple sets at a specific RM load. For example, if a client reached repetition failure after six repetitions with 80 kg in the bench press, the 6RM load is 80 kg. The RM method should be applied with caution as consistently training to failure could induce excessive fatigue and be counterproductive to future training sessions or other training goals (see Chapter 13).

Both %1RM and RM are effective methods to programme for improving strength (Thompson et al., 2020); however, these methods do not consider an individual's daily fluctuation in strength due to cumulative fatigue and other factors (e.g., sleep, nutrition and motivation). For example, a client experiencing muscle soreness and lack of sleep is unlikely to perform at peak capacity for a session planned to involve near maximal loads.

Subjective intensity

Using subjective intensity methods, discussed below, enables training to be modified to accommodate the client's current perceived capacity in an effort to optimise fatigue management and reduce injury risk (Carroll et al., 2018; Helms et al., 2016). A potential disadvantage of subjective intensity methods can be undershooting what a client can achieve, or training at an intensity that exceeds the client's recovery capacity before the next session. Stated differently, it is possible that a client's perceived capability or elected intensity could result in training at a suboptimal intensity.

Rating of perceived exertion (RPE)

The RPE-based method of programming involves selecting a load for an exercise that corresponds to a certain perceived exertion on a scale of 1–10 (see Figure 7.3). A target RPE for a single set can be prescribed for a certain number of repetitions in this model. The RPE should be 10 when repetition

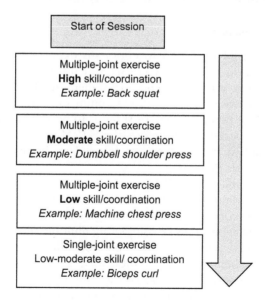

Figure 7.3 Resistance training exercise order sequencing.

failure (i.e., no additional repetitions can be completed) occurs; however, this does not always transpire in practice. For example, participants in one study reported RPE scores below 10 when they reached repetition failure. Yet, they were able to accurately gauge the number of additional repetitions they could have completed at the end of a set – known as 'repetitions in reserve' (Hackett et al., 2012).

Repetitions in reserve (RIR)

The concept of intentionally completing sets a certain number of repetitions away from repetition failure is referred to as repetitions in reserve (RIR) (Zourdos et al., 2016). Conceptually, RIR is the inverse of RPE on a scale of 1–10. For example, an RPE of 9 (see Figure 7.4) should correspond to an RIR rating of 1 (Zourdos et al., 2016). When used consistently, the RIR method appears to offer better accuracy than RPE and is becoming a practical and widely adopted method of prescribing RT intensity (Helms et al., 2016).

Calculating resistance training volume

Volume in RT is defined as the total amount of work completed for an exercise, in a training session, or over an extended period of time (Schoenfeld et al., 2019). The method for calculating and prescribing volume should be standardised and consistent over time to understand the dose-response

Rating of perceived exertion (RPE)	Descriptor	Repetitions in Reserve (RIR)
1	Little to no effort	
2		
3-4	Light effort	
5-6		4-6
7		3
7.5		2-3
8		2
8.5		1-2
9		1
9.5		*
10	Maximum effort	0

Figure 7.4 Scale for rating of perceived exertion (RPE) for resistance exercise. *No further repetitions but could increase load. Values in the RPE column correspond to the RIR or perceived level of exertion indicated in the description column. Descriptions of perceived exertion are associated with the number of repetitions in reserve (RIR).

Reproduced with permission from Zourdos et al. (2016).

Table 7.6 The volume-load method

Exercise	Load (kg)	Repetitions	Sets	Volume-load (kg)	Average intensity (kg)	RIR
Back squat	60	8	1	480	60	7
	100	5	5	2500	100	3
Leg press	150	8	1	1200	150	8
	200	10	3	6000	200	3

relationship between the volume of training and an adaptive outcome (e.g., hypertrophy). A common method to quantify volume is the volume-load (VL) method, which combines the volume (total repetitions) and load lifted. For example, the VL from 3 × 10 repetitions with 100 kg is 3000 kg. Dividing the VL by the repetition volume allows the average intensity of load for an exercise or training session to be calculated (average intensity = VL (kg)/total repetitions).

A disadvantage of the VL method is that meaningful comparisons in VL between sessions cannot be made when different exercises are used. Exclusively focusing on VL does not consider the complexity or neuromuscular demand of an exercise, and the client's intensity of effort (e.g., RIR), which could lead to misleading inferences. For example, in Table 7.6, the higher VL from the leg press suggests the training stress was more significant than the squat. However, the leg press and squat were performed with a similar RIR (i.e., a similar intensity of effort). To facilitate comparing the volume between different programmes, researchers and practitioners often quantify volume based on the number of 'hard sets' completed (Krieger, 2009, 2010; Schoenfeld et al., 2017).

Hard sets

Hard sets (aka working sets) are the sets performed after warm-up sets that contribute to the objectives of the exercise (e.g., stimulating hypertrophy). For example, the warm-up sets on the squat and leg-press exercises in Table 7.6 were performed at an intensity of >5 RIR and were not classified as hard sets. Only the hard sets (i.e., <4 RIR) were counted, which means more (5) hard sets were completed in the squat versus the leg press (3). Trainers may elect to prescribe and monitor training volume by specifying/recording the number of hard sets completed per muscle group during a training session or across a week.

Designing a training session focused on hypertrophy

Exercise selection for hypertrophy training sessions

Tissues, such as muscle and tendon, have a limited adaptive capacity. For this reason, a finite training volume can be performed for a given movement or muscle within a single training session that elicits adaptation (i.e., a volume threshold). Considering this, dedicating an entire session to training a single muscle group (e.g., a chest day) is generally inefficient. Training multiple muscle groups using various exercises within a session is recommended for hypertrophy training (Schoenfeld et al., 2015). Exercise selection should be guided by factors, such as the client's individual characteristics, equipment and time availability. Since mechanical tension is the primary signal that promotes muscle growth, exercises for hypertrophy should be considered based upon the degree of tension experienced in the target muscle/s along with the relative safety of the exercise for the client. Both free weight and machine-based exercises can be intelligently included in programs aimed at hypertrophy.

Prescribing intensity for hypertrophy training sessions

Training with relatively light or heavy loads can result in similar muscle growth over several weeks, provided sets are taken to (or close to) the point of repetition failure (see Chapter 13). However, there appears to be a minimum load necessary to produce significant hypertrophic responses, even when sets are performed to failure. Lasevicius et al. (2018) found that training with loads between 40 and 80% 1RM to failure produced similar muscle growth after 12 weeks of training; however, training with 20% 1RM resulted in only ~1/2 of the growth compared to the 40–80% 1RM conditions. In the same study, participants were able to complete ~30 repetitions with 40% of their 1RM (Lasevicius et al., 2018). Therefore, a load that can be lifted for ~5–30 repetitions/set (i.e., 40–80% 1RM) is appropriate for sessions focused on hypertrophy. Evidence suggests that almost all the fibres in a muscle are recruited to contract within ~4 repetitions of muscular failure (Sundstrup et al., 2012). Therefore, ending sets between 1 and 4 RIR (see above) is logical.

Prescribing volume hypertrophy training sessions

There is a relationship between the number of hard sets (see above) completed per week and muscle growth, where more hard sets produce more muscle growth, to a point (Krieger, 2010; Schoenfeld et al., 2017). However, the muscle protein synthetic response to a bout of RT is finite and more training volume will not increase it further (Ogasawara et al., 2017). In other words, it appears that a 'volume threshold' exists where extra training volume (above an individual's volume threshold) does not elicit any benefit. For instance, training a single muscle group for more than ~10 challenging sets in a single session may result in diminishing or negative returns in some individuals (Damas et al., 2019; Ogasawara et al., 2017).

Research also indicates that performing up to ~20 sets per week per muscle is proximal to a maximally effective volume in some young resistance-trained individuals, although some individuals may require less or more volume for optimal results (Roberts et al., 2018; Scarpelli et al., 2020). Haun et al. (2018) reported that increasing set-volume from 20 to 32 sets/week/muscle from week 3 to 6 of a training program resulted in a *dampened* increase in lean body mass compared to the increase observed when set-volume was increased from 10 to 20 sets/week/muscle from week 1 to 3 of the study. However, loads used throughout the study were relatively light (~60%1RM) and training was not completed to the point of repetition failure. Using heavier loads and training closer to (or to) failure can generate more fatigue and may reduce the number of sets necessary to stimulate maximal muscle growth. These variables (load, proximity to failure), rest between exercises, and other factors should ultimately influence training volume allocation to better ensure a client is completing a safe and effective amount of volume. Although more research is necessary in various training contexts, limited research suggests completing over 30 sets/week/muscle may not result in additional muscle growth, at least in some individuals (Haun et al., 2018).

Setting the initial training dose for hypertrophy

Beginning a hypertrophy training programme at an individualised volume, based on recent historical training (e.g., ~20% more than recent training), has been shown to produce more hypertrophy compared to a non-individualised (~20 sets per week) approach (Scarpelli et al., 2020). Therefore, week one of a new hypertrophy training cycle should depend on recent historical training and individual factors. Since more set-volume appears to enhance growth to a point (Schoenfeld et al., 2019), an example of an approach is to begin a training cycle at approximately 6–8 sets/muscle/week and increase the set-volume by 1–2 sets per week up to a maximally effective dose followed by a recovery (aka de-load) week. Additionally, a training cycle aimed at hypertrophy could be designed that targets an appropriate number of hard sets (e.g., ~15–25) to complete each week of a multi-week cycle and overload could be applied by judiciously targeting an increase in the load used for an exercise, the total number of repetitions completed for an exercise, or a combination of both.

Should hypertrophy sessions include advanced methods?

The use of advanced methods, such as supersets (see Chapter 13), may be warranted to apply progressive overload. Moreover, advanced methods can increase metabolite accumulation, a possible mechanism for hypertrophy (see Chapter 13). However, using advanced methods that encourage training to failure should be programmed carefully to manage fatigue and reduce the risk of injury.

Designing a training session focused on maximum strength development

Exercise selection for maximum strength development training sessions

Maximum strength denotes the maximum amount of force that can be produced during a lift or against a certain resistance. Although strength and hypertrophy are not entirely exclusive of one another, a training session focused on improving maximum strength should involve different considerations than training for hypertrophy. Exercises for strength training can be categorised and ordered as main, associate, assistance, and pre-habilitation exercises – this is the MAAP method (see Table 7.7). Strength training sessions should generally include 1–2 exercises from each (MAAP) category for a total of ~6–8 exercises in a session or possibly fewer depending on the client's circumstances.

Main denotes exercises that are the most important exercises in a programme; for example, the top three exercises in which strength is primarily sought. Associate exercises involve a similar portion of the main exercise or are a direct variation of the main exercise. For example, a dumbbell bench press could be considered an associate exercise to the bench press. An assistance exercise is an exercise that involves similar muscles to the main exercise but involves a markedly different movement pattern. For example, a dumbbell chest fly would be an assistance exercise for the bench press as it is different from a kinetic and kinematic perspective but involves similar musculature (e.g., pectorals and anterior deltoids). Pre-habilitation and core exercises are included in a programme to help prevent injuries, address asymmetries, develop a well-rounded physique, and enhance core strength and stability.

Exercise order for maximum strength development training sessions

Acute fatigue sustained from exercises early in a session can reduce the performance of exercises done later in a session (Simão et al., 2010, 2012). Consequently, over several weeks, exercises completed early in training

Table 7.7 Example exercise selection using the MAAP method

	Main exercise	*Associate exercise*	*Assistance exercise*	*Pre-habilitation or core exercise*
Session 1	Low barbell squat	Low barbell squat from Pins (pin squat)	Dumbbell rear-foot elevated split squat	Dead bugs Pallof press
Session 2	Conventional barbell Deadlift	Barbell Rack pull from Knee	Lat Pulldown	Standing cable Crunch

sessions tend to exhibit greater improvements in strength than exercises completed later in a session (Dias et al., 2010). Therefore, the most important exercises related to the client's goals and exercises involving a greater risk of injury should be prioritised early within a training session (see Figure 7.1). This 'priority' approach enables more quality repetitions of the priority exercises to be performed than performing an exercise towards the end of a training session (Sforzo & Touey, 1996).

The pre-exhaust method

In contrast to performing compound exercises followed by isolation exercises, a technique used by bodybuilders known as 'pre-exhaustion' (PE) is sometimes implemented. The PE method involves performing isolation exercises before a compound exercise. For instance, performing dumbbell flys before the bench press. The objective of PE is to fatigue the smaller, synergistic muscles, so the larger muscles are required to generate greater forces during the compound exercise to compensate for the fatigued smaller muscles (Fisher et al., 2014). However, PE is not recommended for maximum strength training, as the acute fatigue from an isolation exercise likely reduces the individual's capacity to perform the compound exercise (Augustsson et al., 2003).

Intensity for maximum strength development training sessions

Scientific literature suggests that consistently training within an intensity range of 75–90% 1RM is optimal to improve maximal strength (see Chapter 13); this corresponds to ~3–10 repetitions per set, on average. Any of the intensity prescription methods discussed (%1RM, RM, RPE, RIR) can be used for maximal strength programmes. The %1RM method has proven to be effective for improving maximum strength (Thompson et al., 2020). However, emerging evidence suggests using a perceived exertion method (RPE or RIR) is a viable alternative to the %1RM and RM methods (Helms et al., 2018).

Prescribing volume for maximum strength development training sessions

The priority of strength-focused programmes is progressing the absolute intensity of load rather than progressing training volume alone (see Chapter 13). Performing more than one set of an exercise in a session produces superior improvements in strength. Therefore, beginning a strength training programme at ~2–4 sets per exercise per session at an intensity between 75 and 90% 1RM and progressing absolute intensity by ~2–5% each week is a reasonable starting point.

*Prescribing inter-set rest intervals for maximum strength
development training sessions*

Rest intervals of ~3–5 minutes between hard sets facilitate psychological and physiological recovery, enabling the lifter to recover his/her force generation capacity (see Chapter 13). Shorter (1–2 minutes) rest periods may not permit the adequate recovery of physiological processes, such as the re-establishment of muscle blood flow and oxygen delivery, and restoration of muscle phosphocreatine stores (Harris et al., 1976; Willardson, 2008).

Summary

Each training session should be designed according to the training session's objective within the context of the client's long-term goal(s). Exercise selection, the sequence of exercises, and the prescription of intensity, volume, and rest intervals should be guided by the client's ability and goals, the trainer's judgement, and scientific research. The calculation of both intensity and volume is important when designing, monitoring, and evaluating training. The method to calculate volume and intensity varies depending on the type (i.e., endurance or resistance) of training and a combination of approaches can be used. Objective and subjective training data should be consistently logged to monitor and evaluate the client's responses to training.

References

Abadie, B. (1996). Effect of viewing the RPE scale on the ability to make ratings of perceived exertion. *Perceptual and Motor Skills, 83*(1), 317–318.
Ainsworth, B., Haskell, W., Herrmann, S., et al. (2011). 2011 compendium of physical activities: a second update of codes and MET values. *Medicine and Science in Sports and Exercise, 43*(8), 1575–1581.
Arena, R., Myers, J., & Kaminsky, L. (2016). Revisiting age-predicted maximal heart rate: can it be used as a valid measure of effort? *American Heart Journal, 173*, 49–56.
Areta, J., Burke, L., Camera, D., et al. (2014). Reduced resting skeletal muscle protein synthesis is rescued by resistance exercise and protein ingestion following short-term energy deficit. *American journal of physiology. Endocrinology and metabolism, 306*(8), E989–E997.
Augustsson, J., Thomeé, R., Hörnstedt, P., et al. (2003). Effect of pre-exhaustion exercise on lower-extremity muscle activation during a leg press exercise. *Journal of Strength and Conditioning Research, 17*(2), 411–416.
Baar, K. (2014). Using molecular biology to maximize concurrent training. *Sports Medicine, 44*(2), S117–S125.
Bannister, E. (1991). Modeling elite athletic performance. In *Physiological testing of elite athletes* (pp. 403–424). Human Kinetics.
Borg, G. (1982). Psychophysical basis of perceived exertion. *Medicine and Science in Sports and Exercise, 14*, 371–381.
Borg, G. (1998). *Borg's perceived exertion and pain scales.* Human Kinetics.

Carroll, K., Bernards, J., Bazyler, C., et al. (2018). Divergent performance outcomes following resistance training using repetition maximums or relative intensity. *International Journal of Sports Physiology and Performance*, 1–28.

Chen, M., Fan, X., & Moe, S. (2002). Criterion-related validity of the Borg ratings of perceived exertion scale in healthy individuals: a meta-analysis. *Journal of Sports Sciences*, *20*(11), 873–899.

Christou, D., & Seals, D. (2008). Decreased maximal heart rate with aging is related to reduced β-adrenergic responsiveness but is largely explained by a reduction in intrinsic heart rate. *Journal of Applied Physiology*, *105*(1), 24–29.

Damas, F., Angleri, V., Phillips, S., et al. (2019). Myofibrillar protein synthesis and muscle hypertrophy individualised responses to systematically changing resistance training variables in trained young men. *Journal of Applied Physiology*, *127*(3), 806–815.

Dias, I., de Salles, B., Novaes, J., et al. (2010). Influence of exercise order on maximum strength in untrained young men. *Journal of Science and Medicine in Sport/ Sports Medicine Australia*, *13*(1), 65–69.

Fisher, J., Carlson, L., Steele, J., et al. (2014). The effects of pre-exhaustion, exercise order, and rest intervals in a full-body resistance training intervention. *Applied Physiology, Nutrition, and Metabolism*, *39*(11), 1265–1270.

Foster C. (1998). Monitoring training in athletes with reference to overtraining syndrome. *Medicine and Science in sports and Exercise*, *30*(7), 1164–1168.

Foster, C., Florhaug, J., Franklin, J., et al. (2001). A new approach to monitoring exercise training. *Journal of Strength and Conditioning Research*, *15*(1), 109–115.

Foster, C., Porcari, J., Anderson, J., et al. (2008). The Talk Test as a marker of exercise training intensity. *Journal of Cardiopulmonary Rehabilitation and Prevention*, *28*(1), 24–30.

Fox, S., Naughton, J., & Haskell, W. (1971). Physical activity and the prevention of coronary heart disease. *Annals of Clinical Research*, *3*(6), 404–432.

Grgic, J., Schoenfeld, B., Skrepnik, M., et al. (2018). Effects of rest interval duration in resistance training on measures of muscular strength: a systematic review. *Sports Medicine*, *48*(1), 137–151.

Garber, C., Blissmer, B., Deschenes, M., et al. (2011). American College of sports medicine position stand. Quantity and quality of exercise for developing and maintaining cardiorespiratory, musculoskeletal, and neuromotor fitness in apparently healthy adults: guidance for prescribing exercise. *Medicine and Science in Sports and Exercise*, *43*(7), 1334–1359.

Gellish, R., Goslin, B., Olson, R., et al. (2007). Longitudinal modeling of the relationship between age and maximal heart rate. *Medicine and Science in Sports and Exercise*, *39*(5), 822–829.

Hackett, D., Johnson, N., & Halaki, M., et al. (2012). A novel scale to assess resistance-exercise effort. *Journal of Sports Sciences*, *30*(13), 1405–1413.

Harris, R., Edwards, R., Hultman, E., et al. (1976). The time course of phosphorylcreatine resynthesis during recovery of the quadriceps muscle in man. *European Journal of Physiology*, *367*(2), 137–142.

Haun, C., Vann, C., Mobley, C., et al. (2018). Effects of graded whey supplementation during extreme-volume resistance training. *Frontiers in Nutrition*, *5*, 84.

Helms, E., Byrnes, R., Cooke, D., et al. (2018). RPE vs. Percentage 1RM loading in periodized programs matched for sets and repetitions. *Frontiers in Physiology*, *9*, 247.

Helms, E., Cronin, J., Storey, A., et al. (2016). Application of the repetitions in reserve-based rating of perceived exertion scale for resistance training. *Strength and Conditioning Journal, 38*(4), 42–49.

Hickson, R. (1980). Interference of strength development by simultaneously training for strength and endurance. *European Journal of Applied Physiology and Occupational Physiology, 45*(2–3), 255–263.

Jetté, M., Sidney, K., & Blümchen, G. (1990). Metabolic equivalents (METS) in exercise testing, exercise prescription, and evaluation of functional capacity. *Clinical Cardiology, 13*(8), 555–565.

Karvonen, M., Kentala, E., & Mustala, O. (1957). The effects of training on heart rate: a longitudinal study. *Annales Medicinae Experimentalis Et Biologiae Fenniae, 35*(3), 307–315.

Kazior, Z., Willis, S., Moberg, M., et al. (2016). Endurance exercise enhances the effect of strength training on muscle fiber size and protein expression of Akt and mTOR. *PLoS ONE, 11*(2), 1–18.

Kim, M., Sujkowski, A., Namkoong, S., et al. (2020). SESTRINs are evolutionarily conserved mediators of exercise benefits. *Nature Communications, 11*(1), 1–14.

Kraemer, W., Patton, J., & Gordon, S. (1995). Compatibility of high-intensity strength and endurance training on hormonal and skeletal muscle adaptations. *Journal of Applied Physiology, 78*(3), 976–989.

Krieger, J. (2009). Single versus multiple sets of resistance exercise: a meta-regression. *Journal of Strength and Conditioning Research/National Strength & Conditioning Association, 23*(6), 1890–1901.

Krieger, J. (2010). Single vs. multiple sets of resistance exercise for muscle hypertrophy: a meta-analysis. *Journal of Strength and Conditioning Research/National Strength & Conditioning Association, 24*(4), 1150–1159.

Lasevicius, T., Ugrinowitsch, C., Schoenfeld, B., et al. (2018). Effects of different intensities of resistance training with equated volume load on muscle strength and hypertrophy. *European Journal of Sport Science, 18*(6), 772–780.

Manzi, V., Iellamo, F., Impellizzeri, F., et al. (2009). Relation between individualized training impulses and performance in distance runners. *Medicine and Science in Sports and Exercise, 41*(11), 2090–2096.

Melanson, E., & Freedson, P. (1996). Physical activity assessment: a review of methods. *Critical Reviews in Food Science and Nutrition, 36*(5), 385–396.

Myers, T., Schneider, M., Schmale, M., et al. (2015). Whole-body aerobic resistance training circuit improves aerobic fitness and muscle strength in sedentary young females. *Journal of Strength and Conditioning Research, 29*(6), 1592–1600.

Nalbandian, M., & Takeda, M. (2016). Lactate as a signaling molecule that regulates exercise-induced adaptations. *Biology, 5*(4).

Nes, B., Janszky, I., Wisløff, U., et al. (2013). Age-predicted maximal heart rate in healthy subjects: the HUNT fitness study. *Scandinavian Journal of Medicine & Science in Sports, 23*(6), 697–704.

Nunes, J., Grgic, J., Cunha, P., et al. (2020). What influence does resistance exercise order have on muscular strength gains and muscle hypertrophy? A systematic review and meta-analysis. *European Journal of Sport Science*, 1–9. Advance online publication.

Nuuttila, O.-P., Kyröläinen, H., & Häkkinen, K., (2020). Acute physiological responses to four running sessions performed at different intensity zones. *International Journal of Sports Medicine.* Online ahead of print.

Ogasawara, R., Arihara, Y., Takegaki, J., et al. (2017). Relationship between exercise volume and muscle protein synthesis in a rat model of resistance exercise. *Journal of Applied Physiology, 123*(4), 710–716.

Persinger, R., Foster, C., & Gibson, M. (2004). Consistency of the Talk Test for exercise prescription. *Medicine and Science in Sports and Exercise, 36*(9), 1632–1636.

Rhea, M., Alvar, B., Burkett, L., et al. (2003). A meta-analysis to determine the dose response for strength development. *Medicine and Science in Sports and Exercise, 35*(3), 456–464.

Roberts, M., Haun, C., Mobley, C., et al. (2018). Physiological differences between low versus high skeletal muscle hypertrophic responders to resistance exercise training: current perspectives and future research directions. *Frontiers in Physiology, 9*, 834.

Scarpelli, M., Nóbrega, S., Santanielo, N., et al. (2020). Muscle hypertrophy response is affected by previous resistance training volume in trained individuals. *Journal of Strength and Conditioning Research*. Online ahead of print.

Schmidt, D., Anderson, K., Graff, M., et al. (2016). The effect of high-intensity circuit training on physical fitness. *The Journal of Sports Medicine and Physical Fitness, 56*(5), 534–540.

Schoenfeld, B., Grgic, J., Haun, C., et al. (2019). Calculating set-volume for the limb muscles with the performance of multi-joint exercises: implications for resistance training prescription. *Sports, 7*(7). https://pubmed.ncbi.nlm.nih.gov/30153194/

Schoenfeld, B., Ogborn, D., & Krieger, J. (2017). Dose-response relationship between weekly resistance training volume and increases in muscle mass: a systematic review and meta-analysis. *Journal of Sports Sciences, 35*(11), 1073–1082.

Schoenfeld, B., Peterson, M., Ogborn, D., et al. (2015). Effects of low- vs. high-load resistance training on muscle strength and hypertrophy in Well-trained men. *Journal of Strength and Conditioning Research/National Strength & Conditioning Association, 29*(10), 2954–2963.

Sforzo, G., & Touey, P. (1996). Manipulating exercise order affects muscular performance during a resistance exercise training session. *Journal of Strength and Conditioning Research, 10*(1), 20.

Simão, R., de Salles, B., Figueiredo, T., et al. (2012). Exercise order in resistance training. *Sports Medicine, 42*(3), 251–265.

Simão, R., Spineti, J., de Salles, B., et al. (2010). Influence of exercise order on maximum strength and muscle thickness in untrained men. *Journal of Sports Science & Medicine, 9*(1), 1–7.

Spina, R. (1999). Cardiovascular adaptations to endurance exercise training in older men and women. *Exercise and Sport Sciences Reviews, 27*, 317–332.

Spineti, J., de Salles, B., Rhea, M., et al. (2010). Influence of exercise order on maximum strength and muscle volume in nonlinear periodized resistance training. *Journal of Strength and Conditioning Research, 24*(11), 2962–2969.

Stagno, K., Thatcher, R., & van Someren, K. (2007). A modified TRIMP to quantify the in-season training load of team sport players. *Journal of Sports Sciences, 25*(6), 629–634.

Sundstrup, E., Jakobsen, M., Andersen, C., et al. (2012). Muscle activation strategies during strength training with heavy loading vs. repetitions to failure. *Journal of Strength and Conditioning Research/National Strength & Conditioning Association, 26*(7), 1897–1903.

Tanaka, H., Monahan, K., & Seals, D. (2001). Age-predicted maximal heart rate revisited. *Journal of the American College of Cardiology, 37*(1), 153–156.

Thompson, S., Rogerson, D., Ruddock, A., et al. (2020). The effectiveness of two methods of prescribing load on maximal strength development: a systematic review. *Sports Medicine, 50*(5), 919–938.

Wang, L., Mascher, H., Psilander, N., et al. (2011). Resistance exercise enhances the molecular signaling of mitochondrial biogenesis induced by endurance exercise in human skeletal muscle. *Journal of Applied Physiology, 111*(5), 1335–1344.

Willardson, J. (2008). A brief review: how much rest between sets? *Strength & Conditioning Journal, 30*(3), 44.

Wilson, J., Marin, P., Rhea, M., et al. (2012). Concurrent training: a meta-analysis examining interference of aerobic and resistance exercises. *The Journal of Strength and Conditioning Research, 26*(8), 2293–2307.

Zourdos, M., Klemp, A., & Dolan, C., et al. (2016). Novel resistance training-specific rating of perceived exertion scale measuring repetitions in reserve. *Journal of Strength and Conditioning Research, 30*(1), 267–275.

8 Long-term programme design (periodisation)

Stuart N. Guppy and G. Gregory Haff

Introduction

When working with both athletes and non-athletes, many factors must be accounted for by the trainer to ensure that clients achieve their goals at the desired time. The appropriate organisation of training is fundamental to achieving the objectives of the training process. The concept of periodisation is widely used by both strength and conditioning professionals and sports coaches and is generally considered to be a cornerstone of the athletic development process (Haff, 2016; Mujika et al., 2018). The principles of periodisation are also applicable to the physical development of non-athletes regardless of whether they are seeking to improve specific physical qualities, such as maximal strength and aerobic capacity, or simply seeking to improve general health and wellness.

Despite the almost ubiquitous belief that long-term planning of training is required to optimally develop physical qualities important for both athletic and non-athletic populations (Mujika et al., 2018), there is confusion regarding what periodisation entails and its role in the training process. This confusion is largely due to the many different interpretations of periodisation within the literature – specifically, the common mislabelling of programming factors (i.e., sets, repetitions, and intensity) as periodisation (Cunanan et al., 2018; DeWeese et al., 2015a). Therefore, the term 'periodisation' has been frequently misapplied throughout both the scientific literature and in applied practice.

This chapter aims to provide an overview of theoretical and practical aspects underpinning the process of designing a long-term training programme. It also aims to clarify some of the common misunderstandings found in the literature when periodisation is explained. Finally, the chapter will provide practical recommendations for the implementation of the long-term programme design process, specifically within the context of non-athletic populations.

DOI: 10.4324/9781003204657-8

The theory of long-term programme design

Periodisation is commonly labelled in the literature as 'linear' or 'nonlinear' (Harries et al., 2015; Kraemer et al., 2015), but the use of these terms represents a fundamental misinterpretation of the concept (DeWeese et al., 2015a; Issurin, 2010; Plisk & Stone, 2003). Graphical representations of the average training intensity and volume performed over the course of an entire training cycle typically appear inversely linear (Baker, 2007; Poliquin, 1988). However, when the classic literature that forms the theoretical and practical basis for periodisation is closely examined, these linear trends mask a considerable degree of variation in the training process at both the mesocycle (i.e., 2–6 weeks of training) and microcycle (i.e., 2–14 days of training) level (Harre, 1982; Matveyev, 1981; Verkhoshansky & Siff, 2009). Moreover, the linear application of training load directly violates a key tenet of the concept of periodisation – namely, the *non-linearity* of the training process (Matveyev, 1981). Furthermore, a linear application of training load likely increases the overall fatigue as well as the monotony and strain associated with the training programme, which are factors that the periodisation of training seeks to mitigate (Carroll et al., 2019; DeWeese et al., 2015a; Painter et al., 2012).

The mislabelling of programming tools and tactics as periodisation also neglects several factors encompassed within the construct. A truly periodised plan considers physical training alongside individual factors, such as nutrition, psychology, recovery, and motor learning (Mota et al., 2019; Mujika et al., 2018). These factors must be carefully integrated and manipulated within the overall training plan to optimise physical and psychological performance during competition (Mujika et al., 2018). For personal training clients seeking improvements in general health and wellness, several factors that influence the training plan (e.g., work schedule, family commitments, and social activities) must be considered. For example, during periods of high work-related stress, the client may have a decreased ability to recover from training (Stults-Kolehmainen et al., 2014). Therefore, training may have to be altered to reduce the likelihood of injury and sickness (Mann et al., 2016).

The periodisation process is not a 'set and forget' method of organising training (Kiely, 2012). Periodisation is malleable to the changing needs and circumstances of the individual (Harre, 1982; Norris & Smith, 2002). There is no universally accepted singular definition of periodisation. However, at its most basic level, periodisation and the process of long-term programme design is a method of organising training to more easily plan the development of specific training targets (Bompa & Haff, 2009). Considerable thought should be applied to this process so that the training performed by the client has a logical flow, rather than a random selection of ends and means. In the context of this book, periodisation should be thought of as an overall planning construct that seeks to logically sequence and integrate the physiological and psychological stressors experienced by the client. The objective of periodisation is to optimise health and performance outcomes, regardless of how those outcomes are measured (DeWeese et al., 2013; Mujika et al., 2018).

Periodisation of training with non-athlete populations

Within the athletic development domain, which periodisation is commonly studied and described, the logical and sequential integration of training allows sporting form to be raised at specific time-points to optimise per-formance during competition (Haff, 2016; Matveyev, 1981). A large part of periodisation is dictated by the structure and duration of the competitive period. Although developing a periodised plan for non-athletes typically does not revolve around a rigid and well-defined competitive schedule, the central tenets of periodisation still apply (Stone et al., 2007). Training must still be 'nonlinear', with cyclical variations in training focus, volume, and intensity that allow for the development of specific physical qualities aligned with the client's goals (Stone et al., 2007; Thibaudeau, 2006). Regardless of whether the trainer is designing a long-term training plan for athletes or non-athletes, the training history of the individual will dic-tate the duration of training phases targeting general and specific fitness qualities, as well as the complexity of training means used (Bompa & Haff, 2009; Coffey & Hawley, 2017).

Common models of periodisation

Several training models have been proposed and successfully implemented into practice within the periodisation literature. Many of the differences between these models are subtle and most commonly relate to a confu-sion of the term's periodisation and programming (Cunanan et al., 2018; DeWeese et al., 2015a). However, if only the models for the overall planning of training are considered, rather than methods of manipulating program-ming tactics, there are three primary models of periodisation: (1) parallel models, (2) sequential models, and (3) emphasis models.

Parallel models

Careful examination of the classic periodisation literature reveals that many of these models target the simultaneous development of multiple training factors (see Figure 8.1) (e.g., strength, power, endurance, and speed), which can be trained within an individual training session, train-ing day, series of training days, or microcycle (Haff, 2017). Due to the focus on simultaneously developing multiple training factors, this approach to

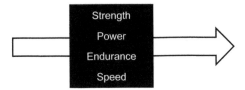

Figure 8.1 Example parallel model of periodisation.

periodisation should be referred to as the parallel model of periodisation (Bompa & Buzzichelli, 2015).

Personal trainers commonly use the parallel model of periodisation to develop multiple fitness components that underpin overall health and fitness. While this model has many benefits, it does have its limitations. Foremost among these limitations is that a greater training volume or load is required to improve any fitness components, which requires an increase in overall training load (Haff, 2017). Since clients have a finite training tolerance, the need to increase volume, intensity, or overall training load will eventually exceed the client's ability to adequately recover from the training stimulus (Issurin, 2010). If this threshold is chronically exceeded, stagnation or even reversal of adaptation may occur (Bompa & Haff, 2009; Thompson et al., 2020). While the parallel model may work well with relatively untrained clients, its limitations may make it less beneficial for more trained clients who require a greater or more targeted training stimulus to continue developing specific components of fitness.

Sequential or block models

With sequential or block periodisation models, the training targets are sequenced over time to expose the client to higher training loads and intensities (see Figure 8.2) (Haff, 2017).

Sequential models typically produce more significant improvements in muscular strength, power, and body composition than parallel models (Harris et al., 2000). While sequential periodisation is a useful planning tool, it is possible that, as the client moves through the sequence of training blocks, detraining effects occur for the factors that are not being trained (Haff, 2017). Specifically, as the time dedicated to an individual training

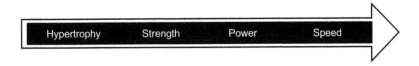

Figure 8.2 Example sequential model of periodisation.

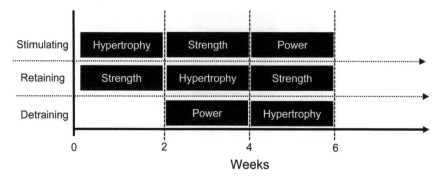

Figure 8.3 Example emphasis model of periodisation.

target increases, without returning to previously developed training factors, there is greater potential for detraining responses to occur.

Emphasis models

The emphasis, or pendulum, periodisation model is a blending of the parallel and sequential periodisation models where aspects of both models are employed (Bompa & Buzzichelli, 2015; Haff, 2017). This model is perhaps ideal for personal training as it allows multiple training factors to be sequenced over time. In an emphasis model, the training targets are classified as either being stimulated, retained, or detrained. As such, the client may train multiple targets (i.e., parallel model) with varying degrees of emphasis, which change every 2 weeks (i.e., sequential model) (see Figure 8.3).

A good example of an emphasis model was proposed by Poliquin (1988), who recommended rotating between 2-week blocks of resistance training that focuses on hypertrophy and strength development (see Table 8.1). The programme presented in Table 8.1 is based upon Poliquin's principles and is more reflective of a programming strategy than a model of periodisation. However, the example demonstrates how programming strategies can be manipulated to align with an emphasis model of periodisation for resistance training. This type of strategy allows for frequent variation and the development of multiple training targets over time.

The long-term programme design process

Multiple phases of assessment and planning are required to develop a long-term training programme. The first phase requires the trainer to establish a clear understanding of the client's goals and aims (Plisk, 2016). Once established, this understanding allows the trainer to determine the physiological and psychological factors that must be targeted to design a programme that meets the client's goals. The most common method of

Table 8.1 Example parallel model for strength training

Week	Main sets			Down sets			Emphasis	
	Sets	Reps	Intensity (% RM)	Sets	Reps	Intensity (% RM)	Primary	Secondar
1	3	10–12	70–75%				Hypertrophy	Strength
2								
3	5	4–6	82–88%	1	10–12	70–75%	Strength	Hypertrophy
4								
5	4	8–10	75–78%				Hypertrophy	Strength
6								
7	5	3–5	85–90%	1	8–10	75–78%	Strength	Hypertrophy
8								
9	4	5–7	80–85%				Hypertrophy	Strength
10								
11	6	2–3	90–95%	1	5–7	80–85%	Strength	Hypertrophy
12								

RM = repetition maximum. For example, if the 10 RM on an exercise was 30 kg, sets of 10 would be performed with a load of 21 kg (70% of 30 kg = 21 kg). Down-sets = sets that are completed after the targeted sets with reduced load. These are typically used to create smooth transitions between phases of a periodised training plan.

aligning the training programme with the goals of the client is through testing of physical capacities and the development of a thorough needs analysis (see Chapter 10). The needs analysis allows the trainer to assess the client's capacities against normative values established within the sports or health sciences literature (Thibaudeau, 2006). In conjunction with the client (see Chapter 3), the trainer can then construct a long-term training plan.

In the context of athletic populations, the long-term plan is commonly termed the annual plan or macrocycle and typically includes the entirety of the preparatory, competitive, and transition periods (Haff & Haff, 2012). Traditionally, the length of these periods is primarily dictated by the competitive schedule and rules imposed by governing bodies for each sport. In the context of non-athletic populations, the length of the macrocycle is dependent on the goal of the client. For example, for a client seeking to improve body composition before a wedding or holiday, the length of the macrocycle is defined solely by the time remaining between the start of training and the event itself. This scenario would entail a preparatory period that was of identical length to the macrocycle, further sub-divided into phases of general and specific preparation.

Different training targets are focussed on the general and specific phase. The overarching goal of the general preparatory phase is to develop basic bio-motor abilities and establish an adequate level of work capacity (Bompa & Haff, 2009). This improvement in work capacity is then capitalised on and expanded during the specific preparation phase, which is characterised by an increase in the specificity of the training means used, along with the intensities and volumes prescribed (Bompa & Haff, 2009). As outlined previously, it may be advantageous to structure the general and specific phases concurrently in some situations, with varying levels of relative emphasis applied for each training target.

Constructing the mesocycle plan

Once the overarching long-term programme outline has been constructed in accordance with the goals of the client, the trainer must structure training in a logical and sequential manner that develops the physical qualities deemed important for achieving the established goals (Haff, 2016). This requires the further subdivision of the training programme into smaller 'chunks' or 'blocks' called mesocycles, which typically last between 2 and 6 weeks (Haff & Haff, 2012). Each mesocycle has primary and secondary foci that seek to build on previously developed physical qualities. For example, a traditional programme seeking to improve maximal strength (see Chapter 13) may adopt a sequential pattern of targeting hypertrophy/strength-endurance followed by a 'strength' block of training. The hypertrophy/strength-endurance block would be used to raise work capacity and develop morphological factors that support future training in the 'strength block'. The 'strength' block would be used to target increases in maximal strength. After completing the hypertrophy and strength blocks of training, a third 'block' is programmed to mitigate the accumulated fatigue and allow the fitness developed in the preceding two blocks to be realised (Stone et al., 1982).

Traditionally, mesocycles have been constructed over four weeks of training, largely due to the convenience of aligning mesocycle lengths with calendar months. However, the work and social schedules of non-athletes may not allow this structure. Instead, it may be more appropriate for clients with shift or variable work and life schedules to use a block structure similar to those suggested by Poliquin (1988) and Baker (1998), where the emphasis is alternated on a bi- or tri-weekly basis. This model allows for enough stability in the training process to ensure positive adaptation occurs (Thompson et al., 2020). Furthermore, the relatively frequent variation in training focus may improve adherence to the programme by maintaining a degree of novelty and variation, which could improve the probability of achieving the client's goals (Baz-Valle et al., 2019; Poliquin, 1988).

Types of mesocycle

Regardless of duration, mesocycles are primarily classified as an accumulation, transmutation, or realisation mesocycle (Issurin, 2010). Accumulation mesocycles entail concentrated training loads to develop the client's overall work capacity. Due to the concentrated loading applied to a limited number of physical qualities during accumulation mesocycles, the fatigue accumulated during this mesocycle is greatest and takes the longest to dissipate through planned variation in training.

The transmutation mesocycle follows the accumulation mesocycle. In this mesocycle, basic physical qualities developed in the accumulation mesocycle are enhanced further through the use of more specific training means (Haff & Haff, 2012; Issurin, 2010). The transmutation cycle normally involves an increase in training intensity and, in the case of strength development, special and specific strength exercises are introduced (Verkhoshansky & Verkhoshansky, 2011). Although rarely implemented when working with non-athletic or clinical populations, the final mesocycle within a training cycle is the realisation (or peaking) mesocycle. Within the context of athletes, the goal of this mesocycle is to allow fatigue to dissipate and sporting form to increase in time for an event or competition (Haff, 2014; Issurin, 2015). The realisation phase is characterised by marked reductions in training load, and the implementation of training means that are highly specific to the athlete's sport.

The microcycle

Once the mesocycle structure and targets have been decided, the microcycles can be designed. For scheduling simplicity, microcycles have typically been defined as a week or seven days of training (Bompa & Haff, 2009; Issurin, 2015), but they can be less than a week where needed. Week-long microcycle lengths have traditionally been used due to the structure and scheduling of work, education, and social life, which are normally constructed from Monday to Sunday or Sunday to Saturday (Issurin, 2015). As such, the trainer must frequently consult with the client when designing the microcycle, as it should conform to the client's circumstances rather than a rigid, pre-determined pattern.

While variation in training targets is applied at the mesocycle level, most variation in the training process occurs at the microcycle level through the manipulation of programming factors, such as volume, intensity, rest duration, exercise selection, and exercise order. At the microcycle level, the concepts of periodisation and programming are most closely aligned. The practitioner must use scientific and practical knowledge to prescribe training stimuli at the appropriate magnitude and place, which requires knowledge of the time-course of recovery from each form of training, along with the compatibility of each training target (Issurin, 2016). For example, suppose the client's primary goal is to improve maximal strength alongside a secondary goal of overall improvements in general health and wellness. In that case, it may be prudent to separate resistance and endurance training to reduce the potential 'interference effect' discussed in Chapter 7 (Coffey & Hawley, 2017; Robineau et al., 2016). Similarly, performing resistance training exercises to failure (see Chapter 13) can result in an elongated recovery from the accumulated fatigue (Gonzalez-Badillo et al., 2016); therefore, the trainer has to appropriately modulate training intensity to ensure stagnation or declines in performance do not occur (Carroll et al., 2019; Thompson et al., 2020). Most commonly, training intensity has been controlled through the implementation of 'heavy' and 'light' days (DeWeese et al., 2015b), with the variation in training intensity on the 'light' day accounting for fatigue generated earlier in the microcycle while still providing sufficient training stimulus.

The role of monitoring in long-term programme design

As discussed in Chapter 5, the implementation of an ongoing testing and monitoring regime facilitates the process of long-term programme design (Comfort et al., 2019; Cunanan et al., 2018). Without testing or monitoring, it is difficult to ensure that the athlete or client is undergoing the desired adaptations in response to the imposed training stimulus, nor is it possible to logically plan future training interventions that maximise performance outcomes at the required time-point (Haff & Haff, 2012; Sands & Stone, 2005).

Summary

Long-term programme design allows for the logical and sequential development of physiological and psychological qualities in a manner that is appropriate to the client's training history and goals. When considered in the context of clients seeking improvements in general health and wellness, this entails accounting for work, family, social commitments or stressors alongside the acute and chronic physiological responses to the training process. Long-term programme design requires considerable thought and planning on the part of the trainer. The long-term programme is not rigid and must remain malleable in response to the client's changing circumstances. Finally, there is no optimal long-term programme design model, as the process is specific to the client's circumstances.

References

Baker, D. (1998). Applying the in-season periodisation of strength and power training to football. *Strength and Conditioning Journal, 20*(2), 18–27.

Baker, D. (2007). Cycle-length variants in periodised strength/power training. *Strength and Conditioning Journal, 29*(4), 10–17.

Baz-Valle, E., Schoenfeld, B., Torres-Unda, J., et al. (2019). The effects of exercise variation in muscle thickness, maximal strength and motivation in resistance trained men. *PLoS One, 14*(12), e0226989.

Bompa, T., & Buzzichelli, C. (2015). Periodisation as planning and programming of sport training. In *Periodization training for sports* (pp. 87–95). Human Kinetics.

Bompa, T., & Haff, G. (2009). *Periodisation: theory and methodology of training* (5th ed.). Human Kinetics.

Carroll, K., Bernards, J., Bazyler, C., et al. (2019). Divergent performance outcomes following resistance training using repetition maximums or relative intensity. *International Journal of Sports Physiology and Performance*, *14*(1), 46–54.

Coffey, V., & Hawley, J. (2017). Concurrent exercise training: do opposites distract? *Journal of Physiology*, *595*(9), 2883–2896.

Comfort, P., Jones, P., & Hornsby, W. (2019). Structured testing vs. continual monitoring. In P. Comfort, P. A. Jones, & J. J. McMahon (Eds.), *Performance assessment in strength and conditioning* (pp. 42–50). Routledge.

Cunanan, A., DeWeese, B., Wagle, J., et al. (2018). The general adaptation syndrome: a foundation for the concept of periodisation. *Sports Medicine*, *48*(4), 787–797.

DeWeese, B. H., Gray, H. S., Sams, M. L., Scruggs, S. K., & Serrano, A. J. (2013). Revising the definition of periodisation: merging historical principles with modern concern. *Olympic Coach Magazine*, *24*(1), 5–19.

DeWeese, B. H., Hornsby, G., Stone, M., et al. (2015a). The training process: planning for strength-power training in track and field. Part 1: theoretical aspects. *Journal of Sport and Health Science*, *4*(4), 308–317.

DeWeese, B., Hornsby, G., & Stone, M. (2015b). The training process: planning for strength-power training in track and field. Part 2: practical and applied aspects. *Journal of Sport and Health Science*, *4*(4), 318–324.

Gonzalez-Badillo, J., Rodriguez-Rosell, D., Sanchez-Medina, L., et al. (2016). Short-term recovery following resistance exercise leading or not to failure. *International Journal of Sports Medicine*, *37*(4), 295–304.

Haff, G. (2014). Peaking for competition in individual sports. In D. Joyce & D. Lewindon (Eds.), *High-performance training for sports* (pp. 291–300). Human Kinetics.

Haff, G. (2016). The essentials of periodisation. In I. Jeffreys & J. Moody (Eds.), *Strength and conditioning for sports performance* (pp. 404–448). Routledge.

Haff, G. (2017). Periodisation and power integration. In M. McGuigan (Ed.), *Developing power* (pp. 33–62). Human Kinetics.

Haff, G., & Haff, E. (2012). Training integration and periodisation. In R. Hoffman (Ed.), *NSCA's guide to program design* (pp. 209–254). Human Kinetics.

Harre, D. (1982). *Principles of sports training*. Sportverlag.

Harries, S., Lubans, D., & Callister, R. (2015). Systematic review and meta-analysis of linear and undulating periodised resistance training programs on muscular strength. *Journal of Strength and Conditioning Research*, *29*(4), 1113–1125.

Harris, G., Stone, M., O'Bryant, H., et al. (2000). Short-term performance effects of high-power, high-force, or combined weight-training methods. *Journal of Strength and Conditioning Research*, *14*(1), 14–20.

Issurin, V. (2015). Microcycles, mesocycles and training stages. In *Building the modern athlete: scientific advancements & training innovations* (pp. 270–319). Ultimate Athlete Concepts.

Issurin, V. (2010). New horizons for the methodology and physiology of training periodisation. *Sports Medicine*, *40*(3), 189–206.

Issurin, V. (2016). Benefits and limitations of block periodised training approaches to athlete's preparation: a review. *Sports Medicine*, *46*(3), 329–338.

Kiely, J. (2012). Periodisation paradigms in the 21st century: evidence-led or tradition-driven. *International Journal of Sports Physiology and Performance*, *7*, 242–250.

Kraemer, W., Torine, J., Dudley, J., et al. (2015). Nonlinear periodisation: insights for use in collegiate and professional American football resistance training programs. *Strength and Conditioning Journal, 37*(6), 17–36.

Langan-Evans, C., Morton, J., & Close, G. (2019). Body composition assessment. In P. Comfort, P. A. Jones, & J. J. McMahon (Eds.), *Performance assessment in strength and conditioning* (pp. 240–274). Routledge.

Mann, J., Bryant, K., Johnstone, B., et al. (2016). Effect of physical and academic stress on illness and injury in division I college football players. *Journal of Strength and Conditioning Research, 30*(1), 20–25.

Matveyev, L. (1981). *Fundamentals of sports training.* Progress Publishers.

Mota, J., Nuckols, G., & Smith-Ryan, A. E. (2019). Nutritional periodisation: application for the strength athlete. *Strength and Conditioning Journal, 41*(5), 69–78.

Mujika, I., Halson, S., Bourke, L., et al. (2018). An integrated, multifactorial approach to periodisation for optimal performance in individual and team sports. *International Journal of Sports Physiology and Performance, 13*(5), 538–561.

Norris, S., & Smith, D. (2002). Planning, periodisation, and sequencing of training and competition: the rationale for a completely planned, optimally executed training and competition program, supported by a multidisciplinary team. In M. Kellmann (Ed.), *Enhancing recovery: preventing underperformance in athletes* (pp. 121–141). Human Kinetics.

Painter, K., Haff, G., Ramsey, M., et al. (2012). Strength gains: block vs daily undulating periodisation weight-training among track and field athletes. *International Journal of Sports Physiology and Performance, 7*(2), 161–169.

Plisk, S. (2016). Effective needs analysis and functional training principles. In I. Jeffreys & J. Moody (Eds.), *Strength and conditioning for sports performance* (pp. 181–200). Routledge.

Plisk, S., & Stone, M. (2003). Periodisation strategies. *Strength and Conditioning Journal, 25*(6), 19–37.

Poliquin, C. (1988). Five steps to increasing the effectiveness of your strength training program. *NSCA Journal, 10*(3), 34–39.

Robineau, J., Barbault, N., Piscione, J., et al. (2016). Specific training effects of concurrent aerobic and strength exercises depend on recovery duration. *Journal of Strength and Conditioning Research, 30*(3), 672–683.

Sands, W., & Stone, M. (2005). Are you progressing and how would you know? *Olympic Coach, 17*(4), 4–10.

Stone, M., O'Bryant, H., Garhammer, J., et al. (1982). A theoretical model of strength training. *NSCA Journal, 4*(4), 36–39.

Stone, M., Stone, M., & Sands, W. (2007). *Principles and practice of resistance training.* Human Kinetics.

Stults-Kolehmainen, M., Bartholomew, J., & Sinha, R. (2014). Chronic psychological stress impairs recovery of muscular function and somatic sensations over a 96-hour period. *Journal of Strength and Conditioning Research, 28*(7), 2007–2017.

Thibaudeau, C. (2006). *The black book of training secrets.* F. Lepine Publishing.

Thompson, S., Rogerson, D., Ruddock, A., et al. (2020). The effectiveness of two methods of prescribing load on maximal strength development: a systematic review. *Sports Medicine, 50*(5), 919–938.

Verkhoshansky, Y., & Siff, M. (2009). *Supertraining* (6th ed.). Verkhoshansky SSTM.

Verkhoshansky, Y., & Verkhoshansky, N. (2011). *Special strength training manual for coaches.* Verkhoshansky SSTM.

9   The warm-up

Ian Jeffreys

Walk around any gym, sports field, or park and it is almost inevitable that most exercisers will attempt some form of warm-up before training. It seems that few aspects of training are as universally accepted as the need to warm-up. Given that the warm-up is widely accepted, it might seem intuitive there would be a wealth of published literature on the rationale for a warm-up and how to do it; yet, this is not the case. It seems that most warm-up practice is based on dogma and historical precedence rather than scientific investigation.

For decades, warm-ups have been designed using a two-phased structure, involving a general phase followed by a specific phase. However, more recently, a greater variety of warm-up approaches have been used. Many coaches and trainers recognise that a warm-up is a powerful tool, but designing an optimal warm-up requires blending scientific knowledge with an understanding of the unique needs of the individual.

Do we need to warm-up?

Given that much of the traditional thinking concerning warm-up was based on historical precedence and dogma, the first step in considering how best to warm-up is to answer the question: is a warm-up required? Clearly, there must be benefits from a warm-up before it should be adopted. The overarching reason for a warm-up is that the body in its resting state is not prepared for optimal performance, which most people instinctively appreciate. For example, upon waking in the morning, the body takes time to adjust, and physical tasks cannot be performed at an individual's maximum capability. Consequently, the classic goal of a warm-up is to prepare mentally and physically for exercise or competition by moving the body from a state of rest and under-preparedness to a state more conducive to optimal performance. A warm-up is highly likely to confer potential performance benefits on the individual; indeed, a systematic review reported that 79% of the studies included showed improvements in performance after utilising various warm-up protocols

DOI: 10.4324/9781003204657-9

(Fradkin et al., 2010). Consequently, the process of warming up has a scientific basis.

What are the benefits of a warm-up?

Optimising warm-up protocols requires an understanding of the physiological processes that underpin how the body changes after a warm-up and the advantages this confers to performance. Exercise is a stressor on the body; thus, the body will adapt to cope with the stressors being imposed upon it (see Chapter 6). The precise adaptations required will depend upon the inherent characteristics of the stressor and also on the characteristics of the individual. Consequently, the search for a universally optimal warm-up protocol is imprudent. Instead, the aim should be to design contextually appropriate warm-ups that provide the greatest benefits for the individuals concerned.

At the start of physical activity there is a re-distribution of blood to the working muscles to deliver oxygen and remove metabolic bi-products (McArdle et al., 2015). The activity increases the body's (deep body and muscle) temperature, which increases oxygen delivery/extraction whilst also enhancing metabolic reactions (McArdle et al., 2015). The increase in temperature also enhances neural function and disrupts transient connective tissue bonds (Enoka, 2008). Additionally, each muscle contraction will potentiate each subsequent contraction through a process called the 'treppe effect' – a natural form of post-activation potentiation (Marieb, 2001). For simplicity, the effects of a warm-up on subsequent performance can be categorised as temperature-related effects and non-temperature related effects (Bishop, 2003). The physiological responses that potentially enhance performance include:

- Increased blood flow to the working muscles facilitating energy production (Racinais et al., 2017)
- Improved oxygen delivery to the working muscles, where higher temperatures facilitate oxygen transfer (the Bohr effect) (McArdle et al., 2015)
- An enhancement of key metabolic reactions, such as the enzymatic reactions that occur in the muscle mitochondria (McArdle et al., 2015)
- Lowered viscous resistance in muscles and joints allowing for more fluid movement over a greater range of movement (Enoka, 2008)
- Enhanced muscle contraction and relaxation times (Racinais et al., 2017)
- Improvements in the rate and amplitude of force production (Asmussen et al., 1976; Bergh & Ekblom, 1979).

The physiological effects are not mutually exclusive and act as part of the cascade of actions that occur in response to activity – with the type of activity affecting the relative magnitude of each response. Importantly, all of the above effects can have a positive influence on performance across a range of capacities. Moreover, the warm-up can be structured to focus on specific adaptations that are most relevant to the client's planned training.

Injury prevention

Another often proposed reason for warming up is to reduce injury risk (Jeffreys, 2016). Unfortunately, far less is known about this aspect of potential warm-up benefits. However, the available evidence suggests that a well-designed and executed warm-up can confer injury reduction benefits (Fradkin et al., 2006; Shrier, 1999, 2000). Indeed, the same effects that enhance performance would also logically reduce injury risk; for example, a lowered viscous resistance would allow for a greater range of motion, potentially reducing the risk of injury at the outer ranges of motion (Safran et al., 1988).

There is a sound physiological rationale for warming up. Although physiology is important, planning and executing effective warm-ups requires incorporating other considerations. In this way, the warm-up can achieve much more than the benefits highlighted so far. The following section will focus on how best to design and perform a warm-up.

Time efficiency

A challenge for any trainer is that there is often 'so much to do and so little time to do it'. Time is a valuable resource and optimising the effectiveness of time can provide great benefits (Jeffreys, 2019a, 2019b). If a client, training twice a week, spends ten minutes of each session warming up, that is 20 minutes/week and 80 minutes/month of potentially valuable training time. The warm-up occupies considerable time when aggregated across months and years, and this time should not be wasted. To reap the full benefits of a warm-up, efficiency of application is paramount. When an activity can contribute to more than one session or programme goal, it construes a potential benefit to the client and the practitioner (i.e., more can be achieved within the same time). However, the activity must be useful; choosing an activity that fails to address a session or programme aim is a wasted opportunity (Jeffreys, 2019a, 2019b).

Analysing warm-up activities through the lens of what else can be achieved, over and above the required short-term physiological effects, necessitates thinking differently about a warm-up (Jeffreys, 2019a, 2019b).

Thinking differently: from traditional to transformational thinking

The traditional purpose of a warm-up, to prepare someone for an upcoming activity, will always be a key consideration. However, maximising the full benefits requires a shift in thinking from the traditional approach to transformational thinking (see Figure 9.1) (Jeffreys, 2017).

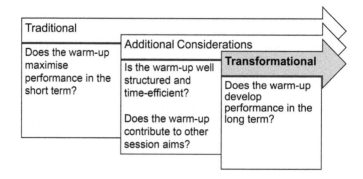

Figure 9.1 Changing the warm-up thought process.

Traditional thinking – does the warm-up maximise performance in the short-term?

Most of the limited warm-up research has investigated the short-term impact of a warm-up intervention on performance, quite often involving a limited number of attempts on one aspect of performance (e.g., jump height or force output) (Jeffreys, 2017). An isolated approach to warm-up research can provide an insight into the types of activities that can be included in the warm-up. Still, the limited perspective of studies should be balanced against broader considerations. The isolated research approach could lead to the erroneous conclusion that there is an optimal warm-up for a given activity. However, this is highly unlikely as many factors influence the direct impact of a warm-up (Jeffreys, 2019a, 2019b).

Any activity will have two potentially confounding effects on performance – this is the fitness/fatigue paradigm (see Chapter 6). The traditional thinking behind the warm-up focused on the fitness effect, where the physiological responses (outlined earlier) confer potentially performance-enhancing effects. However, the physiological responses do not occur in isolation, especially if the warm-up involves an excessive intensity or volume of exercise, as this will also induce some fatigue. The interaction between fitness and fatigue will determine whether the activity enhances or reduces performance. If fitness is greater than fatigue, then performance is enhanced. Conversely, a warm-up that induces more fatigue than fitness will reduce performance. Thus, a warm-up can never be considered in isolation and needs to consider the client's capacities and the nature of the subsequent performance. Isolated studies can be misleading, especially where the research focus is solely on the performance of a single activity post-warm-up. For instance, a warm-up explicitly designed for football players may confer beneficial effects on jump performance but may have induced a degree of fatigue that would preclude this performance from being sustained throughout a match. Consequently, it is essential to analyse the effects of a warm-up in a wider context.

Additional warm-up considerations

Broader considerations (outlined in Figure 9.1) are required if decisions are to be made on a contextual basis that balance the short-term effects with wider considerations that look at the structure, efficiency and holism of the warm-up.

Are the warm-up activities well structured?

Considering how best to layer the various effects of warm-up activities is important when designing a warm-up. Understanding the physiological effects of different activities can help establish effective sequencing and ensure that benefits from one activity can facilitate performance in a subsequent activity. For example, mobility improves by increasing muscle temperature; thus, mobility-based activities are best done after activities that raise body temperature. Similarly, the treppe effect, where muscle contraction force is enhanced by prior muscle activity, can be exploited by gradually increasing the intensity of activities prior to a maximal effort (Marieb, 2001).

Are the activities time-efficient?

Typically, the main focus of a training session will come after the warm-up. Consequently, a warm-up should be structured to achieve the key goals in a time and energy-efficient manner, which requires analysing the efficiency to effectiveness ratio of the activity, and its impact upon the subsequent session. For example, an intervention, such as foam rolling, may elicit a slight performance benefit in a subsequent activity, but the time required to target the various muscle groups effectively could make the overall warm-up time inefficient. Furthermore, other activities that provide more efficient benefits or longer-term advantages might need to be omitted to implement the approach. The consideration of time efficiency can prove a challenge in translating research into effective practice, as the methods used in some studies are not time-efficient and are unlikely to be viable consistently (Jeffreys, 2017).

Do the activities contribute to other session aims?

A warm-up should not focus exclusively on physiological preparation; instead, it should be an integral part of the training session and offer the opportunity to contribute holistically to a client's performance throughout the session. For example, the development of skills, movement patterns

and underpinning capacities that tie in with the main session are beneficial considerations. Rather than being standalone, well-planned warm-ups
can contribute directly to the activities and the goals of the main session
(Jeffreys, 2017, 2019a) and provide a seamless transition between the
warm-up and the main session. However, there are exceptions as occasionally 'separation' of the warm-up goals and main session goals can also be
beneficial (see transformational thinking).

Transformational thinking – developing long-term performance

Careful consideration of the long-term implications of a warm-up beyond
physiological preparation provides new avenues of opportunity. Indeed,
transformational thinking (TT) potentially confers the greatest opportunity to enhance warm-up practice. The concept of TT broadly involves
examining the potential longer-term impact of the activities practiced
in warm-ups beyond the short-term effects. The TT approach provides a
huge range of potential opportunities and adds a different dimension to
the planning process where the warm-up changes from being solely a tool
for short-term preparation into a key tool in overall training effectiveness
(Jeffreys, 2017).

With TT, activities can be chosen as part of the long-term training programme and not simply around the subsequent session's impact. For example, if two activities with similar short-term impacts are considered, the
activity that can provide greater long-term benefits would become the preferred option (even if the short-term effect is not as pronounced). There
are also times when activities with a limited short-term relationship with
the upcoming session need to be included in the warm-up. For example,
the warm-up may be the only opportunity to develop a capacity that may
not be covered in the main session but is essential to the client's general
development. Additionally, activities can be included that contribute to
future training sessions, such as building foundational skills. However, the
concept of separation, mentioned earlier, becomes crucial when adopting
the TT approach.

The RAMP warm-up system

There will never be a singular, universally optimal warm-up. Instead, a
contextual approach is required that considers the clients current capacity,
short- and long-term needs, the upcoming activity, and logistical restric-
tions (e.g., space, equipment, time). Consequently, a flexible structure that
can be adapted to accommodate all of these variables is required – this is
where the RAMP warm-up system is a useful construct (Jeffreys, 2007).

The RAMP system was developed to address the issues associated with
traditional warm-ups and provide a structure around which all of the various thought processes could merge (Jeffreys, 2007). The RAMP system is

built around the physiological processes outlined previously and so maintains the integrity of these processes. However, the RAMP system includes additional and transformational processes, ensuring that all potential considerations are factored into the warm-up design (Jeffreys, 2019a).

The RAMP warm-up is a sequenced structure of three phases that build successively upon the effects of each phase to prepare a client for performance. The diverse training inputs lead to multiple short, medium and long term performance goals (Jeffreys, 2007). Critically, each phase and the activities within them have a clear goal, and several goals can be incorporated into any warm-up. Therefore, the RAMP structure is different to the traditional general and specific warm-up, where the focus is almost totally on physiological preparation. The three phases of the RAMP warm-up are:

1 **R**aise
2 **A**ctivate and **M**obilise
3 **P**otentiate

Raise

The body at rest is not prepared for activity and needs to undergo a period of 'priming' where physiological processes are triggered that prepare the body for subsequent activity – essentially the body needs to start to move. In this unprepared state, activities that are initially low intensity, low complexity and of relatively low amplitude should be selected (Jeffreys, 2019a). As the body starts to move, there is an increase in blood flow and oxygen delivery to the working muscles, increasing muscle and deep body temperature. Additionally, the rise in temperature will decrease the viscosity of the muscles resulting in more efficient movement. Ideally, increases of muscle temperature of approximately 3–4°C are thought to be optimal to elicit these warm-up effects (Faulkner et al., 2013; Mohr et al., 2004); however, this will be dependent on the clients initial starting temperature and the environmental conditions. Increased muscle temperature could also increase power output, where an approximate 4% increase in power output per 1°C has previously been observed (Sargeant, 1987).

Any general activity can elicit an increase in blood flow and temperature. However, the RAMP process involves a deeper consideration regarding the activities applied to produce the physiological effects and how best to structure the activities; this requires consideration of both the upcoming session and the client's long-term training goals. For example, suppose a footballer is going to be training sprinting acceleration in the main session. In that case, the *raise phase* activities can focus on activities that work on the technical aspects of running, such as ankling (See Figure 9.2). For a client who will be performing plyometrics in future training sessions, relevant activities (e.g., low amplitude jumps and landing techniques) could

Exercise	Repetitions
1. Run Forward and backpedal return	4
2. Ankling	4
3. Dribble runs	4
4. 'A' skips	4
5. 'B' skips	3
6. Rhythm low hurdle runs	5 x 20 metres

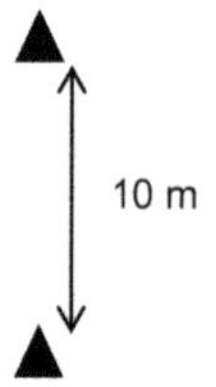

▲
↑
10 m
↓
▲

Instructions: Exercise 2 - 5 = walk back after 10 metres. The goal is developing technique and rhythm, not speed. There is a buildup of intensity during the phase but no run should be performed above 80% of maximal intensity.

Figure 9.2 Raise phase based on developing the running technique for a footballer.

be deployed in the *raise phase* of the current sessions to develop the key skills of plyometrics before they are required. In summary, each activity is planned to elicit the required physiological effect and to achieve a targeted objective. This approach facilitates an extensive increase in the amount of dedicated practise devoted to developing capacities that contribute to the client's wider goals without a net increase in training time (Jeffreys, 2019a).

Most *raise phase* activities are built around either developing specific movement patterns or building specific skills. For example, when working with athletes, the *raise phase* can be achieved by integrating skill-based activities (e.g., ball handling drills for rugby players). In other cases, the raise can be achieved by focusing on movement patterns and the underlying capacities that underpin these. The *raise phase* is progressive in the short and longer-term. In the short-term intensities and amplitudes of movements can be gradually increased to elicit greater physiological effects and enhance the training experience. In the longer term, the movements and skills utilised can be progressed, where the activity builds over time along with the client's capacities. Figure 9.2 shows a *raise phase* warm-up focusing on developing running technique and rhythm for a footballer (or any client wishing to improve running technique).

Activate and mobilise

The physiological effects of the *raise phase*, especially the temperature-related effects, will produce the ideal conditions to enable a client to move fluidly through a greater range of motion. Warm-ups have traditionally included stretching activities; however, what makes the activation and mobilisation phase so different is intention. Once ubiquitous, the role of SS in a warm-up has been questioned and is possibly the biggest area of debate within the topic of warm-ups in recent times. Much of this debate has been due to several research papers and reviews that have questioned the role of SS in a warm-up (Shrier, 2004a; Simic et al., 2013).

A primary reason for SS during warm-up is to reduce muscle stiffness and increase range of motion, thus reducing the potential incidence of activity-related injuries (Hadala & Barrios, 2009). However, no consistent link has been shown between SS during the warm-up and injury prevention (Hart, 2005; Herbert & Gabriel, 2002; Shrier, 1999; Thacker et al., 2004). Consequently, if SS does not reduce the likelihood of injury, then the discussion needs to shift to how SS contributes to performance in the upcoming session and the client's goals.

Research indicates that specific SS protocols can decrease performance indicators, such as speed, power, and jump height (Shrier, 2004a, 2004b). Indeed, when the aim of the main training session is to maximise explosive performance, it has been suggested that SS as the sole activity in a warm-up should be avoided (Simic, 2013). Studies that have investigated the effects of SS on various indices of performance suggest that there may be a negative effect on some explosive performance indices (Hough et al., 2009; Simic et al., 2013) or that performance is unlikely to be affected unless the stretch is held for over 60 seconds (Kay & Blazevich, 2012). As a result, performing SS to enhance acute performance is not generally supported. However, this does not mean SS should always be excluded. A case could be made for SS if the individuals ROM could be a limiting factor or SS has a psychological benefit; for example, if a client feels SS helps him/her perform better.

When analysed from an efficiency perspective, the role of SS in a warm-up is questionable. Given that many stretches focus on a single muscle group, stretching all of the key muscle groups can require several exercises, which, when held for 15–30 seconds, results in a great deal of time expenditure. Additionally, and critically, the goal of stretching in a warm-up is not generally a chronic increase in flexibility – this is likely to be better achieved through a more targeted and specialist approach via dedicated flexibility sessions.

The inclusion of extensive SS in a warm-up could also dissipate some of the temperature-related gains from the *raise phase*, which could have a pronounced effect on performance (Kilduff et al., 2013). As a result, a mobilisation method that can develop effective movements whilst maintaining the temperature benefits of the *raise phase* is preferred; hence, the focus in this stage is on mobility and activation.

The switch of focus from SS to the wider benefits to be gained from the *activate* and *mobilise phase* is characteristic of the RAMP system's TT. As a result, the overarching question now becomes what wider benefits can this phase provide, over and above appropriate short-term preparation? Consequently, the emphasis switches to mobility and movement quality.

Mobility and movement quality

Mobility differs from flexibility in that it involves the ability to move in and out of positions and not merely the ability to attain a position of stretch

(Cook, 2010). As such, mobility incorporates range of motion, stability and movement control. In short, mobility can enhance overall movement quality, which can provide significant benefits to clients (Jeffreys, 2019a). The activation and mobilisation phase aims to develop mobility skills through training the body to appropriately perform the required action under control via developing appropriate movement patterns. Hence, this phase has two components: activation and mobilisation (Jeffreys, 2007). To achieve the activation and mobilisation focus, movements are always deliberate and do not involve overly ballistic actions (Jeffreys, 2007, 2019a).

Given the focus on movement patterns, the key question then becomes what patterns need to be included in this phase? It is here that the Functional Movement Screen (FMS) can be useful (Cook, 2010). The FMS outlines four primary patterns that underpin effective movement: the squat, lunge, a single leg stance, and a brace. Including one exercise from each of these patterns can develop movement skills and mobilise the lower-body joints. The exercises can also be adapted to activate the muscles of the torso, enhance shoulder mobility and activate the posterior chain musculature. The *activate and mobilise phase* ensures that the desired range of motion is achieved for the upcoming session. Furthermore, fundamental movements involved in everyday life and performance are practised and developed in every session.

Developing a progressive sequence of exercises within each basic movement pattern can ensure a progressive development protocol that can provide appropriate stimuli at a range of performance levels. In this way, progression can be provided both within a session and over the longer term. An activation and mobilisation phase for a beginner and advanced client is outlined in Table 9.1. Through choosing a different exercise from the four-movement patterns, a suitable level of progression and challenge can be provided. Additional exercises can be added as required, which can target individual or activity specific movement patterns.

Table 9.1 Activation and mobilisation phase for a novice and intermediate client

	Novice	*Intermediate*
	Introduce and develop basic capacities in each exercise.	*Continue to develop and challenge each pattern with increasing movement complexity.*
Squat pattern	Squat and step	Moving low squat
Lunge patterns	Basic lunge pattern	Lunge with frontal rotation
Single leg stance	Calf walk with shoulder rotation	Hip flexion to single leg RDL
Brace	Bear crawl	Inchworm with whole body rotation and hand to toe touch

All movements patterns are performed for a distance of 10 metres.

The RAMP system activations also have another potential application based around exercises that focus on enhancing a specific function (aka corrective exercises). Some clients may present with functional limitations around areas such as the shoulder, core, hip and foot. In these instances, specific exercises can be integrated into the phase to improve function. Again, these 'corrective' exercises can be progressively sequenced within every warm-up. Bespoke exercises can also be maintained over the longer term, ensuring that movement patterns are reinforced over time. As with the mobilisation exercises, bespoke exercises should be based around active exercises to ensure temperature-related gains from the *raise phase* are maintained.

Potentiation

Even after well planned and executed RAM phases, the body is still not primed for peak performance, especially when maximal efforts are required. Athletes have instinctively known this for years; sprinters will undertake progressive sprints up to maximum speed, and weightlifters will lift progressively heavier weights during a warm-up. The primary aim of the *potentiation phase* is to exploit the treppe effect (outlined earlier) to ensure the progressive sequence of exercises prepares the client to perform optimally in the main session. The progressive exercise sequence of the *potentiation phase* can be designed to provide benefits beyond preparation for a session. For example, components of performance that involve power and speed are often best trained in an unfatigued state. The *potentiation phase* provides an ideal opportunity to train qualities such as speed and agility and also provide an ideal opportunity to teach skilled aspects of performance, such as lifting techniques.

In the short term, the *potentiation phase* must prepare the client for the key aspects of the main session, especially where high-intensity activities are undertaken. Integrated planning is crucial to provide a seamless progression from the warm-up into the main session. This preparation can be considered from a physiological, biomechanical and skill perspective, which all coalesce in determining the optimal sequence of exercises.

The physiological processes should ideally be achieved through specific exercises that replicate the movement patterns, coordination patterns and ranges of motion (i.e., biomechanics) that will be used in the activities after the warm-up. For example, preparation for a plyometric session is best achieved through a progressive sequence of jumping, landing, skipping, hopping and bounding type activities. The skills to be performed in the session should also be considered within the *potentiation phase*. Specifically, exercises that can contribute to the performance of the required skill should be included. For example, programmes that include Olympic lifts would benefit from including movements within the warm-up that develop the key technical aspects of the lifts (e.g., a snatch balance sequence). These movements can be used as warm-up activities over time to develop the client's skill.

For the novice to plyometric exercises, the focus is on technical development using simple exercises that focus on landing and jumping technique. These exercises have little plyometric action, as the focus is simply on technical preparation for more advanced plyometrics to come later in the programme. The intermediate has developed the technical pre-requisites and can utilise more advanced exercises. Here, the focus is on building the stretch-shortening cycle (SSC) capacity and enhancing ground contact efficiency and effectiveness. As a result, more advanced exercises are chosen that contain both a fast and slow SSC element.

Summary

There is a sound physiological rationale behind warming up. The warm-up increases preparedness to perform physical tasks through several temperature and non-temperature related physiological effects. These effects are specific and therefore choosing the warm-up activities that best achieve the required state is a crucial consideration. However, the physiological effects are only part of a bigger picture. Every warm-up can be a part of the training programme itself, achieving both short and longer-term goals. The RAMP structure uses three key phases: (1) Raise, (2) Activate and Mobilise, and (3) Potentiate. The RAMP structure optimises the physiological processes and integrates bespoke exercises into the warm-up, maximising time efficiency and providing both short- and long-term benefits.

References

Asmussen, E., Bonde-Peterson, F., & Jorgenson, K. (1976). Mechano-elastic properties of human muscles at different temperatures. *Acta Physiologica Scandanavia, 96*, 86–93.

Bergh, U., & Ekblom, B. (1979). Influence of muscle temperature on maximal strength and power output in human muscle. *Acta Physiologica Scandanavia, 107*, 332–337.

Bishop, D. (2003). Warm-up. Potential mechanisms and the effects of passive warm-up on performance. *Sports Medicine, 33*(6), 439–454.

Cook, G. (2010). *Movement: functional movement systems: screening assessment and corrective strategies.* On Target Publications.

Enoka, R. (2008). *Neuromechanics of human movement* (4th ed.). Human Kinetics.

Faulkner, S., Ferguson, R., Gerret, N., et al. (2013) Reducing muscle temperature drop after warm up improves sprint cycling performance. *Medicine and Science in Sports and Exercise*, 45 (2), 359–365.

Fradkin, A., Gabbe, B., & Cameron, P. (2006). Does warming up prevent injury in sport? The evidence from randomised controlled trials. *Journal of Science and Medicine in Sport, 9*(3), 214–220.

Fradkin, A., Zazryn, T., & Smoliga, J. (2010). Effects of warming up on physical performance: a systematic review with meta-analysis. *Journal of Strength and Conditioning Research, 24*(1), 140–148.

Hadala, M., & Barrios, C. (2009). Different strategies for sports injury prevention in an America's cup yachting crew. *Medicine and Science in Sports and Exercise, 41*(8), 1587–1596.

Hart, L. (2005). Effect of stretching on sport injury risk: a review. *Clinical Journal Sport Medicine, 15*(2), 371–378.

Herbert, R., & Gabriel, M. (2002). Effects of stretching before and after exercise on muscle soreness and risk of injury: a systematic review. *British Medical Journal, 325*, 468–470.

Hough, P., Ross, E., & Howatson, G. (2009). Effects of dynamic and static stretching on vertical jump performance and electromyographic activity. *Journal of Strength and Conditioning Research, 23*(2), 507–512.

Jeffreys, I. (2007). Warm-up revisited: the ramp method of optimising warm-ups. *Professional Strength and Conditioning, 6*, 12–18.

Jeffreys, I. (2016). Warm up and stretching. In G. Haff and N. Triplett (Ed.), *Essentials of strength training and conditioning* (4th ed., pp. 317–350). Human Kinetics.

Jeffreys, I. (2017). RAMP warm-ups: more than simply short-term preparation. *Professional Strength and Conditioning, 44*, 17–23.

Jeffreys, I. (2019a). *The warm-up – maximise performance and improve long-term athletic development.* Human Kinetics.

Jeffreys, I. (2019b). The warm-up: a behavioral solution to the challenge of initiating a long-term athlete development program. *Strength and Conditioning Journal, 41*(2), 52–56.

Kay, A., & Blazevich, A. (2012). Effect of acute static stretching on maximal muscle performance: a systematic review. *Medicine and Science in Sports and Exercise, 44*, 154–164.

Kilduff, L., Finn, C., Baker, J., et al. (2013). Preconditioning strategies to enhance physical performance on the day of competition. *International Journal of Sports Physiology and Performance, 8*, 677–681

Marieb, E. (2001). *Human anatomy & physiology* (5th ed.). Benjamin Cummings.

McArdle, W., Katch, F., & Katch, V. (2015). *Exercise physiology: energy, nutrition and human performance* (8th ed.). Lippincott Williams & Wilkins.

Mohr, M., Krustrup, P., Nybo, L., et al. (2004). Muscle temperature and sprint performance during soccer matches—beneficial effect of re-warm up at half time. *Scandinavian Journal of Medicine & Science in Sports, 14*(3), 156–162.

Racinais, S., Cocking, S., & Périard, J. (2017). Sports and environmental temperature: From warming-up to heating-up. *Temperature, 4*(3), 227–257.

Safran, M., Garrett, W., Jr, Seaber, A., et al. (1988). The role of warmup in muscular injury prevention. *The American Journal of Sports Medicine, 16*(2), 123–129.

Sargeant, A. (1987). Effect of muscle temperature on leg extension force and short-term power output in humans. *European Journal of Applied Physiology and Occupational Physiology, 56*(6), 693–698.

Shrier, I. (1999). Stretching before exercise does not reduce the risk of local muscle injury: a critical review of the clinical and basic science literature. *Clinical Journal of Sports Medicine, 9*(4), 221–227.

Shrier, I. (2000). Stretching before exercise: an evidence-based approach. *British Journal of Sports Medicine, 34*(5), 324–325.

Shrier, I. (2004a). Meta-analysis on pre-exercise stretching. *Medicine and Science in Sports and Exercise, 36*(10), 1832.

Shrier, I. (2004b). Does stretching improve performance? A systematic and critical review of the literature. *Clinical Journal of Sports Medicine, 14*(5), 267–273.

Simic, L., Sarabon, N., & Markovic, G. (2013). Does pre-exercise static stretching inhibit maximal muscular performance? A meta-analytical review. *Scandinavian Journal of Medicine & Science in Sports, 23*(2), 131–148.

Thacker, S., Gilchrist, J., Stroup, D., et al. (2004). The impact of stretching on sports injury risk: a systematic review of the literature. *Medicine and Science in Sports and Exercise, 36*(3), 371–378.

10 Endurance training

Paul Hough

Cardiorespiratory fitness (CRF) refers to the cardiovascular and respiratory systems' capacity to provide muscles with oxygen during physical activity (PA). CRF is an essential component of physical fitness due to its strong association with health and performance. Numerous studies demonstrate that regular PA decreases all-cause mortality (Arem et al., 2015; Schnohr et al., 2015) and reduces the risk of developing cardiovascular disease (CVD) (Schuler et al., 2013), type 2 diabetes (Chen et al., 2015), and certain cancers (Jee et al., 2018). Regular PA can also improve mental health (Schuch et al., 2018) and reduce the cognitive decline associated with ageing (Raichlen & Alexander, 2017). Conversely, a sedentary lifestyle is associated with increased cardiometabolic disease and shortened lifespan (Katzmarzyk & Lee, 2012).

Exercise that is performed to improve CRF is known as endurance training, cardiovascular training and cardio training. The term endurance training (ET) will be used throughout this chapter. Regular ET induces numerous physiological adaptations that improve CRF (see Figure 10.1). As with all types of training, an appropriate overload must be consistently applied to improve fitness through carefully manipulating training intensity and volume. This chapter will explore ET techniques that can be used to improve CRF and how ET programmes can be designed to improve health and performance outcomes. Additionally, ET will be revisited in Chapter 14 in the context of training to improve body composition.

Endurance training intensity

Before prescribing ET, it is important to understand how the body produces and transfers energy (i.e., bioenergetics). All metabolic processes are fuelled by a molecule called adenosine triphosphate (ATP). However, there are limited stores of ATP within the body, so it must be continually resynthesised via three energy systems:

- Anaerobic: ATP-Phosphocreatine (PCr) system
- Anaerobic: The glycolytic system (anaerobic glycolysis)
- Aerobic: The oxidative system (oxidative phosphorylation)

DOI: 10.4324/9781003204657-10

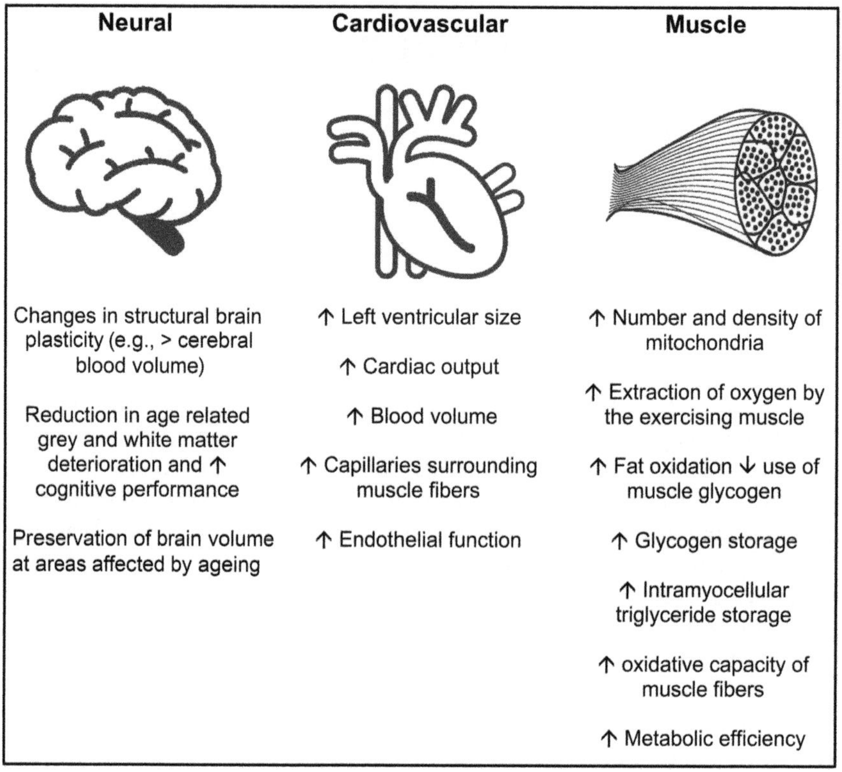

Neural	Cardiovascular	Muscle
Changes in structural brain plasticity (e.g., > cerebral blood volume)	↑ Left ventricular size	↑ Number and density of mitochondria
	↑ Cardiac output	↑ Extraction of oxygen by the exercising muscle
Reduction in age related grey and white matter deterioration and ↑ cognitive performance	↑ Blood volume	↑ Fat oxidation ↓ use of muscle glycogen
	↑ Capillaries surrounding muscle fibers	
Preservation of brain volume at areas affected by ageing	↑ Endothelial function	↑ Glycogen storage
		↑ Intramyocellular triglyceride storage
		↑ oxidative capacity of muscle fibers
		↑ Metabolic efficiency

Figure 10.1 Examples of physiological adaptations to endurance training.

During ET, the energy systems interact to meet the required energy demands of the exercise. The contribution of ATP production from each energy system is dependent on exercise intensity and duration. As intensity increases, the anaerobic systems become more dominant in providing the required ATP (Gastin, 2001). Conversely, as intensity decreases and exercise duration increases, the aerobic (oxidative) system can produce more ATP. For instance, a 100 m sprint predominantly relies on the anaerobic systems, whereas a marathon is almost entirely dependent on the aerobic system.

It is important to exercise at the correct intensity for appropriate durations to stress the aerobic energy system and improve CRF. During high-intensity exercise, the anaerobic contribution to energy production increases and the exercise becomes non-sustainable (i.e., the individual will have to reduce the intensity) due to a combination of fatigue mechanisms. If the exercise intensity is very low, or below the adaptation threshold (see Chapter 6), there will not be a sufficient overload to produce physiological adaptations. Hence, the intensity of ET should be carefully prescribed and monitored (see Chapter 7). Endurance exercise can be categorised into intensity domains to simplify exercise prescription (see Table 10.1).

Intensity domains

Several physiological markers or 'landmarks' have been used to define intensity domains (Burnley & Jones, 2007). The lactate threshold (LT) describes the point where blood lactate begins to increase above resting values. Exercising at an intensity below the LT is defined as moderate-intensity, and exercising above the LT is considered heavy-intensity exercise (see Table 10.1). In the heavy domain, blood lactate concentration and oxygen uptake increase but are generally stable after approximately 10 minutes.

The upper limit of the heavy-intensity domain (see Table 10.1) is considered the maximum sustainable running speed or power output (i.e., intensity) where a metabolic steady-state can be attained. The theoretical threshold between sustainable and non-sustainable exercise is known as the maximal lactate steady state (MLSS) or critical power (CP). The MLSS and CP are measured differently and do not necessarily occur at precisely the same intensity. Nevertheless, exercising above the MLSS or CP corresponds to severe intensity exercise. In the severe domain, there is a gradual increase in oxygen uptake known as the 'VO_2 slow component' (Jones et al., 2011). Exercising in the severe domain is physiologically unsustainable as the VO_2 slow component causes oxygen uptake to increase until VO_{2max} is reached; additionally, central and peripheral fatigue mechanisms reduce the force-generating capacity of the exercising muscles (Black et al., 2017). The intensity domains and corresponding types of ET are outlined in Table 10.1. However, it should be noted that the transition between the domains occurs on a continuum.

Table 10.1 Endurance training intensity domains

Exercise domain	Physiological landmarks	Exercise duration	Training methods
Moderate	LT	4 hours +	MICT
Heavy		~ 3–4 hours	MICT
Severe	MLSS or CP	20–45 minutes	Tempo
		5–10 minutes	Extended intervals
Extreme (maximal)	VO_{2max}	1–5 minutes	HIIT

CP = Critical power; HIIT = High-intensity interval training; LT = Lactate threshold; MICT = Moderate-intensity continuous training; MLSS = Maximal lactate steady state; VO_{2max} = Maximum oxygen uptake.

Is it better to exercise at a high intensity?

High-intensity interval training (HIIT), discussed in Chapter 11, can elicit similar physiological adaptations and improvements in health outcomes as moderate-intensity methods with a lower training time commitment.

However, this does not mean that HIIT is always better than the other types of ET discussed in this chapter. In addition to training time, other factors should be considered when selecting a training method, such as the client's fitness and the desired physiological adaptations. Both training intensity and volume influence cardiorespiratory and skeletal muscle adaptations. Some physiological adaptations are associated with training volume and others with intensity (González-Mohíno et al., 2020; MacInnis & Gibala, 2017). For example, recent research suggests that changes in training volume and intensity can influence the type of mitochondrial adaptations that occur (see Box 10.1).

BOX 10.1

Mitochondrial adaptations to training

David Bishop

Mitochondria are the main site of energy conversion in the cell and are often termed the 'powerhouses' of the cell. Endurance exercise is a potent means to stimulate mitochondrial adaptations (Holloszy, 1967), which can be broadly categorised as an increase in the content (i.e., amount) or function (i.e., the ability to generate energy from oxygen) of the mitochondria in skeletal muscle (Granata et al., 2018a, 2018b). While there is a relationship between greater mitochondrial content and function, there is also evidence that training-induced changes in these two mitochondrial characteristics can be dissociated. Changes in mitochondrial function can occur without changes in mitochondrial content and vice versa (Granata et al., 2016a, 2016b).

There is a debate amongst scientists and coaches about the effects of different training prescriptions on mitochondrial adaptations (Bishop et al., 2019a, 2019b; MacInnis et al., 2019). However, there is general agreement that both high-intensity and high-volume exercise training are effective at increasing mitochondrial content. Nonetheless, the greatest increases in mitochondrial content are typically reported with the largest training volumes (Bishop et al., 2014). In contrast, HIIT appears more effective to increase mitochondrial function (Granata et al., 2018b; MacInnis & Gibala, 2017). Higher-intensity exercise typically results in greater increases in mitochondrial content and function per minute of exercise.

Endurance training methods

Habitual physical activity (taking more steps)

The terms 'physical activity' (PA) and 'exercise' are often used interchangeably, but they are different. PA is 'any bodily movement produced by skeletal muscles that results in energy expenditure' (Caspersen et al., 1985). Therefore, PA encompasses a range of daily tasks such as walking, stair climbing and gardening. Exercise is planned and structured with the objective to maintain or improve a component of fitness (e.g., resistance training). A common reason people cite for not doing regular exercise is 'lack of time' (Justine et al., 2013). However, people with time constraints do not necessarily need to perform conventional methods of ET (discussed below) as as they can achieve health benefits and reduce chronic disease risk by participating in daily PA (Barr-Anderson et al., 2011; Warburton et al., 2006).

Several methods can be used to increase daily PA, such as using stairs instead of escalators, active commuting, and taking walking meetings. For sedentary or moderately active individuals, regular PA can improve CRF and prevent an increase in body fat throughout the lifespan (Celis-Morales et al., 2017). However, daily PA is unlikely to induce significant improvements in CRF amongst active or trained individuals unless specific approaches are used, such as high-intensity exercise 'snacks' (see Chapter 11).

Unlike conventional methods of ET that are simple to measure (e.g., 30 minutes of moderate-intensity running), objectively monitoring PA spread throughout the day used to be difficult. However, the development of wearable activity trackers and mobile apps, enables daily PA levels to be easily monitored, which can improve PA adherence (see Chapter 3). Wearable PA monitors have become more sophisticated and provide a reasonable estimate of daily step counts (Redenius et al., 2019). Therefore, a simple method of increasing PA is to gradually increase the daily step count to achieve a daily or weekly target. Although there are currently no definitive step count targets within most national PA guidelines (see Box 10.3), a reasonable starting point for most clients is achieving over 5000 steps/day as doing less than 5000 steps/day is indicative of sedentary behaviour (Swift et al., 2014).

Moderate-intensity continuous training (MICT)

Moderate-intensity continuous training (MICT) involves performing an exercise continuously for a set time (e.g., 30 minutes) or duration (e.g., 10 km). At the onset of MICT, oxygen consumption increases and begins to plateau after 2–3 minutes. During MICT oxygen consumption is stable, reflecting a balance between the working muscles' energy requirements and the rate at which oxygen is delivered for aerobic ATP production; hence, MICT is also known as 'steady-state' training. Heart rate (HR) and oxygen consumption change at a similar rate during MICT, and HR usually remains relatively stable (within 5 B/min) when a steady-state has been achieved (see Chapter 7).

MICT involves exercising within the moderate-intensity domain (see Table 10.1) and is often used to establish a foundation or 'base' level of CRF. Due to the inverse relationship between volume and intensity, greater volumes of MICT can be performed than high-intensity methods, such as HIIT. There is a dose-response to MICT (discussed later), where performing more MICT (i.e., increasing volume) produces further improvements in physiological adaptations (see Figure 10.1) and CRF. When MICT is programmed relative to the individual's CRF level, it is an effective training method for a range of clients, from novices to elite athletes.

Fartlek training

Fartlek is a Swedish term meaning 'speed play' and involves alternating the intensity throughout the session, combing MICT and interval training techniques (see Figure 10.2). The changes in intensity can be either planned or

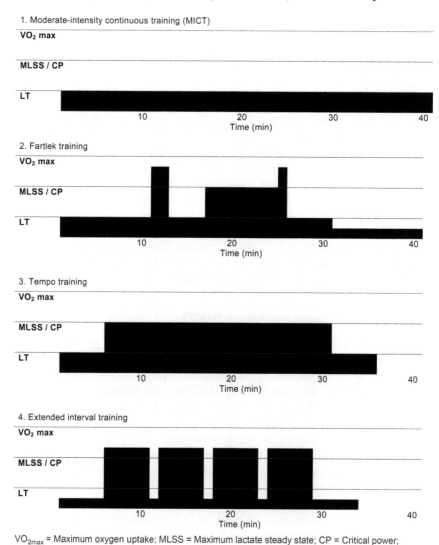

VO_{2max} = Maximum oxygen uptake; MLSS = Maximum lactate steady state; CP = Critical power; LT = Lactate threshold.

Figure 10.2 Endurance training methods.

random. For instance, a runner might plan to run at a moderate intensity for 15 minutes, followed by 15 minutes of hard (severe-intensity) running and 10 minutes at a moderate intensity. Alternatively, random changes in intensity can be applied throughout a Fartlek session using various methods. For example, music can be used to regulate the intensity, where running speed is increased/decreased depending on the track's tempo. However, replicating random Fartlek sessions is problematic as the intensity is not standardised.

Fartlek training can be used to develop the aerobic and anaerobic energy systems, which is advantageous for clients who compete in intermittent, high-intensity sports (e.g., football and rugby). Additionally, some clients may also find the varied nature of Fartlek training more psychologically stimulating and less monotonous than continuous ET.

Tempo/threshold training

Lactate is formed continuously under fully aerobic conditions (see Box 10.2), so an increase in lactate during exercise does not necessarily represent a transition from aerobic to anaerobic metabolism (Brooks, 2020). The previously mentioned MLSS represents the highest exercise intensity where there is a balance between lactate production and lactate removal (i.e., lactate does not significantly increase) (Faude et al., 2009).

BOX 10.2

Lactic acid and fatigue

During fatiguing exercise, excess pyruvate is converted into lactic acid, which dissociates into lactate and hydrogen ions (H^+) causing acidosis (excessive blood acidity) and a disruption of cellular homeostasis (Fitts, 1994). Historically, lactate was thought to play a significant role in the development of muscle fatigue, where an acumination of lactate and acidosis in the muscles was thought to inhibit contractile processes within the muscle. However, there is a longstanding debate if lactate plays a significant role in muscle fatigue or is merely associated with it (Brooks, 2001). Indeed, lactate has beneficial effects. For instance, lactate is used as a fuel source (Brooks, 2020) and may have protective effects during muscle fatigue (Pedersen et al., 2004). Studies where acidosis has been induced have reported limited effects on muscle contractile function, with some scientists suggesting lactate and H^+ production could possibly enhance performance (Cairns, 2006). Furthermore, muscle fatigue is an incredibly complex phenomenon, which originates at numerous sites within the nervous system (Wan et al., 2017) and skeletal muscle (Allen et al., 2008). In summary, the evidence that lactic acid, or more precisely an accumulation of lactate and H^+, is a major cause of skeletal muscle fatigue is inconclusive.

In theory, the MLSS represents an exercise intensity that can be maintained without a significant anaerobic energy contribution (Stegmann & Kindermann, 1982). Tempo training involves exercising at a higher intensity than MICT, near/at the MLSS (see Table 10.1). The objective of tempo training is to improve physiological mechanisms that influence the MLSS, such as increasing the muscles capacity to oxidise lactate and increasing the volume of proteins that transport lactate between cells (Billat et al., 2003; Brooks, 2020; Evertsen et al., 2001).

Unlike MICT, which can be performed for hours, the higher intensity of tempo training (corresponding to the MLSS) can only be maintained for 45–60 minutes (Urhausen et al., 1993). Indeed, exercise performed at an intensity slightly above the MLSS becomes non-sustainable due to the VO_2 slow component (discussed previously) and a combination of fatigue mechanisms (Coates et al., 2003; Fitts, 1994; Wan et al., 2017).

Determining the intensity for tempo training

The gold standard for identifying the MLSS and prescribing the correct tempo intensity is to perform a laboratory exercise test. As laboratory testing is not always feasible, other methods can be used, albeit with less accuracy. The following criteria can be used to estimate an appropriate intensity for tempo training:

• The intensity should feel manageable but challenging. The client should be able to sustain 30 minutes at the selected intensity if they were required
• Talk Test: the client is unable to hold a conversation
• Rating of perceived exertion ~13–16 (Borg RPE Scale)
• Intensity ~80–90% heart rate reserve (see Chapter 7)

Extended interval training

Extended interval training involves exercising within the severe intensity domain (see Table 10.1); it is different from HIIT (see Chapter 11) as the intervals are longer and performed at a lower intensity (see Figure 10.2). Instead of performing a continuous tempo session (discussed previously), short (30–90 seconds) active recovery periods are taken between intervals lasting 5–10 minutes (see Figure 10.2). The short recovery periods ensure that HR and oxygen uptake remains elevated. The duration of recovery periods can be predetermined (e.g., one minute) or gauged using perceived recovery or HR methods. For example, beginning the next interval when the client feels sufficiently recovered or if HR falls below 130 B/min.

Extended interval training offers some advantages over tempo training. For instance, the short breaks allow endurance athletes to train at intensities similar or equal to race pace without accumulating excessive fatigue. The interval format also enables higher training volumes to be completed in the severe-intensity domain, possibly producing superior increases in maximum oxygen uptake than MICT (Bacon et al., 2013; Wen et al., 2019, 2011). Additionally, the short rest periods can make extended intervals more tolerable than tempo sessions from a psychological perspective (Bartlett et al., 2011).

Endurance training to improve health

CRF is an independent predictor of CVD risk, CVD mortality, and all-cause mortality (Ekelund et al., 2019; Lee et al., 2010; Schuler et al., 2013). Although CRF is influenced by genetics, age, sex, and health status, the main modifiable determinant of CRF is an individual's habitual level of PA. Worldwide, physical inactivity has been estimated to cause 6–10% of major non-communicable diseases and up to 9% of premature deaths (Lee et al., 2012), which demonstrates the importance of regular PA.

Numerous studies indicate that regular PA significantly improves CRF and markers of CVD risk. For instance, a 2015 meta-analysis, that included 160 randomised clinical trials, showed that regular ET significantly improved CRF and some cardiometabolic biomarkers (Lin et al., 2015). Alongside improving CRF, reducing CVD risk factors and increasing lifespan, regular endurance exercise can be an effective 'medicine' for treating 26 diseases (Pedersen & Saltin, 2015). Simply put, individuals who perform regular PA have higher levels of CRF and a lower risk of premature mortality than less active individuals (Ekelund et al., 2019; Farrell et al., 2020).

In addition to improving cardiorespiratory, metabolic and musculoskeletal health outcomes, regular PA is important for the prevention and management of mental health conditions, such as depression and anxiety. To illustrate, a meta-analysis of prospective cohort studies demonstrated that achieving 150 minutes/week of moderate-vigorous physical activity was protective against developing depression (Schuch et al., 2018).

Minimising sedentary behaviour

Most of the research cited so far has focused on how regular PA (or exercise) improves CRF and reduces all-cause mortality. However, research also suggests that the accumulation of sedentary time is associated with several major chronic disease outcomes, independent of PA levels (Ekelund et al., 2019; Patterson et al., 2018). Put differently, excessive sedentary (sitting) behaviours are associated with negative health outcomes even amongst people achieving the PA guidelines (see Box 10.3). There appears to be an increased risk of CVD mortality amongst individuals who spend more than six hours/day sitting (Patterson et al., 2018). Therefore, even clients who achieve or exceed the PA guidelines should be encouraged to break-up periods of sedentary time. The findings of a meta-analysis demonstrated that the risk of death was greater amongst people who had the lowest level of PA and highest sedentary time than the group who had the highest level of PA and lowest sedentary time (Ekelund et al., 2019). The data also indicated that approximately 30–40 minutes of daily moderate-to-vigorous PA reduced the risk of death from excessive sedentary time (Ekelund et al., 2019).

The following section will provide PA and ET guidelines for improving health, lowering susceptibility to disease (morbidity), and promoting longevity.

BOX 10.3

Physical activity guidelines for adults (19–64 years)

Physical activity guidelines were updated in the USA and UK in 2018 and 2019, respectively. The fundamental PA guidelines regarding duration and intensity of PA for adults are essentially the same between countries. The UK physical activity guidelines are:

- Accumulate at least 150 minutes (2.5 hours) of moderate intensity activity (e.g., brisk walking or cycling) or 75 minutes of vigorous intensity activity (e.g., running); or even shorter durations of very vigorous intensity activity (e.g., HIIT); or a combination of moderate, vigorous and very vigorous intensity activity.
- Minimise the amount of time spent being sedentary and break up long periods of inactivity with light PA, when possible.
- Perform muscle strengthening activities at least two days a week (see Chapter 13).

The latest PA guidelines are broadly similar to the previous guidelines but there is a notable exception regarding PA duration. Previous guidelines recommended that PA could be achieved in a single session (e.g., 5 × 30 minutes) or accumulated in bouts of ≥10 minutes during a day. However, the requirement for a 10-minute bout of activity is no longer included in the UK or US guidelines, as it was concluded that there is no minimum duration of PA required to achieve some health benefits (US Department of Health and Human Services, 2018; UK Chief Medical Officers' [UKCMO] Physical Activity Guidelines, 2019). The PA guidelines emphasise that more PA provides greater health benefits and even small increases in PA can contribute to improved health and quality of life.

What volume of training is necessary to improve cardiorespiratory fitness?

The term 'dose-response' is used within medicine to describe the relationship between the quantity and effect a drug has; it is studied to formulate an appropriate threshold and optimal dosage of a drug. The dose-response concept has been applied within PA research to address the questions: 'what is the minimal amount of PA that achieves health benefits?' and 'is there an optimal dose (volume) of PA for improving health and avoiding disease?'

The findings from randomised controlled trials and epidemiological studies demonstrate there is a dose-response relationship between the volume of PA and mortality risk, and health benefits (see Figure 10.3). Increasing the volume of PA improves health/fitness and decreases all-cause mortality risk (Church et al., 2007; Lee, 2007). The health benefits associated with regular PA increase as the volume of PA increases, whereby more PA is better, up to a point (see Box 10.4). Arem et al. (2015) complied data from six studies involving 661,137 men and women (age 21–98 years) to quantify the dose-response relationship between leisure time physical activity (LTPA) and mortality. The authors concluded that achieving the PA guidelines (see Box 10.1) was associated with nearly the maximum longevity benefit and doing significantly more (750 minutes/week) PA appeared to offer no greater health benefits (Arem et al., 2015).

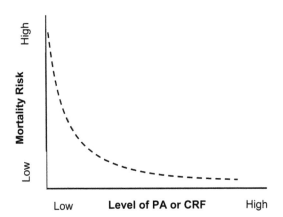

Figure 10.3 The dose-response relationship between physical activity level or cardiorespiratory fitness and mortality.

BOX 10.4

Is too much physical activity bad for you?

The previously mentioned (Arem et al., 2015) study that investigated the link between PA and mortality also investigated if there is an upper limit of PA, whereby too much PA could be detrimental to health. The researchers concluded that high levels of PA are not harmful to health, even when ten times the recommended (150 minutes/week) is performed. Conversely, other studies amongst athletes have suggested that substantial volumes of exercise, performed over several years, may have negative effects on the structure and function of the heart (Andersen et al., 2013; Eijsvogels et al., 2016; Wilson et al., 2011) and could lead to orthopaedic issues, such as osteoarthritis (Michaëlsson et al., 2011).

The discrepancy between studies investigating the effect of PA volume and health outcomes is related to the different types of study design. The meta-analysis of Arem et al. (2015) combined PA data from the general population; whereas studies suggesting that substantial volumes of PA are detrimental to health have focused on specific cardiovascular and orthopaedic health outcomes amongst athletes. In some cases, exceptionally high volumes of ET performed by endurance athletes may have long-term negative health outcomes (Eijsvogels et al., 2016). However, as discussed in Chapter 2, the findings of studies are usually limited to the populations who were studied (e.g., similar age, performing the same activity at comparable volumes). The substantial volume of ET required to induce negative effects will be beyond what most clients are willing or capable of doing. Thus, clients who exceed the PA guidelines should not be discouraged.

Is there a minimum effective does of physical activity?

Research indicates the health benefits of PA are more significant for sedentary or less active (<30 minutes PA/week) individuals. Furthermore, doing less than the recommended 150 minutes/week of PA can still lead to improvements in cardiometabolic and mental health outcomes (Church et al., 2007; Mammen & Faulkner, 2013; Wen et al., 2011) and reduce mortality (Hupin et al., 2015). For instance, a study involving over 55,000 adults (age 18–100 years) found that running for 5–10 minutes/day (<51 minutes/week) was associated with markedly reduced risks of death from all causes and CVD (Lee et al., 2014).

Step counts

The development of wearable devices, such as Smart Watches, enables people to quantify their daily PA by measuring step counts. Steps can be accumulated throughout the day during personal and occupational chores, shopping,

CASE STUDY 10.1

Achieving physical activity guidelines

Teresa (age 45) is currently sedentary and has been advised by her doctor that following the PA guidelines will improve her general health. However, during the initial consultation with her trainer, Teresa demonstrated signs of low self-efficacy and ambivalence (see Chapter 3) as she believed 150 minutes PA per week was unfeasible, and she could not attend the gym more than twice per week. Teresa was also sceptical that a small amount of PA would have any effect on her health.

According to the PA guidelines, Teresa should aim to accumulate 150 minutes of moderate PA throughout the week. However, in this scenario, it is important for the trainer to adopt a collaborative approach and respect Teresa's autonomy (see Chapter 3). Based on Teresa's beliefs, it would have been unwise and potentially counterproductive to devise a rigid exercise programme for her. Instead, during the client consultation, her trainer highlighted that the PA guidelines are not absolute thresholds (i.e., health benefits can be achieved by doing less than 150 minutes/week PA) and that PA can be incorporated into daily tasks, outside of the gym. After developing her understanding of the difference between PA and exercise, and recognising that any PA is better than none, Teresa decided to walk for 20 minutes on at least five days per week.

transportation, etc. Unlike metrics, such as MET/minutes, step counts are simple to understand, can be modified to suit individual needs, and are useful for monitoring progress (Kraus et al., 2019). Therefore, step counts have become a practical method for exercise professionals to prescribe and monitor their client's PA outside of the gym (Brickwood et al., 2019).

How many daily steps are recommended to improve health outcomes?

There is no current consensus regarding the optimal number of daily steps required to achieve health benefits for the general population (Hall et al., 2020). A target of 10,000 steps/day is commonly recommended (Le Masurier et al., 2003); this target was thought to originate from a 1960s Japanese pedometer named 'Manpo-kei, which translates to '10,000 steps meter' (Hatano, 1993). Given that 10,000 steps/day is a widely known and often recommended target, there is surprisingly little scientific basis for it. Indeed, recent evidence indicates that health benefits can be achieved by taking less than 10,000 steps/day (Hall et al., 2020).

Based on the dose-response relationship, it is likely that a higher daily step count produces better health outcomes than a lower daily step count; this notion was supported by a large cohort study of elderly women, where the participants who averaged approximately 4400 steps/day had significantly lower mortality rates (4.3 years after the study) than the participants with a lower (2700) step count (Lee et al., 2019). Furthermore, a recent systematic review of 17 studies, involving over 30,000 adults, indicated that walking an extra 1000 steps/day can lower the risk of CVD and all-cause mortality (Hall et al., 2020). Increasing step count by approximately 2000 steps/day also appears to lower the risk of developing Type 2 Diabetes (Kraus et al., 2018), although further research is required in this area.

Achieving a daily step count between 7000 and 9000 steps may result in health benefits that are similar to achieving the PA guidelines outlined in Box 10.3 (Kraus et al., 2019); hence, a step count of 7000 steps/day has been recommended for healthy adults (Garber et al., 2011). However, as with all exercise recommendations, step targets should be individualised based on the client's health/fitness status and goals. As discussed in Chapter 3, trainers should avoid setting arbitrary goals, as failure to attain these can promote negative feelings (Goodyear et al., 2019). A target of 7000–10,000 steps/day could improve health outcomes amongst sedentary or moderately active clients; conversely, it might be inappropriate or impossible for clients with clinical conditions and/or disabilities.

What intensity of training is necessary to improve cardiorespiratory fitness?

PA guidelines are usually based on two intensity descriptors: moderate and vigorous (ACSM, 2017; Garber et al., 2011). The scientific definition of moderate and vigorous intensity PA requires a basic understanding of metabolic equivalents (METs), introduced in Chapter 7. Moderate intensity PA corresponds to 3–5.9 METs and vigorous PA is ≥6 METs (Garber et al., 2011). Recent PA guidelines have recognised that using METs to define PA intensity lacks practicality. Therefore, moderate and vigorous activities are differentiated by the Talk Test (see Chapter 7), where "being able to talk but not sing indicates moderate-intensity activity, while having difficulty talking without pausing is a sign of vigorous activity" (UKCMO, 2019). The moderate and vigorous descriptors can also be expressed relative to age-adjusted HR training zones (see Chapter 7). However, caution should be applied when using standardised training zones, as percentages of HR (maximum and reserve) vary in relation to individual metabolic thresholds (Meyer et al., 1999). Therefore, HR should be used in conjunction with the Talk Test and RPE (see Chapter 7).

In general, performing vigorous or very vigorous exercise appears to convey greater health benefits compared to light-moderate intensity exercise (Lee & Paffenbarger, 2000; Swain & Franklin, 2006). However, vigorous intensity exercise does not always produce superior outcomes than moderate -intensity exercise. For example, Fisher et al. (2015) reported that MICT led to a greater improvement in CRF compared to vigorous

BOX 10.5

How quickly does cardiorespiratory fitness improve?

Most studies assess CRF by measuring maximum oxygen uptake ($VO_{2\,max}$). There is considerable variation in the rate at which $VO_{2\,max}$ improves following ET as factors such as genetics, age, body mass and starting level of CRF influence how an individual will respond to an ET programme. Individuals with low levels of CRF tend to experience the greatest improvements in VO_{2max}; this was demonstrated in a classic study by Hickson et al. (1977), where eight participants performed an intensive ET programme consisting of a combination of high-intensity cycling and running, 6 days/week for 10 weeks. The participants were a mix of sedentary ($n = 2$), athletic ($n = 2$) and recreationally active ($n = 4$) adults (age 20–42). The findings showed that VO_{2max} increased on a weekly basis (average 0.12 L/min) and the participants VO_{2max} improved by 44% on average. As expected, the two sedentary participants, with the lowest fitness to begin, experienced the largest improvements (52% and 53%) in VO_{2max}. The Hickson study demonstrates that CRF can improve on a weekly basis with regular, intensive training. However, the volume and intensity of training applied in this study is unrealistic and hazardous for individuals with a limited training background.

exercise, although the weekly duration of the MICT was five times longer (five vs. one hour) (Fisher et al., 2015). As discussed in Chapter 11, HIIT is a more time-efficient approach for improving CRF than MICT. However, time-efficiency is not the only consideration when designing a training programme (see Chapters 3 and 11).

An optimum ET intensity to reduce mortality risk or improve CRF has not been defined, as the intensity required to stimulate adaptations is dependent on the client's level of CRF and circumstances. Initially, sedentary clients with low levels of CRF may benefit from light-intensity ET(~30–39% heart rate reserve), whereas recreationally active clients would benefit from moderate or vigorous-intensity ET. In accordance with the principle of progressive overload (see Chapter 6), as a client's CRF improves, higher intensity training techniques are usually required to elicit further improvements. For example, trained clients can benefit from utilising tempo, extended interval training, and HIIT (Swain & Franklin, 2002).

What endurance training methods are appropriate for improving health outcomes?

In general, the MICT approach is recommended for clients with health-related goals as this method is simple to prescribe and monitor, and has been shown to improve CRF across a range of populations (Church et al., 2007; Hupin et al., 2015; Lee et al., 2014). However, as the client's fitness improves, other methods such as Fartlek, extended interval training, and HIIT can be incorporated to provide a sufficient overload, introduce variation, and prevent monotony.

Progressing endurance training

The rate of progression of any training programme should be based on the client's response to the previous training stimulus, programme goals and circumstances. The ET programme can be progressed by increasing one of the acute programme variables (e.g., volume, intensity) and following a systematic, long-term approach (see Chapter 8). For health-related ET programmes, the training volume can be gradually increased to ensure the client is consistently achieving or exceeding 150 minutes/week. Volume can be increased by doing more daily PA, increasing training duration, increasing frequency (sessions/week), or a combination of these.

Although there is no universal recommendation, a 10% increase in ET volume applied every 2–3 weeks is sensible and realistic for most clients. Where clients are unable or reluctant to increase training volume, training intensity can gradually be increased using an appropriate intensity monitoring method (see Chapter 7). Finally, when progressing an ET programme, it is prudent to increase one variable (volume or intensity) at a time to avoid an inappropriate overload, which could cause injury or reduce adherence.

Endurance training to improve health summary

- CRF is an independent predictor of CVD risk and all-cause mortality. Regular PA or structured exercise (i.e., ET) improves CRF.
- There is a dose-response to PA, where more PA leads to greater improvements in health outcomes, up to a point (around 750 minutes/week).
- Regardless of fitness goals, long periods of sedentary behaviour should be minimised, where possible.
- Clients with low CRF can achieve health benefits from increasing daily PA. A simple method for some clients to increase PA is working towards a daily step target.
- To improve health outcomes most adults should follow the PA guidelines outlined in Box 10.3.
- There is not an optimum intensity of ET for health benefits. Sedentary clients with low levels of CRF may benefit from exercising at a light-intensity. A progressive increase in relative intensity is required as fitness improves.
- Several ET methods can be programmed based on the client's goals, preferences and circumstances. The MICT approach is simple to prescribe and monitor, and is effective in enhancing CRF across a range of populations.

- The ET programme can be progressed by increasing volume, intensity and frequency. It is prudent to increase one variable at a time to avoid an inappropriate overload.
- Relative training intensity should be carefully increased as a client's fitness improves. A gradual (~10%) increase in ET volume applied every 2–3 weeks is sensible and realistic for most clients.

Endurance training for performance

Athletes competing in endurance (e.g., cycling and running) and intermittent (e.g., football and tennis) sports require a high level of CRF. Typically, clients wishing to improve CRF for a sport or event will have some ET background. However, if this is not the case, they can benefit from performing MICT and Fartlek methods before transitioning to performance focused ET. There is no specific reference point when a client should transition from a general ET programme to a performance orientated programme. However, a six-week period of MICT, Fartlek and extended interval training will prepare the client for more performance focused ET. Assuming the client has achieved an appropriate base level of CRF, the focus of the training programme should gradually transition to improve sport-specific fitness. Firstly, a needs analysis of the client's sport should be conducted (see Box 10.6).

Needs analysis

A needs analysis involves a systematic approach in identifying the physiological requirements of the sport to design an appropriate ET programme. The programme must include the appropriate types of training that will enhance performance. Some sports require a combination of physiological qualities (e.g., aerobic, anaerobic, neuromuscular). Therefore, an understanding of the bioenergetic demands of the client's sport should be established before designing a training programme (see Box 10.3). The complexity of the needs analysis is largely dictated by the sport. For example, the needs analysis for team sport athletes is usually more complex than endurance sports as, alongside the general physiological demands of the sport, the athlete's position and team tactics must be considered.

The demands of the sport will often guide the prescription of specific types of ET. For example, MICT is appropriate in sports involving long durations of steady-state activity (e.g., distance running) whereas athletes competing in sports involving intermittent, high-intensity efforts (e.g., rugby) benefit from Fartlek and HIIT methods. As with all training prescription, there is no universally recommended programme. Most athletes will benefit from a combination of ET and HIIT (see Chapter 11) approaches to optimise sport-specific fitness.

BOX 10.6

Example needs analysis

The following example outlines a basic needs analysis for a client who is training for a marathon.

Step 1. What does the sport involve?
  The marathon is a long-distance running event. The objective is to complete 26.2 miles in the quickest possible time. Oxidative phosphorylation is the primary metabolic pathway that is utilised (Coyle, 1995). Therefore, marathon performance is dependent on physiological variables related to the aerobic energy system.

Step 2. What are the physiological demands of the sport?
  The key physiological parameters related to marathon performance include VO_{2max}, running economy (RE), fractional utilisation (FE), and the LT (Coyle, 1995; Jones & Carter, 2000). Research indicates that VO_{2max}, RE and the LT explain >70% of the between-subject variance in long-distance running performance (di Prampero et al., 1986). Consequently, a marathon focused training programme should be designed to improve these physiological parameters (Jones & Carter, 2000; Pate & Branch, 1992). Furthermore, RE is proportional to body mass, meaning the athlete must achieve and maintain a relatively low body mass (Bergh et al., 1991).

Step 3. Fitness assessment
  The client's current level of fitness should be assessed using appropriate assessments (see Chapter 5). For a runner, fitness could be gauged through a recent personal best time alongside specific assessments to establish his/her strengths and weaknesses.

Step 4. Programme design
  Following steps 1–3, the trainer can design an individualised training programme using the approaches outlined in Chapters 7 and 8.

Endurance training distribution: how much training should be hard versus easy?
Alex Hutchinson and Paul Hough

Training intensity and volume cannot be increased simultaneously as increasing intensity means less total training volume can be accumulated without injury or exhaustion. Similarly, high training volumes necessitate reducing intensity.

Intensity

A gradual increase in training intensity is required to stimulate physiological adaptations related to endurance performance (Londeree, 1997).

Therefore, methods of increasing exercise intensity, such as tempo training and HIIT are often incorporated within athletic training programmes. However, increases in intensity should be systematically planned, considering the demands of the athlete's sport, lifestyle and the competition period (see Chapter 8). For example, when designing an ET programme for a team sport athlete, any increase in training intensity should be considered alongside the demands of other physical and technical training; the purpose of this is to ensure other sessions are not adversely affected and the risk of injury due to fatigue is minimised.

Endurance training zones

As many as seven ET zones can be delineated based on metabolic factors such as VO_{2max}, blood lactate, and HR. In practice, three zones, based on physiological landmarks (see Table 10.1), are usually sufficient: zone 1 (Z1) is below the first lactate or ventilatory threshold; zone 3 (Z3) is above MLSS and zone 2 (Z2) is between the two thresholds (Kenneally et al., 2020).

While some athletes may undergo regular physiological testing to identify the HRs corresponding to the zones above, a simpler, practical approach for training prescription uses the Talk Test (see Chapter 7). For example, if a client can talk comfortably in complete sentences, she is probably in Z1; if she can talk in short phrases, she is in Z2 (approximately 14–16 on a 6–20 RPE scale). Finally, if a client is only able to speak one or two words, this is indicative she is in Z3 (see Figure 10.4).

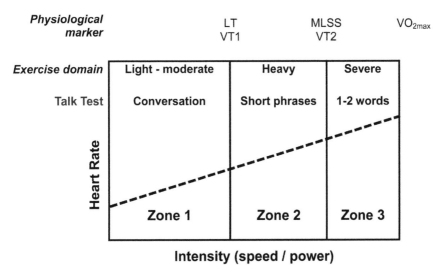

LT = Lactate threshold; VT1 = Ventilatory threshold 1; MLSS = Maximum lactate steady state; VT2 = Ventilatory threshold 2; VO_{2max} = Maximum oxygen uptake.

Figure 10.4 The three-zone training model.

Volume

As with ET for health, there appears to be a dose-response where higher training volumes lead to greater improvements in fitness, up to a point (Costill, 1986). Indeed, a progressive increase in training volume is strongly associated with improved performance in endurance sports (Costill, 1986; Tjelta, 2016). The client's trainability (see Chapter 6) dictates that the rate of improvement in fitness declines as the athlete engages in more training (i.e., a novice athlete will experience a faster relative improvement in CRF than an experienced athlete). Furthermore, as training volume and intensity are increased, appropriate recovery periods are required to facilitate adaptation (see Chapters 6 and 18).

There is scarce literature regarding the optimal training volume or intensity for improving CRF amongst trained individuals, although the training volumes of high-level endurance athletes have been documented by coaches and sport scientists. For example, the typical training volume of high-level marathon runners is around 170–200 km/week (Costill, 1986; Tjelta, 2016). However, it is misguided to simply replicate the training volume of high-level athletes, as the physiological adaptations to ET are based on an interaction between training volume, frequency, intensity, and the athlete's ability to recover from training. Excessive training volumes and/or insufficient recovery can hinder performance (Halson & Jeukendrup, 2004; McKenzie, 1999). Conversely, an insufficient training stimulus and/or too much recovery can lead to lack of progress or detraining (see Chapter 6). Therefore, as a client's fitness improves, the organisation of ET becomes more important to elicit further improvements in fitness.

Training distribution

An intricate and individualised training programme, which achieves the correct balance between overload and recovery, is required for trained athletes to make further improvements in fitness and performance; hence, training programme design is sometimes referred to as an art rather than an exact science. The training distribution indicates what proportion of the overall training is done in different intensity zones. Optimising training distribution is an attempt to plan how much training is done at different intensities to maximise the overall training stimulus.

Elite athlete training patterns

A common training distribution observed among elite endurance athletes is polarised training, which refers to a plan that includes roughly 80% in Z1, little or no time in Z2, and 20% in Z3 (see Figure 10.3) (Stöggl, T., & Sperlich, 2015; Treff et al., 2019). This pattern has been documented in successful athletes across a variety of endurance sports (Seiler & Kjerland, 2006). In addition, in randomised trials that have assigned athletes to train using various training distributions, polarised training has generally resulted in the greatest improvements in performance and fitness (Hydren & Cohen, 2015).

Another common training distribution is the threshold model, which involves a heavy emphasis on Z2 training. Although it is nearly the opposite of polarised training, world-class athletes, such as former marathon world-record holders Paula Radcliffe and Steve Jones, have employed threshold training—a reminder of the difficulty of formulating one-size-fits-all training rules. This also appears to be the model that many people adopt intuitively if they are not following a specific training plan, with more than half their training in Z2 or Z3 (Gilman & Wells, 1993).

Finally, the pyramidal model includes 70–80% in Z1, 10–20% in Z2, and 5–10% in Z3 (Treff et al., 2019). Recent studies have found that the same training plan can be classified as polarised or pyramid depending on whether the distribution is calculated based on training speeds or physiological parameters (e.g., HR), which do not respond instantly to changes in pace (Kenneally et al., 2020). As a result, polarised and pyramid training are often grouped together as consisting of roughly 80% in Z1 and 20% in Z2 and Z3, with the majority of Z1 training considered to be the most important characteristic for improving endurance performance (Esteve-Lanao et al., 2005; Warden & Fitzgerald, 2018).

Recreational athlete and fitness patterns

Polarised and pyramid training appear to be an effective way of balancing volume and intensity in athletes who train between 10–15 hours/week. However, it is less clear that the same logic applies for lower training loads, where theoretically a higher proportion of high-intensity training could be tolerated. Nonetheless, studies demonstrate greater performance gains with polarised training compared to threshold training in sub-elite endurance runners (Esteve-Lanao et al., 2005; Neale et al., 2014), recreational cyclists training six hours a week (Neal et al., 2013) and recreational runners training four hours a week (Muñoz et al., 2014). However, the training loads applied within studies are likely to be higher and/or more intense than many fitness-oriented clients would pursue, compared to amateur endurance athletes. Fitness and health markers can be improved with other training distributions such as HIIT (a mix of Z1 and Z3 with a low total volume) or high-volume training entirely in Z1 (Hydren & Cohen, 2015). Therefore, the distribution of training does not seem to be as important for clients with general health and fitness goals as it is for athletes. The training distribution for clients focused on health/fitness should be based on factors such as recovery from previous exercise, time efficiency, motivation, and enjoyment.

Endurance training to improve performance summary

- The first step in designing a performance focussed ET programmes is to conduct a needs analysis.
- A needs analysis involves developing a deep knowledge and understanding of the physiological demands of the client's sport to programme appropriate ET methods.
- A gradual increase in volume and relative training intensity is required to stimulate physiological adaptations associated with the client's sport. Increases in volume and intensity should be systematically planned, considering the demands of the athlete's sport, lifestyle and the competition period.
- The physiological adaptations to ET are based on an interaction between training volume, frequency and intensity, as well as the athlete's ability to recover from training. As a client's fitness improves, ongoing, subtle changes to the ET programme are required to provide a sufficient training stress whilst managing fatigue.
- Several ET zones have been developed to facilitate programme design. The three-zone model, based on physiological landmarks, is often used to organise an ET programme.
- The training distribution of endurance athletes is variable but it is common for elite athletes to adopt a polarised training model, where around 80% of training is done at a moderate intensity (zone 1) and 20% at a high-intensity (zone three), which is above the MLSS.
- The distribution of training does not seem to be as important for clients with health and fitness goals (i.e., non-athletes). These client's training should be programmed based on factors such as time efficiency, motivation, and recovery from previous exercise.

References

ACSM. (2017). *ACSM's guidelines for exercise testing and prescription* (10th ed.). Wolters Kluwer.

Allen, D., Lamb, G., & Westerblad, H. (2008). Skeletal muscle fatigue: cellular mechanisms. *Physiological Reviews, 88*(1), 287–332.

Andersen, K., Farahmand, B., Ahlbom, A., et al. (2013). Risk of arrhythmias in 52 755 long-distance cross-country skiers: a cohort study. *European Heart Journal, 34*(47), 3624–3631.

Arem, H., Moore, S., Patel, A., et al. (2015). Leisure time physical activity and mortality: a detailed pooled analysis of the dose-response relationship. *JAMA Internal Medicine, 175*(6), 959–967.

Bacon, A., Carter, R., & Ogle, E. (2013). VO_{2max} trainability and high intensity interval training in humans: a meta-analysis. *PLOS ONE, 8*(9), e73182.

Barr-Anderson, D., AuYoung, M., Whitt-Glover, M., et al. (2011). Integration of short bouts of physical activity into organisational routine a systematic review of the literature. *American Journal of Preventive Medicine, 40*(1), 76–93.

Bartlett, J., Close, G., MacLaren, D., et al. (2011). High-intensity interval running is perceived to be more enjoyable than moderate-intensity continuous exercise: implications for exercise adherence. *Journal of Sports Sciences, 29*(6), 547–553.

Bergh, U., Sjödin, B., Forsberg, A., et al. (1991). The relationship between body mass and oxygen uptake during running in humans. *Medicine and Science in Sports and Exercise, 23*(2), 205–211.

Billat, V., Sirvent, P., Py, G., et al. (2003). The concept of maximal lactate steady state: a bridge between biochemistry, physiology and sport science. *Sports Medicine, 33*(6), 407–426.

Bishop, D., Botella, J., Genders, A., et al. (2019a). High-intensity exercise and mitochondrial biogenesis: current controversies and future research directions. *Physiology, 34*(1), 56–70.

Bishop, D., Botella, J., & Granata, C. (2019b). CrossTalk opposing view: exercise training volume is more important than training intensity to promote increases in mitochondrial content. *The Journal of Physiology, 597*(16), 4115–4118.

Bishop, D., Granata, C., & Eynon, N. (2014). Can we optimise the exercise training prescription to maximise improvements in mitochondria function and content? *Biochimica Et Biophysica Acta, 1840*(4), 1266–1275.

Black, M., Jones, A., Blackwell, J., Bailey, S., et al. (2017). Muscle metabolic and neuromuscular determinants of fatigue during cycling in different exercise intensity domains. *Journal of Applied Physiology, 122*(3), 446–459.

Brickwood, K., Watson, G., O'Brien, J., et al. (2019). Consumer-based wearable activity trackers increase physical activity participation: systematic review and meta-analysis. *JMIR mHealth and uHealth, 7*(4), e11819.

Brooks, G. (2001). Lactate doesn't necessarily cause fatigue: why are we surprised? *The Journal of Physiology, 536*(1), 1.

Brooks, G. (2020). Lactate as a fulcrum of metabolism. *Redox Biology, 35*, 101454.

Burnley, M., & Jones, A. (2007). Oxygen uptake kinetics as a determinant of sports performance. *European Journal of Sport Science, 7*(2), 63–79.

Cairns, S. (2006). Lactic acid and exercise performance: culprit or friend? *Sports Medicine, 36*(4), 279–291.

Caspersen, C. J., Powell, K. E., & Christenson, G. M. (1985). Physical activity, exercise, and physical fitness: definitions and distinctions for health-related research. *Public Health Reports, 100*(2), 126–131.

Celis-Morales, C., Lyall, D., Welsh, P., et al. (2017). Association between active commuting and incident cardiovascular disease, cancer, and mortality: prospective cohort study. *BMJ, 357*.

Chen, L., Pei, J.-H., Kuang, J., et al. (2015). Effect of lifestyle intervention in patients with type 2 diabetes: a meta-analysis. *Metabolism: Clinical and Experimental, 64*(2), 338–347.

Chief Medical Officers for England, Northern Ireland, Scotland and Wales (2019). *UK Chief Medical Officers' Physical Activity Guidelines.*

Church, T., Earnest, C., Skinner, J., et al. (2007). Effects of different doses of physical activity on cardiorespiratory fitness among sedentary, overweight or obese postmenopausal women with elevated blood pressure. *JAMA, 297*(19), 2081.

Coats, E., Rossiter, H., Day, J., et al. (2003). Intensity-dependent tolerance to exercise after attaining VO₂ max in humans. *Journal of Applied Physiology, 95*(2), 483–490.

Costill, D. (1986). *Inside running: basics of sports physiology.* Benchmark Press.

166   *Paul Hough*

Coyle, E. (1995). Integration of the physiological factors determining endurance performance ability. *Exercise and Sport Sciences Reviews, 23*(1), 25–64.

di Prampero, P., Atchou, G., Brückner, J., et al. (1986). The energetics of endurance running. *European Journal of Applied Physiology and Occupational Physiology, 55*(3), 259–266.

Eijsvogels, T., Fernandez, A., & Thompson, P. (2016). Are there deleterious cardiac effects of acute and chronic endurance exercise? *Physiological Reviews, 96*(1), 99–125.

Ekelund, U., Tarp, J., Steene-Johannessen, J., et al. (2019). Dose-response associations between accelerometry measured physical activity and sedentary time and all-cause mortality: systematic review and harmonised meta-analysis. *BMJ, 366*.

Esteve-Lanao, J., Juan, A., Earnest, C., et al. (2005). How do endurance runners actually train? Relationship with competition performance. *Medicine and Science in Sports and Exercise, 37*(3), 496–504.

Evertsen, F., Medbø, J., & Bonen, A. (2001). Effect of training intensity on muscle lactate transporters and lactate threshold of cross-country skiers. *Acta Physiologica Scandinavica, 173*(2), 195–205.

Farrell, S., DeFina, L., Radford, N., et al. (2020). Relevance of fitness to mortality risk in men receiving contemporary medical care. *Journal of the American College of Cardiology, 75*(13), 1538–1547.

Faude, O., Kindermann, W., & Meyer, T. (2009). Lactate threshold concepts: how valid are they? *Sports Medicine, 39*(6), 469–490.

Fisher, G., Brown, A., Bohan Brown, M., et al. (2015). High intensity interval- vs moderate intensity- training for improving cardiometabolic health in overweight or obese males. *PLOS One, 10*(10), e0138853.

Fitts, R. (1994). Cellular mechanisms of muscle fatigue. *Physiological Reviews, 74*(1), 49–94.

Garber, C., Blissmer, B., Deschenes, M., American College of Sports Medicine, et al. (2011). American College of Sports Medicine Position Stand. Quantity and quality of exercise for developing and maintaining cardiorespiratory, musculoskeletal, and neuromotor fitness in apparently healthy adults: guidance for prescribing exercise. *Medicine and Science in Sports and Exercise, 43*(7), 1334–1359.

Gastin, P. (2001). Energy system interaction and relative contribution during maximal exercise. *Sports Medicine, 31*(10), 725–741.

Gilman, M., & Wells, C. (1993). The use of heart rates to monitor exercise intensity in relation to metabolic variables. *International Journal of Sports Medicine, 14*(6), 339–344.

González-Mohíno, F., Santos-Concejero, J., Yustres, I., et al. (2020). The effects of interval and continuous training on the oxygen cost of running in recreational runners: a systematic review and meta-analysis. *Sports Medicine, 50*(2), 283–294.

Goodyear, V., Kerner, C., & Quennerstedt, M. (2019). Young people's uses of wearable healthy lifestyle technologies; surveillance, self-surveillance and resistance. *Sport, Education and Society, 24*(3), 212–225.

Granata, C., Jamnick, N., & Bishop, D. (2018a). Principles of exercise prescription, and how they influence exercise-induced changes of transcription factors and other regulators of mitochondrial biogenesis. *Sports Medicine, 48*(7), 1541–1559.

Granata, C., Jamnick, N., & Bishop, D. (2018b). Training-induced changes in mitochondrial content and respiratory function in human skeletal muscle. *Sports Medicine, 48*(8), 1809–1828.

Granata, C., Oliveira, R., Little, J., et al. (2016a). Training intensity modulates changes in PGC-1α and p53 protein content and mitochondrial respiration, but not markers of mitochondrial content in human skeletal muscle. *FASEB Journal, 30*(2), 959–970.

Granata, C., Oliveira, R., Little, J., et al. (2016b). Mitochondrial adaptations to high-volume exercise training are rapidly reversed after a reduction in training volume in human skeletal muscle. *FASEB Journal, 30*(10), 3413–3423.

Hall, K., Hyde, E., Bassett, D., et al. (2020). Systematic review of the prospective association of daily step counts with risk of mortality, cardiovascular disease, and dysglycemia. *International Journal of Behavioral Nutrition and Physical Activity, 17*(1), 78.

Halson, S., & Jeukendrup, A. (2004). Does overtraining exist? An analysis of over-reaching and overtraining research. *Sports Medicine, 34*(14), 967–981.

Hatano, Y. (1993). Use of the pedometer for promoting daily walking exercise. *Journal of the International Committee on Health, Physical Education and Recreation, 29*, 4–8.

Hickson, R., Bomze, H., & Holloszy, J. (1977). Linear increase in aerobic power induced by a strenuous program of endurance exercise. *Journal of Applied Physiology, 42*(3), 372–376.

Holloszy, J. (1967). Biochemical adaptations in muscle. Effects of exercise on mito-chondrial oxygen uptake and respiratory enzyme activity in skeletal muscle. *The Journal of Biological Chemistry, 242*(9), 2278–2282.

Hupin, D., Roche, F., Gremeaux, V., et al. (2015). Even a low-dose of moderate-to-vig-orous physical activity reduces mortality by 22% in adults aged ≥60 years: a system-atic review and meta-analysis. *British Journal of Sports Medicine, 49*(19), 1262–1267.

Hydren, J., & Cohen, B. (2015). Current scientific evidence for a polarised cardio-vascular endurance training model. *Journal of Strength and Conditioning Research, 29*(12), 3523–3530.

Jee, Y., Kim, Y., Jee, S., et al. (2018). Exercise and cancer mortality in Korean men and women: a prospective cohort study. *BMC Public Health, 18*(1), 761.

Jetté, M., Sidney, K., & Blümchen, G. (1990). Metabolic equivalents (METS) in exer-cise testing, exercise prescription, and evaluation of functional capacity. *Clinical Cardiology, 13*(8), 555–565.

Jones, A., & Carter, H. (2000). The effect of endurance training on parameters of aerobic fitness. *Sports Medicine, 29*(6), 373–386.

Jones, A., Grassi, B., Christensen, P., et al. (2011). Slow component of VO_2 kinetics: mechanistic bases and practical applications. *Medicine and Science in Sports and Exercise, 43*(11), 2046–2062.

Justine, M., Azizan, A., Hassan, V., et al. (2013). Barriers to participation in physical activity and exercise among middle-aged and elderly individuals. *Singapore Medical Journal, 54*(10), 581–586.

Katzmarzyk, P., & Lee, I. (2012). Sedentary behaviour and life expectancy in the USA: a cause-deleted life table analysis. *BMJ Open, 2*(4), e000828.

Kenneally, M., Casado, A., Gomez-Ezeiza, J., et al. (2020). Training intensity distri-bution analysis by race pace vs. physiological approach in world-class middle- and long-distance runners. *European Journal of Sport Science, 0*(0), 1–8.

Kraus, W., Janz, K., Powell, K., et al. (2019). Physical activity guidelines advisory com-mittee. Daily step counts for measuring physical activity exposure and its relation to health. *Medicine and Science in Sports and Exercise, 51*(6), 1206–1212.

Kraus, W., Yates, T., Tuomilehto, J., et al. (2018). Relationship between baseline physical activity assessed by pedometer count and new-onset diabetes in the NAVIGATOR trial. *BMJ Open Diabetes Research and Care, 6*(1), e000523.

Le Masurier, G., Sidman, C., & Corbin, C. (2003). Accumulating 10,000 steps: does this meet current physical activity guidelines? *Research Quarterly for Exercise and Sport, 74*(4), 389–394.

Lee, D., Artero, E., Sui, X., et al. (2010). Mortality trends in the general population: the importance of cardiorespiratory fitness. *Journal of Psychopharmacology, 24*(4), 27–35.

Lee, D., Pate, R., Lavie, C., et al. (2014). Leisure-time running reduces all-cause and cardiovascular mortality risk. *Journal of the American College of Cardiology, 64*(5), 472–481.

Lee, I., & Paffenbarger, R. (2000). Associations of light, moderate, and vigorous intensity physical activity with longevity. The Harvard Alumni Health Study. *American Journal of Epidemiology, 151*(3), 293–299.

Lee, I.-M. (2007). Dose-response relation between physical activity and fitness: even a little is good: more is better. *JAMA, 297*(19), 2137–2139.

Lee, I.-M., Shiroma, E., Kamada, M., et al. (2019). Association of step volume and intensity with all-cause mortality in older women. *JAMA Internal Medicine, 179*(8), 1105–1112

Lee, I.-M., Shiroma, E., Lobelo, F., Puska, P., et al. (2012). Impact of physical inactivity on the world's major non-communicable diseases. *Lancet, 380*(9838), 219–229.

Lin, X., Zhang, X., Guo, J., et al. (2015). Effects of exercise training on cardiorespiratory fitness and biomarkers of cardiometabolic health: a systematic review and meta-analysis of randomised controlled trials. *Journal of the American Heart Association, 4*(7).

Londeree B. (1997). Effect of training on lactate/ventilatory thresholds: a meta-analysis. *Medicine and Science in Sports and Exercise, 29*(6), 837–843.

MacInnis, M., & Gibala, M. (2017). Physiological adaptations to interval training and the role of exercise intensity. *The Journal of Physiology, 595*(9), 2915–2930.

MacInnis, M., Skelly, L., & Gibala, M. (2019). CrossTalk proposal: exercise training intensity is more important than volume to promote increases in human skeletal muscle mitochondrial content. *The Journal of Physiology, 597*(16), 4111–4113.

Mammen, G., & Faulkner, G. (2013). Physical activity and the prevention of depression: a systematic review of prospective studies. *American Journal of Preventive Medicine, 45*(5), 649–657.

McKenzie, D. (1999). Markers of excessive exercise. *Canadian Journal of Applied Physiology, 24*(1), 66–73.

Meyer, T., Gabriel, H., & Kindermann, W. (1999). Is determination of exercise intensities as percentages of VO_{2max} or HR_{max} adequate? *Medicine and Science in Sports and Exercise, 31*(9), 1342–1345.

Michaëlsson, K., Byberg, L., Ahlbom, A., et al. (2011). Risk of severe knee and hip osteoarthritis in relation to level of physical exercise: a prospective cohort study of long-distance skiers in Sweden. *PLOS One, 6*(3), e18339.

Muñoz, I., Seiler, S., Bautista, J., et al. (2014). Does polarized training improve performance in recreational runners? *International Journal of Sports Physiology and Performance, 9*(2), 265–272.

Neal, I., Seiler, S., Bautista, J., et al. (2014). Does polarised training improve performance in recreational runners? *International Journal of Sports Physiology and Performance, 9*(2), 265–272.

Neal, C., Hunter, A., Brennan, L., et al. (2013). Six weeks of a polarised training-intensity distribution leads to greater physiological and performance adaptations than a threshold model in trained cyclists. *Journal of Applied Physiology, 114*(4), 461–471.

Pate, R., & Branch, J. (1992). Training for endurance sport. *Medicine and Science in Sports and Exercise, 24*(9), S340–343.

Patterson, R., McNamara, E., Tainio, M., et al. (2018). Sedentary behaviour and risk of all-cause, cardiovascular and cancer mortality, and incident type 2 diabetes: a systematic review and dose response meta-analysis. *European Journal of Epidemiology, 33*(9), 811–829.

Pedersen, B., & Saltin, B. (2015). Exercise as medicine—evidence for prescribing exercise as therapy in 26 different chronic diseases. *Scandinavian Journal of Medicine & Science in Sports, 25*(3), 1–72.

Pedersen, T., Nielsen, O., Lamb, G., et al. (2004). Intracellular acidosis enhances the excitability of working muscle. *Science, 305*(5687), 1144–1147.

Raichlen, D., & Alexander, G. (2017). Adaptive capacity: an evolutionary neuroscience model linking exercise, cognition, and brain health. *Trends in Neurosciences, 40*(7), 408–421.

Redenius, N., Kim, Y., & Byun, W. (2019). Concurrent validity of the Fitbit for assessing sedentary behavior and moderate-to-vigorous physical activity. *BMC Medical Research Methodology, 19*(1), 29.

Schnohr, P., O'Keefe, J., Marott, J., et al. (2015). Dose of jogging and long-term mortality: the Copenhagen City heart study. *Journal of the American College of Cardiology, 65*(5), 411–419.

Schuch, F., Vancampfort, D., Firth, J., et al. (2018). Physical activity and incident depression: a meta-analysis of prospective cohort studies. *The American Journal of Psychiatry, 175*(7), 631–648.

Schuler, G., Adams, V., & Goto, Y. (2013). Role of exercise in the prevention of cardiovascular disease: results, mechanisms, and new perspectives. *European Heart Journal, 34*(24), 1790–1799.

Seiler, K., & Kjerland, G. (2006). Quantifying training intensity distribution in elite endurance athletes: Is there evidence for an 'optimal' distribution? *Scandinavian Journal of Medicine & Science in Sports, 16*(1), 49–56.

Stegmann, H., & Kindermann, W. (1982). Comparison of prolonged exercise tests at the individual anaerobic threshold and the fixed anaerobic threshold of 4 mmol.l(−1) lactate. *International Journal of Sports Medicine, 3*(2), 105–110.

Stöggl, T., & Sperlich, B. (2015). The training intensity distribution among well-trained and elite endurance athletes. *Frontiers in Physiology, 6*, 295.

Swain, D., & Franklin, B. (2002). VO_2 reserve and the minimal intensity for improving cardiorespiratory fitness. *Medicine and Science in Sports and Exercise, 34*(1), 152–157.

Swain, D., & Franklin, B. (2006). Comparison of cardioprotective benefits of vigorous versus moderate intensity aerobic exercise. *The American Journal of Cardiology, 97*(1), 141–147.

Swift, D., Johannsen, N., Lavie, C., et al. (2014). The role of exercise and physical activity in weight loss and maintenance. *Progress in Cardiovascular Diseases, 56*(4), 441–447.

Tjelta, L. (2016). The training of international level distance runners. *International Journal of Sports Science & Coaching, 11*(1), 122–134.

Treff, G., Winkert, K., Sareban, M., et al. (2019). The polarisation-index: a simple calculation to distinguish polarised from non-polarised training intensity distributions. *Frontiers in Physiology, 10.*

Urhausen, A., Coen, B., Weiler, B., et al. (1993). Individual anaerobic threshold and maximum lactate steady state. *International Journal of Sports Medicine, 14*(3), 134–139.

US Department of Health and Human Services. (2018). *Physical activity guidelines for Americans* (2nd ed.).

Wan, J., Qin, Z., Wang, P., et al. (2017). Muscle fatigue: general understanding and treatment. *Experimental & Molecular Medicine, 49*(10), e384–e384.

Warburton, D., Nicol, C., & Bredin, S. (2006). Health benefits of physical activity: the evidence. *Canadian Medical Association Journal, 174*(6), 801–809.

Warden, D., & Fitzgerald, M. (2018). *80/20 Triathlon.* Da Capo Lifelong Books.

Wen, C. P., Wai, J., Tsai, M., et al. (2011). Minimum amount of physical activity for reduced mortality and extended life expectancy: a prospective cohort study. *Lancet, 378*(9798), 1244–1253.

Wen, D., Utesch, T., Wu, J., et al. (2019). Effects of different protocols of high intensity interval training for VO2max improvements in adults: A meta-analysis of randomised controlled trials. *Journal of Science and Medicine in Sport, 22*(8), 941–947.

Wilson, M., O'Hanlon, R., Prasad, S., et al. (2011). Diverse patterns of myocardial fibrosis in lifelong, veteran endurance athletes. *Journal of Applied Physiology, 110*(6), 1622–1626.

11 High-intensity interval training

Paul Hough

High-intensity interval training (HIIT) involves brief, intermittent bouts of high-intensity exercise interspersed by periods of rest or low-intensity exercise. Athletes competing in endurance and team sports have traditionally used HIIT to enhance athletic performance (Bilat, 2001). Over the past 20 years, numerous studies amongst non-athletic populations show that bouts of high-intensity exercise can provide a greater physiological stimulus and adaptations than moderate-intensity continuous training (MICT). HIIT induces physiological adaptations, such as the growth and division of mitochondria (mitochondrial biogenesis), increased stroke volume, and improved vascular function (Batacan et al., 2017; Milanović et al., 2015; Torma et al., 2019). The physiological adaptations associated with HIIT enhance several outcomes, including cardiorespiratory fitness (CRF), exercise performance, skeletal muscle oxidative capacity, and insulin sensitivity.

What is 'high-intensity' exercise?

High-intensity exercise could be interpreted as training 'all-out' with maximal (100%) effort; however, not all HIIT involves working at this intensity. Therefore, it is important to classify what constitutes high-intensity exercise. In this chapter, high-intensity refers to exercise performed at an intensity above the maximal lactate steady-state (MLSS) or critical speed/power (see Chapter 10); this exercise intensity is non-sustainable (i.e., it can only be done for short periods). In practice, high-intensity exercise is associated with a higher rating of perceived exertion (RPE), fatigue and acute discomfort compared to moderate-intensity exercise. The term 'maximal' is used to define exercise that elicits the maximum oxygen uptake (VO_{2max}). Supramaximal refers to an exercise intensity performed above VO_{2max} (see Figure 11.1), including all-out efforts (e.g., sprinting).

DOI: 10.4324/9781003204657-11

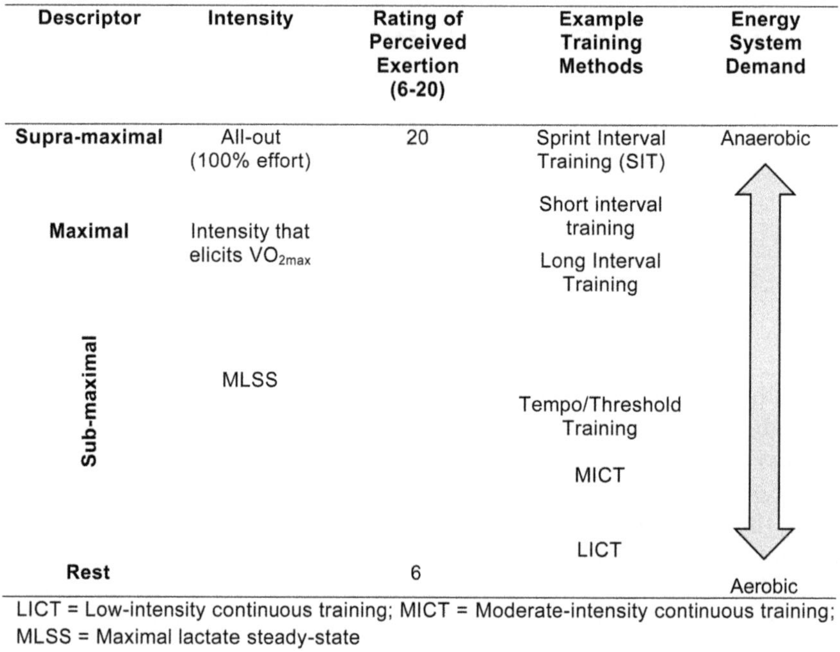

Descriptor	Intensity	Rating of Perceived Exertion (6-20)	Example Training Methods	Energy System Demand
Supra-maximal	All-out (100% effort)	20	Sprint Interval Training (SIT)	Anaerobic
Maximal	Intensity that elicits VO_{2max}		Short interval training / Long Interval Training	
Sub-maximal	MLSS		Tempo/Threshold Training / MICT	
Rest		6	LICT	Aerobic

LICT = Low-intensity continuous training; MICT = Moderate-intensity continuous training; MLSS = Maximal lactate steady-state

Figure 11.1 Training intensity classifications.

HIIT types

The contribution of energy production via the energy systems and the strain on the neuromuscular and musculoskeletal systems varies depending on the HIIT protocol (Laursen & Buchheit, 2019). For example, manipulating the intensity, duration, and the number of work intervals can profoundly change the physiological stimulus. Most HIIT protocols will stress several physiological systems (see Figure 11.2), which means HIIT sessions are more challenging to design than MICT or tempo training (see Chapter 10). Six HIIT types have been classified based on the energy system demand, neuromuscular load, and musculoskeletal strain. The classification of HIIT types enables trainers to design protocols that precisely target specific physiological systems. The six types of HIIT are:

Type 1: aerobic metabolic, with high demands placed on the oxygen (O_2) transport and utilisation systems (cardiorespiratory system and oxidative muscle fibres).
Type 2: metabolic as type 1 but with a greater degree of neuromuscular strain.
Type 3: metabolic as type 1 with a large anaerobic glycolytic energy contribution but limited neuromuscular strain.
Type 4: metabolic as type 3 but a high neuromuscular strain;

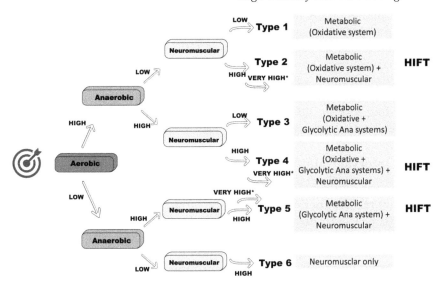

Figure 11.2 Types of HIIT (Leduc et al., 2020).

Type 5: limited aerobic response but with a large anaerobic glycolytic energy contribution and high neuromuscular strain.

Type 6: a very high neuromuscular strain (e.g., speed and power training).

HIIT formats

Before designing a HIIT session, it is important to identify the physiological adaptations required (see Figure 11.2), as this will determine the format of HIIT and the acute variables (e.g., interval intensity/duration and recovery type/duration) that are most appropriate. Twelve variables can be manipulated to target specific HIIT types (Laursen & Buchheit, 2019): (1, 2) work bout intensity and duration, (3, 4) recovery period intensity and duration, (5) number of intervals, (6) number of interval bout series, and (7, 8) the between-series recovery duration and intensity. The eight variables account for the ninth variable: (9) total work performed. Other factors also play a role in the physiological outcome of a HIIT session. These are: (10) the environment (heat and altitude), and (11) the client's nutrition practices. The final (but not least important) variable that can be manipulated is the exercise mode (i.e., type).

Five formats of HIIT have been used by coaches and studied within the literature to target the physiological responses identified in Figure 11.2. The five formats of HIIT are (1) short intervals; (2) long intervals; (3) repeated sprint training; (4) sprint interval training (SIT); (5) game based HIIT (Laursen & Buchheit, 2019). A recent (6th) HIIT format named 'high-intensity functional training' (HIFT) will be discussed later (see Figure 11.2).

Combinations of the six formats of HIIT can be implemented with advanced trainees and athletes. However, some HIIT formats (e.g., repeated sprint and game-based) are not usually applicable for clients training to improve non-specific fitness. Therefore, for simplicity, the proceeding section will focus on (1) SIT, (2) long interval training, and (3) short interval training.

Sprint interval training (SIT)

SIT involves supramaximal (all-out) work periods lasting 10–30 seconds with long recovery periods ≥5 times the duration of the work bout (Sloth et al., 2013). The relatively long rest-periods are required, as a short recovery time following a supramaximal effort may not allow sufficient recovery of the anaerobic energy systems. Therefore, the ability to produce ATP (see Chapter 10) rapidly will decline, causing a reduction in exercise intensity (Bogdanis et al., 1996). Early SIT studies involved 3–4 × 30-second bouts of cycling on a cycle ergometer (i.e., multiple Wingate tests). Due to the short periods of high-intensity exercise, SIT is also referred to within the scientific literature as 'low volume HIIT'.

Long and short interval training

The distinguishing factor between SIT and short and long interval training is the exercise intensity. SIT protocols involve supramaximal (all-out) work periods, which place a high demand on the anaerobic energy pathways. Short and long interval training has been termed aerobic interval training (Conraads et al., 2015; Hough, 2017) as the longer duration (and lower intensity) of long intervals place a greater demand on the aerobic energy system (Withers et al., 1991). In short interval training, the brief rest/recovery periods do not allow for sufficient recovery of the anaerobic systems. Consequently, the aerobic contribution to the energy supply increases with repeated intervals (Parolin et al., 1999).

Long interval training

Long interval training broadly involves extended work periods of 2–4 minutes performed at an intensity equivalent to 80–95% VO_{2max} interspersed with 2–4 minutes of active recovery. Long interval training usually involves a total of 4–6 intervals (Kessler et al., 2012).

Short interval training

Short interval training involves work periods of 15–60 seconds performed at 90–170% VO_{2max}. There are two important distinctions between short interval training and SIT. Firstly, the work periods in short interval train-ing are not performed at a supramaximal intensity (as they are in SIT). Secondly, the rest/recovery periods are equal to or slightly less than the work period. Therefore, cardiorespiratory responses (e.g., heart rate (HR) and oxygen uptake) remain elevated, and the aerobic contribution to ATP resynthesis is higher in short interval training than SIT. Passive recovery (no exercise) periods are usually required to allow the required intensity to be maintained. An example of a short interval training pro-tocol was implemented in a classic study by Tabata et al. (1996). The par-ticipants performed 7–8, 20-second intervals interspersed with 10-second recovery periods; this seminal study lead to the popular 'Tabata training' protocol.

Monitoring intensity

Prescribing and regulating the intensity of sprint intervals is simple as each interval is performed 'all-out' without pacing (see Figure 11.1). Long and short intervals are performed at an intensity of around ≥80–95% VO_{2max} and 90–170% VO_{2max}, respectively. Thus, laboratory-studies have prescribed HIIT relative to participants VO_{2max}. However, measuring oxy-gen uptake is not practical in gym settings. Therefore, other intensity pre-scription methods have been used, such as the speed or power associated with $\dot{V}O_{2max}$ (v/p$\dot{V}O_{2max}$ or maximal aerobic speed [MAS]) and anaerobic speed reserve (Laursen & Buchiet, 2019). These methods require testing or specialist equipment. Most trainers use RPE and HR to guide HIIT sessions (see Chapter 7). However, both RPE and HR methods are associ-ated with limitations during HIIT, which will briefly be discussed.

At the beginning of high-intensity exercise, HR does not correspond with the individuals speed or power output, as there is a lag in the HR response. Although a target HR (e.g., 90% HR_{max}) can be achieved during long intervals, the brief duration of both sprint and short intervals is usu-ally insufficient to achieve a target HR. Therefore, RPE and, ideally, speed or power measures should be used in conjunction with HR. For example, short intervals on a rowing ergometer could be prescribed based on a per-centage of the client's average power achieved during a 500-meter all-out effort (sprint) and an RPE of 15–18.

Using RPE to prescribe the intensity of HIIT is practical as it can be used during different modes of exercise, does not require equipment, and allows the client to self-regulate the intensity based on physiological and psychological inputs. Some studies have reported RPE is a viable method to regulate HIIT (Ciolac et al., 2015; Viana et al., 2019), whereas others have not (Jabbour & Majed, 2018). This discrepancy is not surprising as numerous factors (e.g., age, interval number/duration, and fitness level) influence RPE. Therefore, RPE should be used in conjunction with speed/power and HR (Aamot et al., 2014).

HIIT summary

- High-intensity exercise corresponds to an intensity above the MLSS or critical speed/power; this intensity is non-sustainable.
- HIIT involves brief, intermittent bouts of high-intensity exercise interspersed with periods of rest or low-intensity exercise.
- HIIT can produce significant improvements in CRF, vascular function, and muscle metabolism with a lower time commitment than MICT.
- HIIT has been classified into six types based on the energy system demand, neuromuscular load, and musculoskeletal strain. Type 1 places high demands on the aerobic oxidative system. Type 6 imposes a very high neuromuscular strain and minimal aerobic involvement.
- Six HIIT formats can be used to target the desired physiological responses and adaptations. These are (1) Sprint; (2) Long; and (3) short intervals; (4) repeated sprints; (5) game-based HIIT; and (6) High-intensity functional training.
- Several HIIT variables can be manipulated. The key variables are interval intensity and duration, rest interval intensity and duration, exercise modality, and the number of repetitions.
- Practical methods to prescribe and monitor the intensity of HIIT are HR, rating of perceived exertion and speed/power.

HIIT for health

Low levels of CRF are associated with a higher incidence of cardiovascular disease, type 2 diabetes, and some cancers. Improvements in CRF amongst sedentary individuals can reduce all-cause mortality risk by up to 40% (Blair et al., 1995). Numerous studies demonstrate that regular HIIT improves CRF, blood glucose homeostasis, and cardiovascular function amongst healthy adults (Milanović et al., 2015; Ramos et al., 2015; Weston et al., 2014). Furthermore, HIIT can improve health outcomes in populations with type 2 diabetes, coronary artery disease, heart failure, metabolic syndrome and obesity (Gibala et al., 2012).

The health and fitness benefits of HIIT can be achieved with less training time than MICT. For example, 15 minutes of high-intensity exercise spread across six HIIT sessions can enhance skeletal muscle oxidative capacity and endurance performance (Gibala & McGee, 2008). Therefore, HIIT is considered a more time-efficient training method than MICT (Gibala et al., 2012; Milanović et al., 2015), which is attractive from an exercise promotion perspective as 'lack of time' is a commonly cited barrier to engaging in regular exercise (Pagnan et al., 2017).

Despite numerous studies demonstrating that HIIT improves various health outcomes with less time commitment to MICT, it was not previously recommended within physical activity guidelines (Department of Health [DH], 2011). However, the scientific evidence that HIIT can be as (or more) effective than MICT for improving health outcomes was acknowledged in the latest United Kingdom physical activity guidelines. Consequently, HIIT is now considered a viable exercise option for the general population (UK Chief Medical Officers' [UKCMO] Physical Activity Guidelines, 2019).

Physiological adaptations

The improvements in VO_{2max} following HIIT can be attributed to both central and peripheral adaptations, such as an increase in stroke volume (Trilk et al., 2011) and up-regulation of mitochondrial enzymes, which could improve muscle oxidative capacity (Burgomaster et al., 2008; Gibala & McGee, 2008). HIIT can also improve metabolic health outcomes, such as glycemic control and insulin sensitivity (Jelleyman et al., 2015; Little et al., 2011). The physiological adaptations that occur following HIIT are influenced by the HIIT protocol used (see Figure 11.3). For example, the

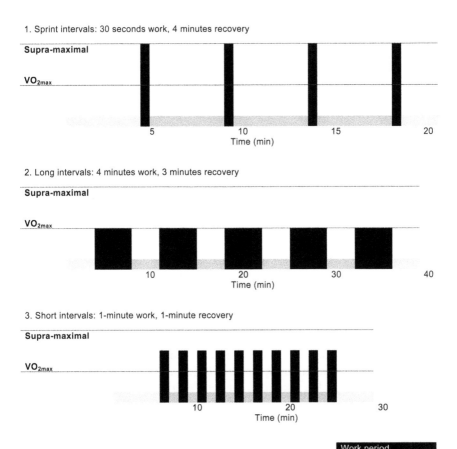

Figure 11.3 Example HIIT protocols.

high level of type II muscle fibre recruitment during SIT and short intervals may produce greater oxidative adaptations in these fibres than long intervals (Burgomaster et al., 2008; Ma et al., 2013). In contrast, long intervals may provide a more significant stimulus for central adaptations, such as enhanced cardiac output (Macpherson et al., 2011).

Is HIIT appropriate for sedentary or minimally active people?

Studies in patients with cardiac and metabolic diseases show that 8–12-week HIIT programmes are safe and can elicit improvements in cardio-metabolic risk factors such as, blood lipid profile, blood pressure, and body composition (Kessler et al., 2012). However, the feasibility of HIIT as an exercise strategy for the general public has been questioned for several reasons (Biddle & Batterham, 2015). For example, affect responses (i.e., feelings or emotions) experienced during exercise could influence future behaviour (e.g., adherence) (Rhodes & Kates, 2015). High-intensity exercise has been associated with more negative psychological effects than MICT, such as increased ratings of discomfort and reduced feelings of pleasure (Ekkekakis et al., 2011). Therefore, some researchers have suggested that adherence to HIIT could be poor amongst individuals who perceive HIIT (particularly SIT) to be more unpleasant than MICT (Biddle & Batterham, 2015; Hardcastle et al., 2014). In contrast, there is some evidence that HIIT provides some psychological advantages over MICT, such as lower ratings of exertion during training than MICT, that could improve exercise adherence (Bartlett et al., 2011; Kilpatrick et al., 2015).

Is HIIT more enjoyable than moderate-intensity continuous training?

Recent systematic reviews investigating the affective responses to different exercise intensities have produced somewhat confusing findings (Niven et al., 2020; Oliveira et al., 2013). Participants typically perceive HIIT as less pleasant than MICT during and after the exercise (Niven et al., 2020). However, the body of evidence indicates that most participants rated HIIT as more enjoyable than MICT overall (Niven et al., 2020; Oliveira et al., 2013). The emotional responses to HIIT reported within the literature vary due to dissimilarities between studies (e.g., different populations and the HIIT protocols). For example, the rest periods during HIIT allow cognitive and physical recovery, which could reduce perceived exertion and increase enjoyment; however, this psychological benefit reduces as work periods are extended (Price & Moss, 2007). Therefore, short intervals may offer psychological advantages compared to long intervals, which could potentially promote exercise adherence (Kilpatrick et al., 2015).

Is HIIT better for long-term adherence to exercise?

It is unclear if HIIT is better for long-term adherence to training than MICT, as exercise intensity is not the only determinant of exercise adherence (Thiel et al., 2018). Other factors, such as access to facilities, self-efficacy (see Chapter 3), and social support, influence psychological responses to exercise and adherence. It is not possible to predict how each client will respond to HIIT psychologically and if HIIT will promote better adherence than MICT or vice versa. Therefore, trainers should determine the client's psychological responses to HIIT and consider his/her preferences when designing the training programme.

Sprint interval training

All three (sprint, long, and short interval) forms of HIIT can improve CRF amongst healthy, trained and untrained individuals, and clinical populations (Milanović et al., 2015; Rognmo et al., 2004). Despite the short duration work periods, similar or superior improvements in maximal oxygen uptake (VO_{2max}) and muscle oxidative capacity have been reported following SIT compared to MICT (Astorino et al., 2013; Whyte et al., 2010). For example, similar improvements in muscle metabolism and exercise performance were reported following SIT (135 minutes), which was considerably shorter than the MICT (630 minutes) programme (Burgomaster et al., 2008).

How can sprinting improve cardiorespiratory fitness?

During a supramaximal 30 second sprint on a cycle ergometer, most ATP is produced anaerobically – approximately 25–30% from the phosphagen system and 65–70% from glycolysis (Bogdanis et al., 1995; Withers et al., 1991). However, the supply of ATP from aerobic metabolism significantly increases during each successive sprint, even when sprints are separated by 2–4 minute recovery periods (Bogdanis et al., 1996; Buchheit et al., 2012). The greater aerobic involvement with successive sprints promotes fatigue-resistant adaptations and partly explains how a period of SIT can improve CRF (see Table 11.1).

Is sprint interval training actually time-efficient?

A meta-analysis of 34 studies reported that a 2–12 week period of SIT significantly improves CRF (Vollaard et al., 2017). Within the meta-analysis, many of the studies used protocols consisting of 4–6 supramaximal repetitions lasting 30 seconds (Vollard et al., 2017). Although the total duration of the work bouts was 2–9 minutes, the total session duration (including the warm-up, rest periods and cool-down) could be 30 minutes, which is similar to the duration of a MICT session. Furthermore, 30 seconds of supramaximal intensity exercise is physiologically and psychologically

Table 11.1 Examples of high-intensity interval training interventions that have improved health outcomes

Outcomes	Population/Study	Protocols Work periods	Intensity	Rest periods	Rest intensity	Study duration
Long and short interval training						
↑ VO_{2max} ↓ Systolic blood pressure → Fasting glucose → Glucose control	Untrained men (Nybo et al., 2010)	5 × 2 minutes (run)	95% HR_{max}	2 minutes	Not specified	12 weeks
↑ Mitochondrial proteins ↑ Glucose control	Diabetic adults (Little et al., 2011)	10 × 60 seconds (cycle)	90% HR_{max}	60 seconds	Cycling at 50 watts	2 weeks
↑ VO_2 peak ↑ Exercise performance (500 kcal cycle test)	Overweight/Obese men (Boyd et al., 2013)	8–10 × 60 seconds (cycle)	100% max aerobic power	60 seconds	Unloaded cycling	3 weeks
↑ Muscle oxidative capacity ↑ Insulin sensitivity	Sedentary males & females (Hood et al., 2011)	10 × 60 seconds (cycle)	80%-95% of HR reserve	60 seconds	Not specified	2 weeks
→ Body fat ↑ VO_2 peak ↑ peak power	Obese adults (Tong et al., 2011)	20 × 30 seconds (cycle)	120% Peak aerobic power	60 seconds	Cycling at 20 watts	6 weeks
↑ VO_2 peak ↑ 30 s sprint mean power ↑ Mitochondrial proteins	Young males (Ma et al., 2013)	8 × 20 seconds (cycle)	170% VO_2 peak	10 seconds	Unloaded cycling	4 weeks

(Continued)

Table 11.1 Examples of high-intensity interval training interventions that have improved health outcomes (Continued)

Outcomes	Population/Study	Protocols				Study duration
		Work periods	Intensity	Rest periods	Rest intensity	
Sprint interval training						
↑VO$_2$ peak	Sedentary women (Allison et al., 2017)	3 × 20 seconds (stair climbing)	All-out	2 minutes	Passive rest	6 weeks
↑VO$_2$ peak ↓mean arterial pressure ↓blood glucose concentration (in men)	Overweight/obese men & women (Gillen et al., 2014)	3 × 20 seconds	All-out	2 minutes	Cycling at 50 watts	6 weeks
↓Body fat ↓Fasting insulin ↓Leptin concentration	Untrained young women (Trapp et al., 2008)	8 seconds (60 reps max) (cycle)	All-out	12 seconds	Unloaded cycling 20–30 RPM	15 weeks
↑VO$_2$ peak ↑Insulin action	Young men (Babraj et al., 2009)	4–6 × 30 seconds (cycle)	All-out	4 minutes	Rest or very light	2 weeks

demanding. Consequently, Hardcastle et al. (2014) argued that performing 30–90 minutes/week of SIT is not a viable or attractive alternative to the current moderate-intensity PA guidelines.

Recent studies have applied shorter (10–20 second) or fewer sprint intervals to address the limitations of classic SIT protocols. Promisingly, reducing SIT volume does not reduce the cardiometabolic health benefits reported with longer SIT protocols (Gillen et al., 2014; Hazell et al., 2012). Therefore, classic SIT protocols (4–6 × 30 seconds) are unnecessary; improvements in cardiometabolic outcomes can be achieved with shorter (e.g., 2–3 × 20-second sprints) protocols.

Long and short interval training

Long and short HIIT protocols can be equally or more effective in improving VO_{2max} than MICT (Bacon et al., 2013; Wen et al., 2019). For example, an eight-week study showed that both the short (15 seconds at 90–95% HR_{max}, 15 seconds recovery) and long (4 minutes at 90–95% HR_{max}, 3 minutes recovery) protocols produced greater improvements in VO_{2max} than MICT (45 minutes at 70% HR_{max}) (Helgerud et al., 2007). Similar improvements in CRF following short and long interval protocols have also been consistently replicated in other studies (see Table 11.1).

What is the minimum effective intensity and volume of HIIT?

The intensity of SIT is simple to programme and regulate as the client exercises as hard as possible (all-out) with no pacing (see Figure 11.1). Several long and short HIIT protocols can improve health and performance outcomes, provided the exercise intensity is high enough (Bacon et al., 2013; Conraads et al., 2015; Okura et al., 2003). The positive effects of HIIT appear to decline if the intensity is not significantly greater than MICT. For example, a low intensity (70% peak aerobic power) protocol was less effective than a high intensity (100% peak aerobic power) protocol in enhancing CRF (Boyd et al., 2013). Additionally, an average training HR of 88% HR_{max} for HIIT produced similar VO_{2max} and endothelial function improvements compared to MICT performed at 80% HR_{max} (Conraads et al., 2015). The body of evidence indicates the minimum effective intensity for long and short HIIT is approximately 80–85% VO_{2max}, which broadly corresponds to ≥85–90% of HR_{max} (see Chapter 7).

The volume of HIIT required depends on the client's training status, fitness, adherence, and goals. Research indicates the minimum volume of training required to improve both CRF and muscle oxidative capacity is three minutes/week of SIT (i.e., supramaximal exercise) performed within ten minute training sessions (3 × 10 minutes/week) (Gillen et al., 2014; Metcalfe et al., 2012). A lower volume of HIIT could conceivably be effective amongst sedentary or clinical populations.

Although HIIT protocols can significantly improve CRF, metabolic health, and cardiometabolic risk factors, it is unclear if HIIT is more effective than other endurance training methods (see Chapter 10) in improving these outcomes over a long period (>12 weeks). For instance, a 16-week study involving 81 untrained males reported similar improvements in CRF and cardiometabolic risk factors after MICT and HIIT interventions (Kemmler et al., 2014).

Is HIIT safe?

Various clinical experts have endorsed HIIT as an appropriate and beneficial form of exercise for cardiac patient groups (Mezzani et al., 2013); yet, it has been suggested that HIIT imposes potentially greater health and safety risks than light or moderate-intensity exercise (Kessler et al., 2012). For example, high-intensity exercise increases the relative risk of adverse cardiovascular events, such as acute myocardial infarction, compared to light-intensity activity, particularly amongst individuals with cardiovascular risk factors (Nakamura et al., 2009; Thompson et al., 2007). Examples of contraindications trainers should be aware of include:

- Unstable angina pectoris
- Uncompensated heart failure
- Recent myocardial infarction (<4 weeks)
- Recent coronary artery bypass graft or percutaneous coronary intervention (<12 months)
- Heart disease that limits exercise (valvular, congenital, ischaemic, and hypertrophic cardiomyopathy)
- Complex ventricular arrhythmias or heart block
- Severe chronic obstructive pulmonary, cerebrovascular disease, or uncontrolled peripheral vascular disease
- Uncontrolled diabetes mellitus
- Hypertensive patients with blood pressure >180/110 mmHg (or uncontrolled)
- Severe neuropathy

(Weston et al., 2014)

Previous safety concerns regarding adverse cardiovascular events were based on a lack of adverse events reported during HIIT sessions. However, adverse events in the post-exercise recovery period have not been widely documented. Therefore, Price et al. (2020) conducted a systematic review and meta-analysis to establish if physiological indicators of cardiovascular risk respond similarly to a bout of HIIT compared to MICT. Blood pressure responses to interval exercise were not different than MICT immediately or one hour after exercise; however, reductions in diastolic blood pressure and flow-mediated dilation (indicators of cardiovascular risk) were observed 10–15 minutes after HIIT. The

CASE STUDY 11.1

HIIT for Beginners

Tom is a sedentary, 40-year-old male (28% body fat). Tom's doctor diagnosed him with pre-diabetes and advised him to participate in regular exercise. Tom has limited exercise experience and does not have much time to train due to a hectic work schedule. Thus, HIIT seems like a good option for Tom. However, it is important to consider that HIIT studies with sedentary and clinical populations have been conducted within a controlled and supervised environment. Although, most studies have reported HIIT is generally safe and effective, caution must be applied when prescribing non-supervised HIIT for sedentary populations, as the client could initially find it difficult to achieve the required exercise intensity. Performing MICT before HIIT enables clients to establish an exercise routine (see Chapter 3), practice regulating exercising intensity, and improve CRF. Consequently, Tom's programme includes an introductory period of MICT consisting of 3×20–30 minute cycling sessions/week at 70–75% of HR_{max}. Following 3–4 weeks of MICT, a long interval protocol, consisting of two-minute repetitions ~85% HR_{max} (three minutes of active recovery ~50% HR_{max}) is introduced (Boudou et al., 2003).

latter findings suggest there is a small increase in the risk of cardiovascular events in the initial period following HIIT, particularly SIT, amongst clinical populations (Price et al., 2020). However, collectively, the current evidence indicates that HIIT does not convey higher cardiovascular risk than MICT for apparently healthy individuals (Price et al., 2020).

Although the risk of cardiovascular complications during and after HIIT is low amongst non-clinical populations, the risk of orthopedic injuries could be increased. For instance, injuries have been reported during 12-week studies using SIT (Lunt et al., 2014) and long interval protocols (Nybo et al., 2010). Therefore, caution should be applied when programming HIIT for clients with limited training experience. For these clients it might be prudent to prescribe HIIT at the lower effective intensity (e.g., 85% HR_{max}) or to incorporate a period of MICT before introducing HIIT (see Case Study 11.1). This transitional approach to HIIT can be programmed by subdividing the training programme into MICT and HIIT mesocycles (see Chapter 8).

Is HIIT practical for the general population?

Although HIIT has been demonstrated to induce several health benefits within laboratory-based studies, less is known about its effectiveness outside of the laboratory in the real-world. As previously discussed, questions regarding affective responses, self-regulation, and adherence to HIIT have led some to argue that HIIT is not a feasible long-term exercise strategy for sedentary populations. Most HIIT studies have been laboratory-based, often using specialised equipment. Moreover, participants are often provided with guidance, supervision, and encouragement during the training. It is unclear if unsupervised HIIT in real-world settings can produce the same magnitude of improvements in health and fitness outcomes as those reported in laboratory studies. For example, only modest improvements in CRF were reported following a walking/jogging HIIT study within a community park setting (Lunt et al., 2014). The authors speculated that the small improvement in CRF compared to previous studies was due to a reduced adherence to the training programme.

The participants compliance to supervised HIIT is usually high under supervised conditions (Weston et al., 2014). However, studies have reported mixed findings regarding the compliance and adherence to long-term unsupervised HIIT (Blackwell et al., 2017; Moholdt et al., 2011; Scott et al., 2019). At present, the long-term benefits or potential disadvantages of unsupervised HIIT are currently unknown in sedentary populations, as most studies have not included long-term follow-up assessments.

High-intensity snacks

Some people do not have access to an ergometer, gym or the perceived time to perform the type of HIIT protocols conducted in laboratory-based studies. Recent studies have addressed this issue by implementing HIIT using basic bodyweight exercises (discussed later) or stairs (Allison et al., 2017). Studies have also investigated the efficacy of incorporating bouts of high-intensity exercise throughout the day, (aka exercise snacks) instead of performing a conventional training session (Francois et al., 2014). For example, in a six-week SIT study participants performed 3×20 second sprint intervals of stair climbing (three days/week), which resulted in a 12% improvement in CRF (Allison et al., 2017). Emerging research suggests performing small blocks (snacks) of high-intensity exercise can enhance CRF and leg strength amongst untrained participants, but the long-term feasibility and efficacy has not been determined (Jenkins et al., 2019; Little et al., 2019; Wun et al., 2020).

Bodyweight HIIT

Performing HIIT using bodyweight exercises (aka calisthenics) has become popular within the fitness industry. The creators of bodyweight HIIT protocols often claim that bodyweight HIIT improves fitness and body composition, but most of these claims are based on HIIT laboratory-research. Extrapolating the results of HIIT studies to bodyweight training is problematic as most HIIT studies have been supervised by researchers using calibrated ergometers. There is currently a lack of empirical evidence that bodyweight HIIT significantly improves body composition. Indeed, the evidence that any form of HIIT improves body composition is not convincing (see Chapter 14).

How does bodyweight HIIT compare to conventional HIIT?

Most bodyweight HIIT protocols adopt a SIT approach, requiring the exerciser to perform as many repetitions as possible (AMRAP) within a short period (usually 10–30 seconds). Research indicates bodyweight HIIT can improve CRF and muscular performance amongst sedentary and recreationally active individuals (see Table 11.2). Although bodyweight exercises using multiple muscle groups, such as squats, impose a physiological stress, it is questionable if they can elicit the same magnitude of physiological stress compared to intervals using conventional exercise modes (e.g., running or cycling). For example, Gist et al. (2014) reported that performing 30 seconds of burpees (a full-body exercise) as fast as possible resulted in physiological responses at the lower intensity range (78% VO_{2peak}, 85%HR_{max}, peak RPE = 14.5) reported in previous HIIT studies. Performing bodyweight HIIT could, therefore, be sufficient for maintaining CRF amongst active or trained individuals. However, there is insufficient evidence that bodyweight HIIT improves components of fitness amongst trained individuals. The body of evidence suggests that trained individuals or athletes benefit from performing HIIT using conventional exercises (e.g., running and cycling). Emerging research suggests HIFT (discussed later) could also provide an effective training stimulus.

Advantages and disadvantages of bodyweight HIIT

A notable disadvantage of bodyweight HIIT is that the intensity is more difficult to regulate and monitor (see Table 11.3). As discussed previously, the intensity of short intervals cannot be accurately regulated using HR, and the power/speed of bodyweight exercises cannot be precisely monitored; thus, RPE is used to regulate and monitor intensity during bodyweight HIIT. Using RPE alone can make it difficult to calibrate intensity during the work bouts as the RPE reference points or anchors (see Chapter 7) are less obvious for bodyweight exercises than running or cycling. For example, there is a substantial difference in power output and effort, between light spinning (~7–8 RPE) and all-out sprinting (~20 RPE) on a cycle ergometer. Thus, the intensity of SIT on an ergometer is easier to calibrate using RPE compared to bodyweight exercises.

As with resistance training to failure with light loads (see Chapter 13), the initial repetitions of a bodyweight exercise will feel relatively easy for most clients. A significant increase in RPE may only become apparent as muscular and cardiorespiratory fatigue accumulate towards the end of the work bout. Therefore, during bodyweight HIIT, RPE is more influenced by

Table 11.2 Examples of bodyweight high-intensity interval training (HIIT) studies

Population/study	HIIT exercises	Protocol	Frequency & duration	Outcomes
Untrained males (n=5) and females (n=13) (Blackwell et al., 2017)	1. Star-jumps, 2. Squat thrusts, 3. Static sprints	5 × 1 minute Work: 1 minute (AMRAP) Rest: 90 seconds walk	3 days/week Duration: 4 weeks	Compared to lab HIIT and handgrip training groups: Similar ↑ in CRF between lab HIIT and bodyweight HIIT
Moderately trained army cadets; males (n=17) and females (n=9) Gist et al. (2015)	Burpees	5–7 × 30 seconds Work: All-out Rest: 4 minutes walking	3 days/week Duration: 4 weeks	Compared to conventional army training programme: No significant change in aerobic capacity, anaerobic capacity, or Army Physical Fitness Test performance in HIIT or conventional group
Recreationally active females (n=22) (McRae et al., 2012)	One exercise per session: 1. Burpees; 2. Jumping Jacks; 3. Mountain climbers; 4. Squat thrusts	8 × 20 seconds Rest: 10 seconds	4 days/week Duration: 4 weeks	Compared to MICT (30 min run, ~85% HR_{max}) ↑ CRF in HIIT (8%) and MICT (7%) ↑ muscle endurance (leg extensions, chest press, push-ups, sit-ups, and back extensions) in the HIIT group were significantly greater than MICT and control groups
Untrained (obese) males (n=4) and females (n=5) (Scott et al., 2019)	9 exercise pairs (30 seconds of each exercise)	Work: 1 minute @ ≥80% HR_{max} Rest: 10 seconds	Duration: 12 weeks	Compared to lab HIIT and MICT groups: Similar ↑ in capillarisation within the muscle microvascular endothelium No between-group differences
Untrained males (n=9) and females (n=11) (Wilke et al., 2018)	A circuit of 15 Full-body exercises	Work: 20 seconds 'all-out' efforts Rest: 10 seconds Performed for 15 minutes	3 days/week Duration: 12 weeks	Compared to MICT: ↑ maximum strength leg (5%) and shoulder (7.6%) strength ↑ Endurance workload (5.0%) ↑ Motivation to exercise

AMRAP = As many repetitions as possible; CRF = Cardiorespiratory fitness; MICT = Moderate-intensity continuous training.

Table 11.3 Advantages and disadvantages of bodyweight HIIT

Advantages	Disadvantages
Practicality: can be performed anywhere without equipment.	Intensity regulation: difficult to precisely monitor intensity.
Overload: Simple to provide progressive overload by increasing the duration of the work bouts or number of repetitions.	Overload: • Lack of progression options as fitness improves. • Increasing exercise complexity (e.g., single leg squats) could reduce the systemic physiological stimulus. • Exercises could become easier if bodyweight decreases.
Variation: numerous exercises can be used in different combinations, which provides a novel physiological stimulus, which could prevent monotony.	Variation: too much variation could make it difficult to monitor progress.
Enjoyment: can be done within a group setting, which could improve motivation and adherence.	Enjoyment: Routines that are too challenging could be demotivating and reduce self-efficacy (see Chapter 3).
Technique: Simple bodyweight exercises (e.g., step-ups) can be learnt easily.	Technique: More technically demanding exercises (e.g., burpees) become difficult to perform correctly when fatigued, which could reduce the physiological demand and increase injury risk.

the duration of the work bout compared to simple, cyclical exercises, such as running or cycling. Finally, bodyweight HIIT typically involves sprint (all-out) intervals where each exercise is performed with maximal effort. However, bodyweight exercises, particularly complex ones (e.g., burpees), require an element of pacing to maintain the correct technique.

HIIT for improving health and fitness summary

- Various HIIT protocols induce both central and peripheral adaptations that improve CRF.
- Well-designed and supervised HIIT programmes are safe and can elicit similar improvements in cardio-metabolic risk factors compared to MICT; these improvements have been demonstrated within healthy and clinical populations.
- The intensity threshold to elicit the benefits of long and short HIIT is approximately $\geq 80-85\%$ VO_{2max} or $\geq 85-90\%$ HR_{max}.
- An optimal volume of HIIT has not been identified. A ten minute SIT protocol consisting of a total of 60 seconds of supramaximal exercise performed three times per week (i.e., 30 minutes/week) can induce positive physiological adaptations.

- Performing short blocks (aka snacks) of high-intensity exercise during daily living (e.g., climbing stairs quickly) may improve CRF if performed regularly.
- Bodyweight HIIT can induce improvements in both CRF and muscular performance amongst sedentary and recreationally active individuals.
- There is insufficient evidence that bodyweight HIIT improves components of fitness or body composition amongst trained individuals, such as athletes.

High-intensity functional training (HIFT) – Insights from CrossFit practices
C. Leduc, P.B. Laursen, and M. Buchheit

A specific variation of HIIT, named high-intensity functional training (HIFT), more commonly known as CrossFit™, has recently become popular internationally (Feito et al., 2018). Generic HIIT can be programmed to target specific levels of metabolic (i.e., aerobic and anaerobic systems) and neuromuscular stress (Laursen & Buchheit, 2019). Conversely, HIFT requires high levels of aerobic, anaerobic, and neuromuscular demands simultaneously, which can help to develop a range of physical qualities (Feito et al., 2018). Traditional HIIT uses cyclical activities (e.g., cycling, rowing, running, and swimming); HIFT integrates technical exercises from sports such as Olympic weightlifting and gymnastics, making it a novel approach that could potentially be used to prepare athletes for sports performance (Feito et al., 2018).

Despite the growing popularity of HIFT, there is a lack of scientific research concerning both the acute and chronic responses to it (Claudino et al., 2018), which is required for optimal programming. More precisely, the acute physiological responses, in terms of the metabolic and neuromuscular demands associated with HIFT training sessions, are not yet completely understood. Such evidence would help to define the desired physiological targets of a training session (see Figure 11.2). Without this information, trainers cannot be certain they are applying the appropriate stimulus with HIFT to produce the desired training responses.

The following section will describe the acute metabolic (oxidative and anaerobic contribution) and neuromuscular responses to HIFT, in order to classify those exercises into one or more of the known HIIT types (See Figure 11.2). An overview on how key variables can be manipulated to target specific physiological goals will also be provided.

Typical exercises and acute responses of HIFT

Typical HIFT exercises

HIFT is generally performed using three exercise modalities: Olympic weightlifting, gymnastics, and cyclical exercises, such as running and cycling

(CrossFit™, 2020). These modalities can either be performed in isolation or combined to form specific session patterns (e.g., Olympic weightlifting + gymnastics). Within CrossFit™, some of the workouts are used as performance indicators or benchmarks. The CrossFit™ workouts are typically named (e.g., Fran, Cindy, and Grace) for convenience and ease of comparison.

Aerobic, anaerobic, and neuromuscular responses to typical HIFT workout and associated HIIT types

The acute physiological responses to HIFT have not been investigated to the same degree as other HIIT formats. This section will characterise the acute physiological responses to HIFT and highlight how different HIFT sessions may elicit different acute physiological responses (see Figure 11.2 and Table 11.4), which could be considered as a new format of HIIT, adding to established HIIT formats (e.g., short and long intervals).

What variables can be manipulated in HIFT?

Exercise mode

As discussed previously, 12 variables can be manipulated to target specific HIIT types (Laursen & Buchheit, 2019). Exercise mode affects the metabolic and neuromuscular responses to any given workout, but this has not been widely explored in the context of HIIT or HIFT. For example, during running adding changes of direction increases neuromuscular strain (Brughelli et al., 2008). Similarly, it is also apparent that jumping during the interval likely increases the neuromuscular stress in comparison with running only exercises (Laursen & Buchheit, 2019).

HIFT includes a variety of movements, such as Olympic weightlifting and gymnastics, which have received less attention in the literature. Different exercise modalities could elicit similar aerobic ($\approx 90\% HR_{max}$) and anaerobic responses (blood lactate: 10–12 mMol/L), yet the neuromuscular responses for each modality may be distinctly different (see Table 11.4), with Olympic weightlifting and gymnastics exercises inducing a higher neuromuscular load compared with cyclical exercises performed alone (Maté-muñoz et al., 2018). Although these findings are important to consider for trainers considering HIFT, more work is needed to confirm the findings, as few studies have investigated the neuromuscular responses and the rate of lactate accumulation (which is a better indicator of anaerobic contribution) to HIFT.

Exercise mode recommendations

- Gymnastic and Olympic weightlifting exercises increase the neuromuscular load of the workout in comparison with traditional HIIT exercise formats (e.g., running, cycling, rowing).

Table 11.4 Examples of HIFT studies

Study	Population	Session patterns	Session description	Metabolic (oxidative system) responses	Metabolic (glycolytic anaerobic system) responses	Neuromuscular responses	HIIT type (see Figure 11.2)
Fernández et al. (2015)	10 healthy adults	Olympic weightlifting + gymnastics	Fran workout: 21–15–9. The workout consisted of a thruster + pull-ups	~95 % HR_{max}	BLa: 14.5 mmol/L	/	Type 4 (O_2***/An***/N***)
		Gymnastics	Cindy workout: 5 pullups, 10 push-ups, and 15 air-squats in 20 min	~97 % HR_{max}	BLa: 14.0 mmol/L	/	Type 4 (O_2***/An***/N*)
Kliszczewicz et al. (2015)	10 healthy males	Gymnastics	Cindy workout: 5 pullups, 10 push-ups, and 15 air-squats in 20 min	~98 % HR_{max}	/	/	Type 4 (O_2***/A***/N*)
Kliszczewicz et al. (2017)	10 healthy males	Olympic weightlifting	Grace workout: 30 power clean &jerks at 61.4kg using an Olympic barbell for time	~172 B/ min	BLa: 14.3 mmol/L	/	Type 4 (O_2**/A***/N***)
		Olympic weightlifting + metabolic conditioning	15 min AMRAP 250-meter row, 20-kettlebell swings (16 kg), and 15-dumbbell thrusters (13.6 kg)	~170 B/ min	BLa: 13.7 mmol/L	/	Type 4 (O_2**/A**/N**)
Maté-muñoz et al. (2018)	34 healthy men (>6 months of strength training)	Gymnastics	Cindy workout: 5 pullups, 10 push-ups, and 15 air-squats in 20 min	~92 % HR_{max}	BLa: 11.8 mmol/L	Decrease CMJ variables	Type 4 (O_2***/A**/N*)

(Continued)

Table 11.4 Examples of HIFT studies (Continued)

Study	Population	Session patterns	Session description	Metabolic (oxidative system) responses	Metabolic (glycolytic anaerobic system) responses	Neuromuscular responses	HIIT type (see Figure 11.2)
		Metabolic conditioning	AMRAP 4 min as many double-unders as possible in 8 sets of 20 s with 10 s of rest between sets.	~92 % HR_{max}	BLa: 10 mmol/L	No change	Type 4 (O_2***/A**/N*)
		Olympic weightlifting	Maximum number of power-cleans possible in 5 min lifting a load equivalent to 40% of the individual's 1RM	~89 % HR_{max}	BLa: 11.2 mmol/L	Decrease CMJ variables	Type 4 (O_2**/A**/N***)
Tibana et al. (2017)	9 CrossFit athletes	Olympic weightlifting + metabolic conditioning	(a) Five sets of one repetition of snatch from the block at 80% of 1RM with 2–5 min of rest; (b) 3 sets of 5 Touch & Go Snatches (full) at 75% of 5RM with 90 s rest between sets; (C) 3 sets of 60 s of weighted plank hold with 90 s rest; After the third set of the above, 5 min rest was allowed and then endurance conditioning was performed with 10 min of 30 double-unders and 15 power snatches (34 kg).	~86 % HR_{max}	BLa: ≈ 12 mmol/L	Decrease in mean power 5 repetitions of 50% of 1RM back squat	Type 4 (O_2**/A**/N***)

Study	Participants	Sport	Protocol	HR	BLa	Other	HIIT type
Timón et al. (2019)	12 trained men	Gymnastics	Burpees and Toes to Bar increasing repetitions (1–1, 2–2, 3–3....) AMRAP 5 minutes.	~178 B/min	BLa: 13.3 mmol/L	/	Type 4 (O$_2$**/A**/N*)
		Olympic weightlifting	3 rounds for time of 20 Wall Ball (9 kg) and 20 Power Clean (a load of 40% 1RM). All repetitions of the first exercise had to be completed before beginning the next exercise.	~184 B/min	BLa: 18.4 mmol/L	/	Type 4 (O$_2$***/A***/N***)
Chen et al. (2018)	15 well-trained male basketball players	Olympic weightlifting	30 minutes of exercise (20 s work/40 s rest) with 6 exercises × 5 rounds.	/	BLa:13.6 mmol/L	No change in CMJ	Type 4 (O$_2$**/A**/N**)
Williams and Kraemer (2015)	8 men (age 20–23)	Olympic weightlifting	KB-HIIT 12-minute session. 20 s work/10 s rest was repeated for each exercise (a) sumo squat, (b) 2-handed swings, (c) clean and press and (d) sumo deadlift	~149 B/min	/	/	Type 4 (O$_2$**/A/N**)
Wong et al. (2017)	17 (Male = 10, Female = 7) adults	Olympic weightlifting	12 consecutive rounds of the 2-hand KB swing. Each round consisted of 30 s of exercise followed by 30 s rest. Males used a 16 kg KB, and females used an 8 kg KB	~169 B/min	/	/	Type 4 (O$_2$**/A/N**)

HIIT type column: O$_2$ = aerobic; A = anaerobic; N = neuromuscular; * = moderate aerobic, anaerobic, or neuromuscular response; ** = high aerobic, anaerobic or neuromuscular response; *** = very high aerobic, anaerobic or neuromuscular response.

Table key: 1RM = one repetition maximum; AMRAP = as many repetitions as possible; BLa = Blood lactate; KB = Kettlebell.

- While the inclusion of resistance-based exercise is an interesting adjunct, considerations surrounding the appropriate progression and loading are warranted. A primary emphasis should be put on exercise technique first to optimise safety and efficiency.
- HIFT should be separated with adequate recovery periods (>24 hours). Trainers must consider the potential residual fatigue induced by HIFT on subsequent training sessions that require muscular freshness to be performed well (e.g., strength and speed training).

Work intensity and duration

Work intensity is a variable that is not widely manipulated with HIFT, as HIFT applies either a set time to complete a workout or a specific number of sets/repetitions per exercise to finish the workout as fast as possible (see Table 11.4). Most of the movements in HIFT are not cyclical enough to be performed continuously and VO_{2max} cannot be determined through resistance-based exercise. Therefore, in contrast to traditional HIIT formats, HIFT does not use any of the usual prescription methods (e.g., HR, and MAS or power) to determine workout intensity. Additionally, the traditional 1RM prescription method (see Chapter 7) is problematic as some of the movements are not expressed relative to a maximal effort (e.g., push-ups or muscle ups).

Some adjustments of HIFT exercises could be used to control the intensity (e.g., scaled version of benchmark workouts, and velocity-based training), but such adjustments have yet to be investigated. Recently, Tinana et al. (2019) used the RPE to control the response to a HIFT session. The participants were asked to maintain an RPE of six (based on a 0–10 scale) throughout the workout. For the RPE condition, the participants performed less repetitions and had a lower blood lactate concentration compared with an 'all-out' workout condition. Interestingly, the percentage of HR_{max} was similar for both conditions (Tinana et al., 2019). These results suggest that submaximal RPE targets (e.g., 6–8) can be used to manipulate the physiological response of a HIFT session to elicit a large aerobic (type 2) response alongside a lower anaerobic contribution (see Figure 11.2). It is likely (not assessed) that the neuromuscular responses in the Tibana et al. (2019) study followed a similar pattern to the anaerobic response, as less repetitions were performed in the RPE-guided group versus the group maximum effort group.

Regarding the duration of a HIFT session, Kliszczewicz et al. (2017) compared the effect of a short (<5 minute) and long (15 minute) HIFT workout and reported no substantial difference between the two workouts regarding the aerobic and anaerobic responses. This suggests that short and long HIFT sessions may have similar metabolic responses. Despite these interesting results, further work is needed to understand how the work intensity and duration may elicit different metabolic and neuromuscular responses in the context of HIFT.

Work intensity and duration recommendations

- Trainers can consider using RPE to enable clients to autoregulate the intensity HIFT workouts (see Table 11.5). Using an RPE target of 6–8/10 may allow similar aerobic responses than 'all-out' exercises, while decreasing neuromuscular fatigue and keeping the anaerobic glycolytic contribution relatively consistent.
- The duration of the workout should be increased slowly throughout the training cycle to promote movement quality and safety.

Rest interval

Both the duration and intensity of the rest interval are important characteristics of HIIT. Recovery is quicker in a given time period when the work intensity is lower, and recovery is enhanced when the recovery duration is prolonged. Such manipulations directly impact on the repletion of work capacity and the subsequent physiological responses of the HIIT session (Laursen & Buchheit, 2019). Recovery is central to the ability to produce/replicate a sufficient intensity to produce a physiological stimulus and begin the training adaptation process (Bishop et al., 2008). However, in HIFT workouts, the rest interval is generally self-paced (Feito et al., 2018) and only the number of sets and repetitions or the total time of the exercise is prescribed. There is little information available concerning the manipulation of the rest interval during HIFT. HIFT can employ high skill movement patterns, such as weightlifting or gymnastics routine derivatives. Therefore, increasing or decreasing the duration of the recovery period could be important to optimise the technical quality of the exercises during HIFT work bouts and, subsequently, the magnitude of the metabolic and neuromuscular response (Mangine et al., 2018). For example, lengthening the rest period would target HIIT type 2 (mainly aerobic and neuromuscular with low or no anaerobic contribution) responses. Conversely, shortening the rest period would likely increase the anaerobic contribution, shifting to HIIT type three or four (see Figure 11.2).

Rest practical recommendations

- A short rest period will likely increase the anaerobic contribution. Conversely, a long rest period will increase the aerobic contribution.
- Including longer rest intervals decreases the rate of muscular fatigue development, which directly helps in maintaining the quality of movements, especially movements involving additional weight.

Table 11.5 Practical recommendations when implementing high-intensity functional training

	Exercise			Recovery			HIIT type (see Figure 11.2)
	Intensity	Duration	Modality	Intensity	Duration	Modality	
General HIIT format	95–125% MAS (80–105% V_{IFT})	10 seconds to 3–4 minutes	Cyclical exercise	Passive or Active ≈55% MAS (40% V_{IFT})	10 seconds to 2 minutes	Passive or Jogging or Walking	Type 1, 2, 3, 4, 5
HIFT	All-out or RPE guided (5–8)	Depends on: Workout prescribed or Time set	Cyclical, weightlifting or gymnastics exercise	Self-paced	Self-selected between repetitions or exercises	Passive	Type 2, 4, 5

MAS = Maximal aerobic speed; V_{IFT} = Final speed at the end of the 30–15 intermittent fitness test; RPE = Rating of perceived exertion.

Is HIFT appropriate for high performance athletes?

The 'toothpaste theory' nicely illustrates a potential issue of using HIFT with elite athletes (Laursen & Buchheit, 2019). The HIFT approach can be likened to squeezing toothpaste only from the middle of the tube (i.e., targeting both metabolic and neuromuscular adaptations simultaneously), which is a useful strategy for generalised conditioning. However, trained athletes require a more focused approach (i.e., separate HIIT, power, strength, and speed work) to get all the 'toothpaste' out (alternatively, squeezing strongly and consistently on just one side, and before the other). More research is necessary to examine the long-term training effect of HIFT in elite athletes, and the possible occurrence of an 'interference effect' (see Chapter 7) on subsequent physiological adaptations and exercise performance following HIFT.

HIFT summary

- HIFT is a relatively new HIIT approach that involves specific exercise modalities, such as gymnastic type exercises or Olympic weightlifting. These exercises increase the neuromuscular load of the sequences (i.e., favouring a HIIT type four response for most of the HIFT sessions).
- Different physiological responses (see Table 11.5) can be targeted by manipulating key variables (e.g., intensity or the duration of the work intervals).
- HIFT requires high levels of both strength and aerobic and anaerobic conditioning, which makes it a potentially time efficient training method. Therefore, HIFT is a viable option when working with clients who have limited training time.
- When used occasionally with higher level athletes, including elites, HIFT offers great training variation in terms of varying biological, physiological, and psychological stimuli, which is probably its main advantage.
- HIFT, must be carefully programmed to avoid excessive fatigue and potential interreference effects (see Chapter 7). The long-term adaptations occurring in elite athletes are unknown and should be the topic of future research.

References

Aamot, I., Karlsen, T., Dalen, H., et al. (2016). Long-term Exercise Adherence After High-intensity Interval Training in Cardiac Rehabilitation: A Randomized Study. *The Journal for Researchers and Clinicians in Physical Therapy*, *21*(1), 54–64.

Allison, M., Baglole, J., Martin, B., et al. (2017). Brief intense stair climbing improves cardiorespiratory fitness. *Medicine and Science in Sports and Exercise*, *49*(2), 298–307.

Astorino, T., Schubert, M., Palumbo, E., et al. (2013). Magnitude and time course of changes in maximal oxygen uptake in response to distinct regimens of chronic interval training in sedentary women. *European Journal of Applied Physiology, 113*(9), 2361–2369.

Babraj, J., Vollaard, N., Keast, C., et al. (2009). Extremely short duration high intensity interval training substantially improves insulin action in young healthy males. *BMC Endocrine Disorders, 9,* 3.

Bacon, A., Carter, R., Ogle, E., et al. (2013). VO$_{2max}$ trainability and high intensity interval training in humans: a meta-analysis. *PLOS ONE, 8*(9), e73182.

Bartlett, J., Close, G., MacLaren, D., et al. (2011). High-intensity interval running is perceived to be more enjoyable than moderate-intensity continuous exercise: implications for exercise adherence. *Journal of Sports Sciences, 29*(6), 547–553.

Batacan, R., Duncan, M., Dalbo, V., et al. (2017). Effects of high-intensity interval training on cardiometabolic health: A systematic review and meta-analysis of intervention studies. *British Journal of Sports Medicine, 51*(6), 494–503.

Biddle, S., & Batterham, A. (2015). High-intensity interval exercise training for public health: a big HIT or shall we HIT it on the head? *International Journal of Behavioral Nutrition and Physical Activity, 12*(1), 95.

Billat, L. (2001). Interval training for performance: A scientific and empirical practice. Special recommendations for middle- and long-distance running. Part I: aerobic interval training. *Sports Medicine, 31*(1), 13–31.

Bishop, P., Jones, E., & Woods, A. (2008). Recovery from training: a brief review: brief review. *Journal of Strength and Conditioning Research, 22*(3), 1015–1024.

Blackwell, J., Atherton, P., Smith, K., et al. (2017). The efficacy of unsupervised home-based exercise regimens in comparison to supervised laboratory-based exercise training upon cardio-respiratory health facets. *Physiological Reports, 5*(17).

Blair, S., Kohl, H., Barlow, C., et al. (1995). Changes in physical fitness and all-cause mortality. A prospective study of healthy and unhealthy men. *JAMA, 273*(14), 1093–1098.

Bogdanis, G., Nevill, M., Boobis, L., et al. (1996). Contribution of phosphocreatine and aerobic metabolism to energy supply during repeated sprint exercise. *Journal of Applied Physiology, 80*(3), 876–884.

Bogdanis, G., Nevill, M., Boobis, L., et al. (1995). Recovery of power output and muscle metabolites following 30 s of maximal sprint cycling in man. *The Journal of Physiology, 482*(Pt 2), 467–480.

Boudou, P., Sobngwi, E., Mauvais-Jarvis, F., et al. (2003). Absence of exercise-induced variations in adiponectin levels despite decreased abdominal adiposity and improved insulin sensitivity in type 2 diabetic men. *European Journal of Endocrinology, 149*(5), 421–424.

Boyd, J., Simpson, C., Jung, M., et al. (2013). Reducing the intensity and volume of interval training diminishes cardiovascular adaptation but not mitochondrial biogenesis in overweight/obese men. *PLOS ONE, 8*(7), e68091.

Brughelli, M., Cronin, J., Levin, G., et al. (2008). Understanding change of direction ability in sport: a review of resistance training studies. *Sports Medicine, 38*(12), 1045–1063.

Buchheit, M., Abbiss, C., Peiffer, J., et al. (2012). Performance and physiological responses during a sprint interval training session: relationships with muscle oxygenation and pulmonary oxygen uptake kinetics. *European Journal of Applied Physiology, 112*(2), 767–779.

Burgomaster, K., Howarth, K., Phillips, S., et al. (2008). Similar metabolic adaptations during exercise after low volume sprint interval and traditional endurance training in humans. *The Journal of Physiology, 586*(1), 151–160.

Chen, W., Wu, H.-J., Lo, S.-L., et al. (2018). Eight-week battle rope training improves multiple physical fitness dimensions and shooting accuracy in collegiate basketball players. *Journal of Strength and Conditioning Research, 32*(10), 2715–2724.

Chief Medical Officers for England, Northern Ireland, Scotland and Wales (2019). *UK Chief Medical Officers' Physical Activity Guidelines.*

Ciolac, E., Mantuani, S., Neiva, C., et al. (2015). Rating of perceived exertion as a tool for prescribing and self regulating interval training: A pilot study. *Biology of Sport, 32*(2), 103–108.

Claudino, J., Gabbett, T., Bourgeois, F., et al. (2018). CrossFit overview: systematic review and meta-analysis. *Sports Medicine – Open, 4*(11), 1–14.

Conraads, V., Pattyn, N., De Maeyer, C., et al. (2015). Aerobic interval training and continuous training equally improve aerobic exercise capacity in patients with coronary artery disease: the SAINTEX-CAD study. *International Journal of Cardiology, 179,* 203–210.

CrossFit (2020). Level 1 training guide (3rd ed.). http://library.crossfit.com/free/pdf/CFJ_English_Level1_TrainingGuide.pdf

DH (Department of Health) (2011). Start Active, Stay Active: A report on physical activity from the four home countries' Chief Medical Officers.

Ekkekakis, P., Parfitt, G., & Petruzzello, S. (2011). The pleasure and displeasure people feel when they exercise at different intensities. *Sports Medicine, 41*(8), 641–671.

Feito, Y., Heinrich, K., Butcher, S., et al. (2018). High-intensity functional training (HIFT): definition and research implications for improved fitness. *Sports, 6*(76), 1–19.

Fernández Fernández, J., Sabido Solana, R., Moya, D., et al. 2015). Acute physiological responses during crossfit® workouts. *European Journal of Human Movement, 35,* 114–124.

Francois, M., Baldi, J., Manning, P., et al. (2014). 'Exercise snacks' before meals: a novel strategy to improve glycaemic control in individuals with insulin resistance. *Diabetologia, 57*(7), 1437–1445.

Gibala, M., Little, J., MacDonald, M., et al. (2012). Physiological adaptations to low-volume, high-intensity interval training in health and disease. *The Journal of Physiology, 590*(5), 1077–1084.

Gibala, M., & McGee, S. (2008). Metabolic adaptations to short-term high-intensity interval training: a little pain for a lot of gain? *Exercise and Sport Sciences Reviews, 36*(2), 58–63.

Gillen, J., Percival, M., Skelly, L., et al. (2014). Three minutes of all-out intermittent exercise per week increases skeletal muscle oxidative capacity and improves cardiometabolic health. *PLOS ONE, 9*(11), e111489.

Gist, N., Freese, E., & Cureton, K. (2014). Comparison of responses to two high-intensity intermittent exercise protocols. *Journal of Strength and Conditioning Research, 28*(11), 3033–3040.

Gist, N., Freese, E., Ryan, T., et al. (2015). Effects of Low-Volume, High-Intensity Whole-Body Calisthenics on Army ROTC Cadets. *Military Medicine, 180*(5), 492–498.

Hardcastle, S., Ray, H., Beale, L., et al. (2014). Why sprint interval training is inappropriate for a largely sedentary population. *Frontiers in Psychology, 5,* 1505.

Hazell, T., Olver, T., Hamilton, C., et al. (2012). Two minutes of sprint-interval exercise elicits 24-hr oxygen consumption similar to that of 30 min of continuous endurance exercise. *International Journal of Sport Nutrition and Exercise Metabolism, 22*(4), 276–283.

Helgerud, J., Høydal, K., Wang, E., et al. (2007). Aerobic high-intensity intervals improve VO$_{2max}$ more than moderate training. *Medicine and Science in Sports and Exercise, 39*(4), 665–671.

Hood, M., Little, J., Tarnopolsky, M., et al. (2011). Low-volume interval training improves muscle oxidative capacity in sedentary adults. *Medicine and Science in Sports and Exercise, 43*(10), 1849–1856.

Hough, P. (2017). High-intensity interval training. In P. Hough, P., & S. Penn (Eds.). *Advanced Personal Training: science to practice* (pp. 149–164). Routledge.

Jabbour, G., & Majed, L. (2018). Ratings of Perceived Exertion Misclassify Intensities for Sedentary Older Adults During Graded Cycling Test: Effect of Supramaximal High-Intensity Interval Training. *Frontiers in Physiology, 9.*

Jelleyman, C., Yates, T., O'Donovan, G., et al. (2015). The effects of high-intensity interval training on glucose regulation and insulin resistance: a meta-analysis. *Obesity Reviews, 16*(11), 942–961.

Jenkins, E., Nairn, L., Skelly, L., et al. (2019). Do stair climbing exercise "snacks" improve cardiorespiratory fitness? *Applied Physiology, Nutrition, and Metabolism, 44*(6), 681–684.

Kemmler, W., Scharf, M., Lell, M., et al. (2014). High versus moderate intensity running exercise to impact cardiometabolic risk factors: the randomized controlled RUSH-study. *BioMed Research International, 2014,* 843095.

Kessler, H., Sisson, S., & Short, K. (2012). The potential for high-intensity interval training to reduce cardiometabolic disease risk. *Sports Medicine, (42*(6), 489–509.

Kilpatrick, M., Martinez, N., Little, J., et al. (2015). Impact of high-intensity interval duration on perceived exertion. *Medicine and Science in Sports and Exercise, 47*(5), 1038–1045.

Kliszczewicz, B., Buresh, R., Bechke, E., et al. (2017). Metabolic biomarkers following a short and long bout of high-intensity functional training in recreationally trained men. *Journal of Human Sport and Exercise, 12*(3), 710–718.

Laursen, P., & Buchheit, M. (2019). *Science and application of high-intensity interval training*. Human Kinetics.

Leduc, C., Laurssen, P., & Bucheit, M. (2021). High-intensity functional training. In P. Hough, P., & B. Schoenfeld (Eds.). *Advanced Personal Training: science to practice (2nd ed.)*. Routledge.

Little, J., Gillen, J., Percival, M., et al. (2011). Low-volume high-intensity interval training reduces hyperglycemia and increases muscle mitochondrial capacity in patients with type 2 diabetes. *Journal of Applied Physiology, 111*(6), 1554–1560.

Little, J., Langley, J., Lee, M., et al. (2019). Sprint exercise snacks: a novel approach to increase aerobic fitness. *European Journal of Applied Physiology, 119*(5), 1203–1212.

Lunt, H., Draper, N., Marshall, H., et al. (2014). High intensity interval training in a real-world setting: a randomized controlled feasibility study in overweight inactive adults, measuring change in maximal oxygen uptake. *PLOS ONE, 9*(1), e83256.

Ma, J., Scribbans, T., Edgett, B., et al. (2013). Extremely low-volume, high-intensity interval training improves exercise capacity and increases mitochondrial protein content in human skeletal muscle. *Open Journal of Molecular and Integrative Physiology, 3*(4), 720–726.

Macpherson, R., Hazell, T., Olver, T., et al. (2011). Run sprint interval training improves aerobic performance but not maximal cardiac output. *Medicine and Science in Sports and Exercise, 43*(1), 115–122.

Mangine, G., Dusseldorp, T., Feito, Y., et al. (2018). Testosterone and cortisol responses to five high-intensity functional training competition workouts in recreationally active adults. *Sports, 6*(62).

Maté-muñoz, J., Lougedo, J., Barba, M., et al. (2018). Cardiometabolic and muscular fatigue responses to different CrossFit workouts. *Journal of Sports Science and Medicine, 17*(4), 668–679.

Metcalfe, R., Babraj, J., Fawkner, S., et al. (2012). Towards the minimal amount of exercise for improving metabolic health: beneficial effects of reduced-exertion high-intensity interval training. *European Journal of Applied Physiology, 112*(7), 2767–2775.

McRae, G., Payne, A., Zelt, J., et al. (2012). Extremely low volume, whole-body aerobic-resistance training improves aerobic fitness and muscular endurance in females. *Applied Physiology, Nutrition, and Metabolism, 37*(6), 1124–1131.

Mezzani, A., Hamm, L., Jones, A., et al. (2013). Aerobic exercise intensity assessment and prescription in cardiac rehabilitation. *European Journal of Preventive Cardiology, 20*(3), 442–467.

Milanović, Z., Sporiš, G., & Weston, M. (2015). Effectiveness of high-intensity interval training (HIT) and continuous endurance training for VO_{2max} improvements: a systematic review and meta-analysis of controlled trials. *Sports Medicine, 45*(10), 1469–1481.

Moholdt, T., Aamot, I., Granøien, I., et al. (2011). Long-term follow-up after cardiac rehabilitation: a randomized study of usual care exercise training versus aerobic interval training after myocardial infarction. *International Journal of Cardiology, 152*(3), 388–390.

Nakamura, F., Soares-Caldeira, L., Laursen, P., et al. (2009). Cardiac autonomic responses to repeated shuttle sprints. *International Journal of Sports Medicine, 30*(11), 808–813.

Niven, A., Laird, Y., Saunders, D., et al. (2020). A systematic review and meta-analysis of affective responses to acute high intensity interval exercise compared with continuous moderate- and high-intensity exercise. *Health Psychology Review*, 1–34.

Nybo, L., Sundstrup, E., Jakobsen, M., et al. (2010). High-intensity training versus traditional exercise interventions for promoting health. *Medicine and Science in Sports and Exercise, 42*(10), 1951–1958.

Okura, T., Nakata, Y., & Tanaka, K. (2003). Effects of exercise intensity on physical fitness and risk factors for coronary heart disease. *Obesity Research, 11*(9), 1131–1139.

Oliveira, B., Slama, F., Deslandes, A., et al. (2013). Continuous and high-intensity interval training: which promotes higher pleasure? *PLOS ONE, 8*(11).

Pagnan, C., Seidel, A., & MacDermid Wadsworth, S. (2017). I just can't fit it in! Implications of the fit between work and family on health-promoting behaviors. *Journal of Family Issues, 38*(11), 1577–1603.

Parolin, M., Chesley, A., Matsos, M., et al. (1999). Regulation of skeletal muscle glycogen phosphorylase and PDH during maximal intermittent exercise. *The American Journal of Physiology, 277*(5), E890–900.

Price, K., Gordon, B., Bird, S., et al. (2020). Acute cardiovascular responses to interval exercise: a systematic review and meta-analysis. *Journal of Sports Sciences, 38*(9), 970–984.

Price, M., & Moss, P. (2007). The effects of work:rest duration on physiological and perceptual responses during intermittent exercise and performance. *Journal of Sports Sciences, 25*(14), 1613–1621.

Ramos, J., Dalleck, L., Tjonna, A., et al. (2015). The impact of high-intensity interval training versus moderate-intensity continuous training on vascular function: a systematic review and meta-analysis. *Sports Medicine, 45*(5), 679–692.

Rhodes, R., & Kates, A. (2015). Can the affective response to exercise predict future motives and physical activity behavior? A systematic review of published evidence. *Annals of Behavioral Medicine: A Publication of the Society of Behavioral Medicine, 49*(5), 715–731.

Rognmo, Ø, Hetland, E., Helgerud, J., et al. (2004). High intensity aerobic interval exercise is superior to moderate intensity exercise for increasing aerobic capacity in patients with coronary artery disease. *European Journal of Cardiovascular Prevention and Rehabilitation, 11*(3), 216–222.

Scott, S., Shepherd, S., Andrews, R., et al. (2019). A multidisciplinary evaluation of a virtually supervised home-based high-intensity interval training intervention in people with type 1 diabetes. *Diabetes Care, 42*(12), 2330–2333.

Sloth, M., Sloth, D., Overgaard, K., et al. (2013). Effects of sprint interval training on VO_{2max} and aerobic exercise performance: A systematic review and meta-analysis. *Scandinavian Journal of Medicine & Science in Sports, 23*(6).

Tabata, I., Nishimura, K., Kouzaki, M., et al. (1996). Effects of moderate-intensity endurance and high-intensity intermittent training on anaerobic capacity and VO_{2max}. *Medicine and Science in Sports and Exercise, 28*(10), 1327–1330.

Thiel, A., Thedinga, H., Barkhoff, H., et al. (2018). Why are some groups physically active and others not? A contrast group analysis in leisure settings. *BMC Public Health, 18*(1), 377.

Thompson, P., Franklin, B., Balady, G., et al. (2007). Exercise and acute cardiovascular events placing the risks into perspective: a scientific statement from the American heart association council on nutrition, physical activity, and metabolism and the council on clinical cardiology. *Circulation, 115*(17), 2358–2368.

Tibana, R., Vieira, I., Neto, D., et al. (2017). Extreme conditioning program induced acute hypotensive effects are independent of the exercise session intensity. *International Journal of Exercise Science, 10*(8), 1165–1173.

Tibana, R., Sousa, N., Prestes, J., et al. (2019). Is perceived exertion a useful indicator of the metabolic and cardiovascular responses to a metabolic conditioning session of functional fitness? *Sports, 7*(161).

Timón, A., Olcina, G., Camacho-cardeñosa, M., et al. (2019). 48-hour recovery of biochemical parameters and physical performance after two modalities of CrossFit workouts. *Biology of Sport, 36*(3), 283–289.

Trilk, J., Singhal, A., Bigelman, K., et al. (2011). Effect of sprint interval training on circulatory function during exercise in sedentary, overweight/obese women. *European Journal of Applied Physiology, 111*(8), 1591–1597.

Tong, T., Chung, P., Leung, R., et al. (2011). Effects of non-Wingate-based high-intensity interval training on cardiorespiratory fitness and aerobic-based exercise capacity in sedentary subjects: a preliminary study. *Journal of Exercise Science & Fitness, 9*(2), 75–81.

Torma, F., Gombos, Z., Jokai, M., et al. (2019). High intensity interval training and molecular adaptive response of skeletal muscle. *Sports Medicine and Health Science, 1*(1), 24–32.

Trapp, E., Chisholm, D., Freund, J., et al. (2008). The effects of high-intensity intermittent exercise training on fat loss and fasting insulin levels of young women. *International Journal of Obesity (2005), 32*(4), 684–691.

Viana, A., Fernandes, B., Alvarez, C., et al. (2019). Prescribing high-intensity interval exercise by RPE in individuals with type 2 diabetes: Metabolic and hemodynamic responses. *Applied Physiology, Nutrition, and Metabolism, 44*(4), 348–356.

Vollaard, N., Metcalfe, R., & Williams, S. (2017). Effect of number of sprints in an SIT session on change in VO_{2max}: a meta-analysis. *Medicine and Science in Sports and Exercise, 49*(6), 1147–1156.

Wen, D., Utesch, T., Wu, J., et al. (2019). Effects of different protocols of high intensity interval training for VO_{2max} improvements in adults: a meta-analysis of randomised controlled trials. *Journal of Science and Medicine in Sport, 22*(8), 941–947.

Weston, K., Wisløff, U., & Coombes, J. (2014). High-intensity interval training in patients with lifestyle-induced cardiometabolic disease: a systematic review and meta-analysis. *British Journal of Sports Medicine, 48*(16), 1227–1234.

Whyte, L., Gill, J., & Cathcart, A. (2010). Effect of 2 weeks of sprint interval training on health-related outcomes in sedentary overweight/obese men. *Metabolism: Clinical and Experimental, 59*(10), 1421–1428.

Wilke, J., Kaiser, S., Niederer, D., et al. (2019). Effects of high-intensity functional circuit training on motor function and sport motivation in healthy, inactive adults. *Scandinavian Journal of Medicine & Science in Sports, 29*(1), 144–153.

Williams, B., & Kraemer, R. (2015). Comparison of cardiorespiratory and metabolic responses in kettlebell high-intensity interval training versus sprint interval cycling. *Journal of Strength and Conditioning Research, 29*(12), 3317–3325.

Withers, R., Sherman, W., Clark, D., et al. (1991). Muscle metabolism during 30, 60 and 90 s of maximal cycling on an air-braked ergometer. *European Journal of Applied Physiology and Occupational Physiology, 63*(5), 354–362.

Wong, A., Nordvall, M., Walters-Edwards, M., et al. (2021). Cardiac Autonomic and Blood Pressure Responses to an Acute Bout of Kettlebell Exercise. *Journal of Strength and Conditioning Research, 35*(1), S173–S179.

Wun, C., Zhang, M., Ho, B., et al. (2020). Efficacy of a six-week dispersed Wingate-cycle training protocol on peak aerobic power, leg strength, insulin sensitivity, blood lipids and quality of life in healthy adults. *International Journal of Environmental Research and Public Health, 17*(13).

12 Training the core

Marc Surdyka and Sam Spinelli

What is the core?

The core is an important division of the body, providing connection between the upper and lower extremities, stabilising the spine, and allowing for a wide range of movements. There is no single agreed-upon region for the core, but it can generally be thought of as the area between the rib cage and pelvis (Majewski-Schrage et al., 2014). Due to the lack of agreement on its borders, there is variability in the musculature that is assigned to the core. However, using approximate borders, there are a few groups of muscles that can be classified as core muscles (Akuthota et al., 2008; Majewski-Schrage et al., 2014). These are the abdominal muscles, the spinal muscles, the diaphragm, and the pelvic floor muscles (Akuthota et al., 2008; Bliven et al., 2013; Majewski-Schrage et al., 2014). Collectively these groups of muscles form a cylindrical shape that wraps 360 degrees around the mid-section (Akuthota et al., 2008; Bliven et al., 2013; Majewski-Schrage et al., 2014).

What is the role of the core?

The core has a range of different functions that enables efficient movement to occur. The first function of the core is to provide control of the lumbar spine, allowing for a stable unit between the pelvis and rib cage (Bliven et al., 2013; McGill, 2001; Parkhouse & Ball, 2010). This stable unit functions to transfer force from the lower extremities to the upper extremities, and vice versa. This is exhibited in simple activities such as walking, in which the arm and leg actions are synchronised through the core. Furthermore, the creation of tension across the core enables forces to be efficiently transferred during complex activities, such as a boxer's punch where the core transfers the force generated from the legs and hips into the arm and fist (Bliven et al., 2013; McGill, 2001; Parkhouse & Ball, 2010).

DOI: 10.4324/9781003204657-12

The second critical function of the core is to produce movement dynamically, allowing for variable movement patterns and tasks to occur (Parkhouse & Ball, 2010; Robison, 1992; Saal, 1992). This is achieved through the structure of the core, which allows muscles to produce the actions of flexion, extension, rotation, and lateral flexion. These actions can either be performed in isolation or synchronously to produce motion in all three planes (Bliven et al., 2013; McGill, 2001; Parkhouse & Ball, 2010). The actions can also be coordinated with limb movements in order to perform functional activities, such as rotating and reaching across your body while cooking (Parkhouse & Ball, 2010; Robison, 1992; Saal, 1992).

Since there are identical core muscles on each side of the spine and rib cage, these muscles can function together to either create or resist motion (McGill, 2001; Parkhouse & Ball, 2010). The core provides stability and control primarily through coordinated isometric contractions to resist the spine, rib cage, and pelvis from moving, like when deadlifting (McGill, 2001). In contrast, tri-planar movement, the second main function of the core, is achieved through isotonic contractions working cohesively to generate motion, like during a Russian twist (Parkhouse & Ball, 2010).

What is a neutral spine?

The aim of many core exercises is to maintain a neutral spine position (Robison, 1992; Saal, 1992). This concept originated from Panjabi who coined the terms 'neutral position' and 'neutral zone' (Panjabi, 1992a). These are precise terms based on load-displacement measures; essentially, how much force it takes to move the spinal segments (Panjabi, 1992a). However, the current understanding is that the neutral spine is essentially the midpoint between maximum lumbar flexion and extension (O'Sullivan et al., 2010; Panjabi, 1992a).

The spine is least able to handle stress when it is at extreme ranges of motion. Therefore, the neutral spine is theorised to be a position in which the spine is at the least risk of injury (Panjabi, 1992a; Robison, 1992; Saal, 1992). However, the neutral spine is not a set specific position, but instead is a range in each direction where there is a reduced degree of challenge to passive structures. In an upright standing position, a small lordosis in the lumbar spine is generally accepted as a neutral spine position (O'Sullivan et al., 2010; Panjabi, 1992a). Throughout different movements such as squatting or hinging activities, the spine begins to go into flexion and loses some lordosis (Burnett et al., 2008; McGill & Marshall, 2012; Vigotsky et al., 2015). However, it is normal for up to 40 degrees of flexion to occur during movements such as squatting, kettlebell swings, and good mornings (Burnett et al., 2008; McGill & Marshall, 2012; Vigotsky et al., 2015).

What is core stability?

Similar to the lack of consensus on what defines 'the core', the term core stability has taken on various interpretations. Many definitions of core stability have stemmed from the early works of Panjabi who classified the stabilisation of the spine into three distinct components: the passive sub-system (vertebrae, discs, and ligaments), the active sub-system (muscles and tendons), and the neural control sub-system (nerves and central nervous system) (Panjabi, 1992b). According to Panjabi, the three sub-systems work synchronously to achieve stability of the lumbar spine around resting spinal position and toward the end ranges of motion (Panjabi, 1992a, 1992b).

Since Panjabi's initial classification of core stability, the active sub-system has often been linked to a seminal paper by Bergmark (1989) who categorised the muscles of this region into local and global systems based on their attachments and actions (Behm et al., 2010b; Bergmark, 1989). The global system includes muscles spanning many segments, such as the superficial erector spinae. Therefore, muscles in the global system are often considered the prime movers of the spine, which are also responsible for adapting to external forces experienced by the body (Behm et al., 2010b; Bergmark, 1989). The local system, with its smaller, deeper muscles (e.g., the multifidus) accommodates intersegmental changes affecting the position and posture of the lumbar spine (Behm et al., 2010b; Bergmark, 1989).

The transverse abdominis (TA) assists with intervertebral stiffness and acts in a feed-forward manner before the initiation of limb movements. It has been suggested that the TA plays the most significant role in maintaining core stability in healthy individuals (Hodges et al., 2003; Hodges & Richardson, 1996, 1997, 1998). However, research indicates that the TA does not act in isolation. The ability to resist unwanted motion is better achieved through bracing all of the muscles of the core as opposed to trying to confine activation to the TA alone through abdominal hollowing (Grenier & McGill, 2007; Morris et al., 2013; Tayashiki et al., 2015).

Before elaborating on the function of the core as it relates to training, it is important to examine the purpose of the core during day-to-day activities. While the trunk musculature is active during sitting, standing and walking, the magnitude of its activity is variable and relatively low overall (Andersson et al., 1996; Cholewicki et al., 1997; Nairn et al., 2013). For example, the mean rectus abdominis and external oblique activity during walking is less than 5% of maximal voluntary contraction (White & McNair, 2002).

Core stability can be thought of as the highly coordinated, conscious or unconscious effort of the passive, active, and neural sub-systems to adequately produce, resist, control, and/or transfer forces and motion to meet the demands of a specific task under continuously changing conditions (Kibler et al., 2006; Moreau et al., 2001; Reed et al., 2012). Through examining all the core literature together, a better framework for attempting to define and explain core stability can be established.

Testing the core

Without unanimously agreed upon definitions of 'core' and 'core stability', standardised testing is inconsistent and lacking (Reed et al., 2012). A vital component of the definition outlined above is that core stability is task-specific. Therefore, the function of the core will vary between walking, sprinting, throwing, jumping, squatting, pressing, and other exercises that might take place within a gym setting.

Commonly employed core assessment tests with normative values exist, such as isometric endurance times for the trunk extensors, flexors, and lateral musculature (Lee, 2018; McGill et al., 1999; Moreau et al., 2001). For example, healthy men and women in their early 20s should be expected to hold a side plank with feet staggered for approximately 80–90 seconds (McGill et al., 1999). However, there is not always a quantifiable transfer from isolated core training to other exercises, activities, or sports (Reed et al., 2012). Therefore, a thorough evaluation of compound exercises (e.g., squats, deadlifts, push-ups, and pull-ups) may be one of the most appropriate means to test the stability of the core.

Training the core

Various classification systems have been developed with the intention of optimising core training by grouping exercises into distinct categories such as mobility, motor control, work capacity, strength and stability exercises (Hibbs et al., 2008; Spencer et al., 2016). Also, as mentioned above, there was previously a significant emphasis on isolated muscle activation for stability that largely stemmed from the field of rehabilitation (Hodges et al., 2003; Hodges & Richardson, 1996, 1997, 1998). However, a simpler solution may exist.

Compound lifts

A broad review of the literature indicates that compound, free-weight exercises serve as, arguably, the best tool for training core stability (Behm et al., 2010a; Martuscello et al., 2013; Wirth et al., 2017). Behm and colleagues (2010a, 2010b) go as far as saying that ground-based free-weight exercises (e.g., back squats, deadlifts, and lifts that involve trunk rotation) should form the foundation of exercises to train the core musculature for all level of clients (i.e., recreational fitness clients to high-performance athletes).

The body functions to complete specific tasks rather than activate singular muscles. During compound lifts, the core is forced to create a stable and rigid base by increasing intra-abdominal pressure and co-contraction of the surrounding musculature (Brown et al., 2006; Georgopoulos, 2000; Lederman, 2010; van Dieën et al., 2003). For example, movements like squats, deadlifts, pull-ups, push-ups, and barbell hip thrusts can elicit high activation of the abdominals, erector spinae, multifidus, and TA (Andersen et al., 2018; Hewit, 2018; Marcolin et al., 2015; Martín-Fuentes et al., 2020; van den Tillaar & Saeterbakken, 2018; Yavuz et al., 2015). These dynamic, multi-joint exercises can also be quantifiably progressed over time to create simultaneous improvements in core stability (Martuscello et al., 2013).

Unstable surfaces

The common narrative for performing exercises on unstable surfaces is that if compound exercises (e.g., squats) on a stable surface are good, then performing them on unstable surfaces is even better. However, scientific research does not support this theory (Behm et al., 2010a, 2010b, 2015; Willardson, 2004; Wirth et al., 2017). Indeed, training on unstable devices should be avoided when the primary training goal is hypertrophy, absolute strength, or power, as force generation, power output and movement velocity are impaired (Behm et al., 2010a, 2010b, 2015; Willardson, 2004; Wirth et al., 2017). Unstable surfaces may serve other purposes, such as rehabilitation of specific injuries, but they should not be used during traditional resistance training exercises to improve core stability.

Unilateral lifts

One of the easiest and most effective ways to increase the stability demands of the core may be to incorporate unilateral movements that create asymmetric loads (Behm et al., 2005; Grenier & McGill, 2007). For example, standing unilateral dumbbell shoulder presses elicit higher EMG activity of the rectus abdominis, external oblique, and erector spinae than seated bilateral dumbbell shoulder presses (Saeterbakken & Fimland, 2012). In addition to standing, Figure 12.1 depicts half kneeling and long-sitting (Z-press) options that induce asymmetrical loads to challenge the core without completely sacrificing the integrity of the movement. Although this concept does not apply uniformly across all exercises, performing a combination of bilateral and unilateral exercises may be an optimal strategy for training the core (Andersen et al., 2019; Saeterbakken et al., 2015; Saeterbakken & Fimland, 2012).

Isolation

Ground-based free weight exercises can be complemented by appropriately dosed movements aimed at targeting the trunk. However, the relatively low abdominal and erector spinae activity produced during exercises like the 'Dying Bug' and 'Bird Dog' may be insufficient for increasing strength in healthy populations (Souza et al., 2001). Therefore, more demanding exercises that are better suited for progressive overload, in one capacity or another, are recommended. For example, a forearm plank with 20%

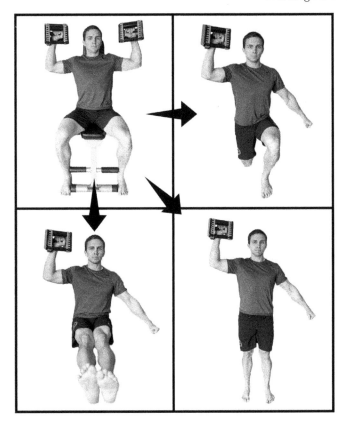

Figure 12.1 Altering base of support and symmetry of load.

of body mass added to the lower back performed to task failure demonstrated similar rectus abdominis and external oblique activity to that of a 6 RM back squat (van den Tillaar & Saeterbakken, 2018). After a baseline of strength is established, an additional load can be applied over time. Moreover, manipulating the position of the arms relative to the torso by placing the elbows at nose level, as opposed to in line with the shoulders, and contracting the gluteal muscles as hard as possible (see Figure 12.2) is another method for increasing the intensity of a standard plank and the overall activation of the abdominals (Schoenfeld et al., 2014).

Task-specific

It is reasonable to assume that core training leads to significant carryover into athletic performance. However, this theory has not been well established (Prieske et al., 2016; Willardson, 2004; Wirth et al., 2017). Indeed, it has been suggested that practising the sport skill on the same surface on

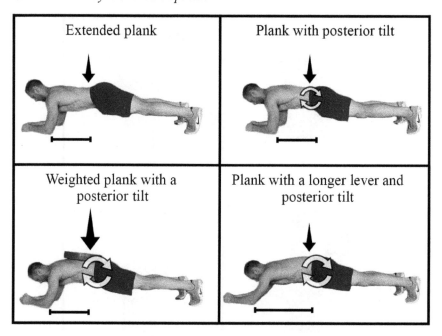

Figure 12.2 Altering cues, lever arm, and magnitude of load.

which the skill is performed during competition is the optimal method to promote increases in balance, proprioception, and core stability for any given sports skill (Willardson, 2004). Traditional resistance training can be utilised to further enhance physical fitness and athletic performance by inducing desirable adaptations, such as improvements in strength and power (Willardson, 2004; Wirth et al., 2017).

Practical application of core training methods

Based on the information above, a hierarchy, or three-tier pyramid, can be constructed to represent how to prioritise training for the core (see Figure 12.3). As in most programs, the foundation consists of stable, compound movements that, in this case, simultaneously elicit sufficient activation of the trunk musculature (Marcolin et al., 2015; Martín-Fuentes et al., 2020; Yavuz et al., 2015). These lifts can be given a higher priority by programming them earlier in the session to better manage fatigue for optimal performance (Farinatti et al., 2013; Miranda et al., 2013; Spineti et al., 2010). In doing so, a greater stimulus for muscle growth and strength adaptations can occur within the context of the overarching plan, while still adequately training the core (Mangine et al., 2015; Sheikholeslami-Vatani et al., 2016).

The second consideration (middle tier) should feature exercises that emphasise resisting trunk motion by using asymmetrical loads. Movements

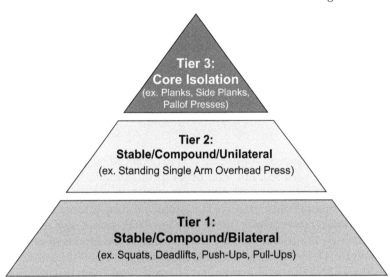

Figure 12.3 Core training pyramid.

like the standing unilateral dumbbell shoulder press, unilateral dumbbell row, offset load lunge (weight in one hand), and unilateral glute bridge allows the appendicular and axial muscles to be challenged collectively (Ekstrom et al., 2007; Saeterbakken et al., 2015; Saeterbakken & Fimland, 2012). As depicted in Figure 12.1, the base of support can be modified to enhance this effect further, assuming that the underlying concepts that drive progressive overload are not sacrificed in the process.

The final tier of the pyramid (see Figure 12.3) features core emphasised, or 'isolation' type movements. Similar to how an upper-body training programme, for example, often transitions from a larger compound movement to smaller isolation type movements (e.g., bench press to tricep extensions), the same principle can be applied with the core (Farinatti et al., 2013; Ogasawara et al., 2013; Ribeiro et al., 2017; Spineti et al., 2010). These more isolated core exercises can be spaced out throughout a programme as there will be overlap between movements for muscles challenged. For example, a front plank and side plank utilises many similar muscles and can be placed on different days (Escamilla et al., 2016; McGill et al., 2009; Schoenfeld et al., 2014).

Based on the functions of the core, it may be beneficial to incorporate isometric and isotonic exercises in all three planes of motion when designing and implementing a comprehensive training programme (see Tables 12.1 and 12.2) (Escamilla et al., 2016; Parkhouse & Ball, 2010). To complement the first tier of the pyramid (see Figure 12.3), this could be performed in one of three ways. The first method would utilise specific core exercises to target weak points in a lift, such as reverse hyperextensions to enhance lumbar erector spinae strength for the deadlift. A contrasting method would strategically pair a trunk flexor dominant movement like a hollow body hold with the deadlift that is a trunk extensor dominant exercise (not necessarily to be performed as a superset). Finally, incorporating a rotational exercise, such as the Pallof press, can increase overall variability.

Terminology

Accurate terminology is important for exercise prescription and when communicating with clients and other professionals. For example, a forearm plank is a sagittal plane, *anti-extension* based exercise that targets the abdominal musculature. If no internal torque from the muscles were generated, the client's pelvis and low back would sag toward the floor, resulting in lumbar extension secondary to the effects of gravity on body weight. Therefore, when a forearm plank is executed correctly, it is deemed an anti-extension manoeuvre, even though the trunk flexors are working.

There are, of course, exceptions to the labelling of exercises in Tables 12.1 and 12.2. For instance, complex exercises, such as bear crawling, involve resisting motion in multiple planes. Therefore, the tables should be used as guidelines rather than definitive rules. Understanding the primary muscles being addressed is also important, while continuing to appreciate that no muscle activates in isolation.

In summary, training the core should follow similar principles as other muscle groups in terms of manipulating variables, such as sets, repetitions, hold times, intensity, moment arms, and frequency (Heaselgrave et al.,

Table 12.1 Isometric core exercise variations

Anti-extension	Anti-flexion	Anti-rotation	Anti-lateral flexion
Dying bug	Superman hold	Pallof press	Side plank
Plank	Reverse hyper hold	Kneeling chops	Suitcase carry
Hollow body hold	Back extension hold	Bird dog	Overhead Pallof press

Table 12.2 Isotonic core exercise variations

Flexion	Extension	Rotation	Lateral flexion
V-Ups	Superman	Med ball side throw	Standing side bend
Hanging leg raises	Reverse hyper	Russian twist	Side plank hip lift
Medicine ball slams	Back extension	Chop and lift	Hanging leg raise with side bend

2019; Schoenfeld et al., 2014, 2016). The core has some unique characteristics, but it does not inherently need to be trained daily, and progressive overload should be employed when possible.

Summary

Although the core has not been universally well-defined, it is mostly agreed upon that it has two primary functions. The first is to help provide a stable base through which forces can be transmitted between the extremities; this is largely achieved via isometric contractions of the core musculature. The second primary function is to perform flexion, extension, rotation, and lateral flexion either in isolation or in coordinated contractions to produce tri-planar movement for functional activities – this is achieved through isotonic contractions of the core musculature. Therefore, a comprehensive programme that targets both the main functions of the core should be implemented to train the core optimally. Compound lifts and unilateral movements with asymmetrical loading significantly challenge the core, and more task-specific, isolated core training can be implemented based on the client's individual needs. A holistic core training programme involves programming exercise options that incorporate various movement and contraction types, which are progressed over time.

References

Akuthota, V., Ferreiro, A., Moore, T., et al. (2008). Core stability exercise principles. *Current Sports Medicine Reports, 7*(1), 39–44.

Andersen, V., Fimland, M., Mo, D., et al. (2018). Electromyographic comparison of barbell deadlift, hex bar deadlift, and hip thrust exercises: a cross-over study. *Journal of Strength and Conditioning Research/National Strength & Conditioning Association, 32*(3), 587–593.

Andersen, V., Fimland, M., & Saeterbakken, A. (2019). Trunk muscle activity in one- and two-armed American kettlebell swing in resistance-trained men. *Sports Medicine International Open, 3*(1), E12–E18.

Andersson, E., Oddsson, L., Grundström, H., et al. (1996). EMG activities of the quadratus lumborum and erector spinae muscles during flexion-relaxation and other motor tasks. *Clinical Biomechanics, 11*(7), 392–400.

Behm, D., Drinkwater, E., Willardson, J., et al. (2010a). Canadian society for exercise physiology position stand: the use of instability to train the core in athletic and nonathletic conditioning. *Applied Physiology, Nutrition, and Metabolism, 35*(1), 109–112.

Behm, D., Drinkwater, E., Willardson, J. M., et al. (2010b). The use of instability to train the core musculature. *Applied Physiology, Nutrition, and Metabolism, 35*(1), 91–108.

Behm, D., Leonard, A., Young, W., et al. (2005). Trunk muscle electromyographic activity with unstable and unilateral exercises. *The Journal of Strength and Conditioning Research, 19*(1), 193–201.

Behm, D., Muehlbauer, T., Kibele, A., et al. (2015). Effects of strength training using unstable surfaces on strength, power and balance performance across the lifespan: a systematic review and meta-analysis. *Sports Medicine, 45*(12), 1645–1669.

Bergmark, A. (1989). Stability of the lumbar spine. A study in mechanical engineering. *Acta Orthopaedica Scandinavica, 230*, 1–54.

Bliven, K., Huxel Bliven, K., & Anderson, B. (2013). Core stability training for injury prevention. *Sports Health: A Multidisciplinary Approach, 5*(6), 514–522.

Brown, S., Vera-Garcia, F., & McGill, S. (2006). Effects of abdominal muscle coactivation on the externally preloaded trunk: variations in motor control and its effect on spine stability. *Spine, 31*(13), E387–E393.

Burnett, A., O'Sullivan, P., Ankarberg, L., et al. (2008). Lower lumbar spine axial rotation is reduced in end-range sagittal postures when compared to a neutral spine posture. *Manual Therapy, 13*(4), 300–306.

Cholewicki, J., Panjabi, M., & Khachatryan, A. (1997). Stabilising function of trunk flexor-extensor muscles around a neutral spine posture. *Spine, 22*(19), 2207–2212.

Ekstrom, R., Donatelli, R., & Carp, K. (2007). Electromyographic analysis of core trunk, hip, and thigh muscles during 9 rehabilitation exercises. *Journal of Orthopaedic & Sports Physical Therapy, 37*(12), 754–762.

Escamilla, R., Lewis, C., Pecson, A., et al. (2016). Muscle activation among supine, prone, and side position exercises with and without a Swiss ball. *Sports Health: A Multidisciplinary Approach, 8*(4), 372–379.

Farinatti, P., da Silva, N., & Monteiro, W. (2013). Influence of exercise order on the number of repetitions, oxygen uptake, and rate of perceived exertion during strength training in younger and older women. *Journal of Strength and Conditioning Research, 27*(3), 776–785.

Georgopoulos, A. (2000). Neural aspects of cognitive motor control. *Current Opinion in Neurobiology, 10*(2), 238–241.

Grenier, S., & McGill, S. (2007). Quantification of lumbar stability by using 2 different abdominal activation strategies. *Archives of Physical Medicine and Rehabilitation, 88*(1), 54–62.

Heaselgrave, S., Blacker, J., Smeuninx, B., et al. (2019). Dose-response relationship of weekly resistance-training volume and frequency on muscular adaptations in trained men. *International Journal of Sports Physiology and Performance, 14*(3), 360–368.

Hewit, J. (2018). A comparison of muscle activation during the pull-up and three alternative pulling exercises. *Journal of Physical Fitness, Medicine & Treatment in Sports, 5*(4), 1–7.

Hibbs, A., Thompson, K., French, D., et al. (2008). Optimising performance by improving core stability and core strength. *Sports Medicine, 38*(12), 995–1008.

Hodges, P., Holm, A., Holm, S., et al. (2003). Intervertebral stiffness of the spine is increased by evoked contraction of transversus abdominis and the diaphragm: in vivo porcine studies. *Spine, 28*(23), 2594–2601.

Hodges, P., & Richardson, C. (1996). Inefficient muscular stabilisation of the lumbar spine associated with low back pain. *Spine, 21*(22), 2640–2650.

Hodges, P., & Richardson, C. (1997). Feed-forward contraction of transversus abdominis is not influenced by the direction of arm movement. *Experimental Brain Research, 114*(2), 362–370.

Hodges, P., & Richardson, C. (1998). Delayed postural contraction of transversus abdominis in low back pain associated with movement of the lower limb. *Journal of Spinal Disorders, 11*(1), 46–56.

Kibler, W., Press, J., & Sciascia, A. (2006). The role of core stability in athletic function. *Sports Medicine, 36*(3), 189–198.

Lederman, E. (2010). The myth of core stability. *Journal of Bodywork and Movement Therapies, 14*(1), 84–98.

Lee, C. (2018). Korean upper extremity performance test for the elderly: normative data and characteristics of upper extremity function of adults and older adults. *American Journal of Occupational Therapy, 72*(4).

Majewski-Schrage, T., Evans, T., & Ragan, B. (2014). Development of a core-stability model: a Delphi approach. *Journal of Sport Rehabilitation, 23*(2), 95–106.

Mangine, G., Hoffman, J., Gonzalez, A., et al. (2015). The effect of training volume and intensity on improvements in muscular strength and size in resistance-trained men. *Physiological Reports, 3*(8). e12472.

Marcolin, G., Petrone, N., Moro, T., et al. (2015). Selective activation of shoulder, trunk, and arm muscles: a comparative analysis of different push-up variants. *Journal of Athletic Training, 50*(11), 1126–1132.

Martín-Fuentes, I., Oliva-Lozano, J., & Muyor, J. (2020). Electromyographic activity in deadlift exercise and its variants. A systematic review. *PLoS One, 15*(2), e0229507.

Martuscello, J., Nuzzo, J., Ashley, C., et al. (2013). Systematic review of core muscle activity during physical fitness exercises. *Journal of Strength and Conditioning Research, 27*(6), 1684–1698.

McGill, S. (2001). Low back stability: from formal description to issues for performance and rehabilitation. *Exercise and Sport Sciences Reviews, 29*(1), 26–31.

McGill, S. M., Childs, A., & Liebenson, C. (1999). Endurance times for low back stabilisation exercises: clinical targets for testing and training from a normal database. *Archives of Physical Medicine and Rehabilitation, 80*(8), 941–944.

McGill, S. M., & Marshall, L. W. (2012). Kettlebell swing, snatch, and bottoms-up carry: back and hip muscle activation, motion, and low back loads. *Journal of Strength and Conditioning Research/National Strength & Conditioning Association, 26*(1), 16–27.

McGill, S., McDermott, A., & Fenwick, C. (2009). Comparison of different strongman events: trunk muscle activation and lumbar spine motion, load, and stiffness. *Journal of Strength and Conditioning Research, 23*(4), 1148–1161.

Miranda, H., Figueiredo, T., Rodrigues, B., et al. (2013). Influence of exercise order on repetition performance among all possible combinations on resistance training. *Research in Sports Medicine, 21*(4), 355–366.

Moreau, C., Green, B., Johnson, C., et al. (2001). Isometric back extension endurance tests: a review of the literature. *Journal of Manipulative and Physiological Therapeutics, 24*(2), 110–122.

Morris, S., Lay, B., & Allison, G. (2013). Transversus abdominis is part of a global not local muscle synergy during arm movement. *Human Movement Science, 32*(5), 1176–1185.

Nairn, B., Chisholm, S., & Drake, J. (2013). What is slumped sitting? A kinematic and electromyographical evaluation. *Manual Therapy, 18*(6), 498–505.

Ogasawara, R., Yasuda, T., Ishii, N., et al. (2013). Comparison of muscle hypertrophy following 6-month of continuous and periodic strength training. *European Journal of Applied Physiology, 113*(4), 975–985.

O'Sullivan, K., O'Dea, P., Dankaerts, W., et al. (2010). Neutral lumbar spine sitting posture in pain-free subjects. *Manual Therapy, 15*(6), 557–561.

Panjabi, M. (1992a). The stabilizing system of the spine. Part II. Neutral zone and instability hypothesis. *Journal of Spinal Disorders, 5*(4), 390–397.

Panjabi, M. (1992b). The stabilizing system of the spine. Part I. Function, dysfunction, adaptation, and enhancement. *Journal of Spinal Disorders, 5*(4), 383–389.

Parkhouse, K., & Ball, N. (2010). Influence of dynamic versus static core exercises on performance in field based fitness tests. *Journal of Bodywork and Movement Therapies, 5*(4), 517–524.

Prieske, O., Muehlbauer, T., & Granacher, U. (2016). The role of trunk muscle strength for physical fitness and athletic performance in trained individuals: a systematic review and meta-analysis. *Sports Medicine, 46*(3), 401–419.

Reed, C., Ford, K., Myer, G., et al. (2012). The effects of isolated and integrated "core stability" training on athletic performance measures. *Sports Medicine, 42*(8), 697–706. https://doi.org/10.1007/bf03262289.

Ribeiro, A., Schoenfeld, B., & Sardinha, L. (2017). Comment on: a review of the acute effects and long-term adaptations of single- and multi-joint exercises during resistance training. *Sports Medicine, 47*(4), 791–793.

Robison, R. (1992). The new back school prescription: stabilisation training. Part I. *Occupational Medicine, 7*(1), 17–31.

Saal, J. (1992). The new back school prescription: stabilization training. Part II. *Occupational Medicine, 7*(1), 33–32.

Saeterbakken, A., Andersen, V., Brudeseth, A., et al. (2015). The effect of performing bi- and unilateral row exercises on core muscle activation. *International Journal of Sports Medicine, 36*(11), 900–905.

Saeterbakken, A., & Fimland, M. (2012). Muscle activity of the core during bilateral, unilateral, seated and standing resistance exercise. *European Journal of Applied Physiology, 112*(5), 1671–1678.

Schoenfeld, B., Contreras, B., Tiryaki-Sonmez, G., et al. (2014). An electromyographic comparison of a modified version of the plank with a long lever and posterior tilt versus the traditional plank exercise. *Sports Biomechanics, 13*(3), 296–306.

Schoenfeld, B., Ogborn, D., & Krieger, J. (2016). Effects of resistance training frequency on measures of muscle hypertrophy: a systematic review and meta-analysis. *Sports Medicine, 46*(11), 1689–1697.

Sheikholeslami-Vatani, D., Ahmadi, S., & Salavati, R. (2016). Comparison of the effects of resistance exercise orders on number of repetitions, serum IGF-1, testosterone and cortisol levels in normal-weight and obese men. *Asian Journal of Sports Medicine, 7*(1), e30503.

Souza, G., Baker, L., & Powers, C. (2001). Electromyographic activity of selected trunk muscles during dynamic spine stabilisation exercises. *Archives of Physical Medicine and Rehabilitation, 82*(11), 1551–1557.

Spencer, S., Wolf, A., & Rushton, A. (2016). Spinal-exercise prescription in sport: classifying physical training and rehabilitation by intention and outcome. *Journal of Athletic Training, 51*(8), 613–628.

Spineti, J., de Salles, B., Rhea, M., et al. (2010). Influence of exercise order on maximum strength and muscle volume in nonlinear periodized resistance training. *Journal of Strength and Conditioning Research, 24*(11), 2962–2969.

Tayashiki, K., Takai, Y., Maeo, S., et al. (2015). Intra-abdominal pressure and trunk muscular activities during abdominal bracing and hollowing. *International Journal of Sports Medicine, 37*(2), 134–143.

van den Tillaar, R., & Saeterbakken, A. (2018). Comparison of core muscle activation between a prone bridge and 6-RM back squats. *Journal of Human Kinetics, 62,* 43–53.

van Dieën, J., Kingma, I., & van der Bug, J. (2003). Evidence for a role of antagonistic cocontraction in controlling trunk stiffness during lifting. *Journal of Biomechanics, 36*(12), 1829–1836.

Vigotsky, A., Harper, E., Ryan, D., et al. (2015). Effects of load on good morning kinematics and EMG activity. *PeerJ, 3,* e708.

White, S., & McNair, P. (2002). Abdominal and erector spinae muscle activity during gait: the use of cluster analysis to identify patterns of activity. *Clinical Biomechanics, 17*(3), 177–184.

Willardson, J. (2004). The effectiveness of resistance exercises performed on unstable equipment. *Strength and Conditioning Journal, 26*(5), 70–74.

Wirth, K., Hartmann, H., Mickel, C., et al. (2017). Core stability in athletes: a critical analysis of current guidelines. *Sports Medicine, 47*(3), 401–414.

Yavuz, H., Erdağ, D., Amca, A., et al. (2015). Kinematic and EMG activities during front and back squat variations in maximum loads. *Journal of Sports Sciences, 33*(10), 1058–1066.

13 Resistance training

Paul Hough

Regular resistance training (RT) improves muscle strength (i.e., the ability of a muscle to produce external force), which is why RT is also known as strength training. Athletes have historically performed RT to improve athletic performance, increase muscle mass, and reduce injury risk (Suchomel et al., 2016). However, increases in strength and muscle mass are not just beneficial for athletes. Regular RT improves physical and mental health and reduces the risk of several chronic diseases (Saeidifard et al., 2019; Stamatakis et al., 2018; Wescott, 2012). Consequently, muscle-strengthening activities are included in global physical activity guidelines for adults, children and seniors (World Health Organization [WHO], 2020). A detailed discussion on RT for improving health follows later in this chapter.

Improvements in strength and health outcomes following RT occur due to a combination of physiological and anatomical adaptations (see Table 13.1), which are dependent on the training stimulus (e.g., intensity and volume). Although a detailed discussion of the physiological adaptations to RT is beyond the scope of this book, a basic understanding of the adaptive mechanisms is required to design bespoke programmes that target specific adaptations and outcomes. The following section will summarise the fundamental mechanisms and processes by which RT causes increases in strength and muscle growth (hypertrophy). Specific programming considerations for improving health, hypertrophy and maximal strength are presented later.

Resistance training adaptations

Neural adaptations

Strength gains can be achieved without significant structural musculoskeletal changes, such as hypertrophy, due to adaptations that occur within the nervous system (Carroll et al., 2019). Indeed, initial improvements in strength at the onset (1–8 weeks) of regular RT occur predominantly due to neural adaptations (see Table 13.1) (Del Vecchio et al., 2019; Škarabot

DOI: 10.4324/9781003204657-13

et al., 2021). Over time there is a gradual increase in hypertrophic factors, which are associated with improvements in strength (Seynnes et al., 2007).

Table 13.1 Principal physiological adaptations to resistance training

Adaptation	Meaning
↑ Motor unit recruitment	An increase in the number of motor units that can be recruited (Folland & Williams, 2007)
↑ Motor unit synchronisation	An increase in the probability of motor units firing at a near-simultaneous discharge rate (Felici et al., 2001)
↑ Rate coding	An increase in the motor unit firing rates (action potentials per unit of time) (Leong et al.,1999)
Changes in corticospinal tract function	Enhanced efficiency of the motor pathways from the central nervous system to the peripheral nervous system (Glover & Baker, 2020; Kidgell et al., 2017)
Muscle fibre hypertrophy	Increased cross-sectional area of a muscle fibre and subsequent increase in size of the muscle as a whole (Folland & Williams, 2007)
Sarcoplasmic hypertrophy	Increased volume of sarcoplasm relative to myofibril protein accretion (Roberts et al., 2020)

Muscle hypertrophy

Skeletal muscle fibres experience growth following regular, progressive RT due to many factors, such as changes in muscle protein turnover, satellite cells and molecular regulatory processes (Sartori et al., 2021; Wackerhage et al., 2019). The protein content of a muscle fibre is determined by the dynamic balance of muscle protein synthesis (MPS) and breakdown, which over time determines whether muscle tissue is maintained, lost or gained. The regulation of protein balance involves a complex series of molecular events within the muscle cells (Sartori et al., 2021). When the rate of MPS exceeds muscle protein breakdown there is a net increase in myofibrillar proteins (Glass, 2005; MacDougall et al., 1984; Phillips, 2014). Over time, a consistent increase in MPS following RT results in the accretion of contractile proteins and corresponding muscle hypertrophy (Coffey & Hawley, 2007; Marcotte et al., 2015). Although the exact mechanisms that regulate hypertrophy are complex and have not been fully clarified (Damas et al., 2016; Wackerhage et al., 2019), the generation of tension within skeletal muscle fibres during RT is fundamental to inducing hypertrophy (see page 241).

Should clients who do not want to increase muscle mass avoid resistance training?

Gains in strength without substantial hypertrophy can occur due to neural adaptations (see Table 13.1). Therefore, clients who do not seek hypertrophy

---

BOX 13.1

Do you need to lift heavy loads to increase muscle size?

Jozo Grgic

When the sets are performed to repetition failure, there is compelling evidence that low-load and high-load resistance training (RT) may produce similar increases in muscle size. For example, a 2017 meta-analysis reported no statistically significant difference between the effects of low-load and high-load RT on muscle hypertrophy (Schoenfeld et al., 2017a). From a mechanistic perspective, comparable hypertrophy experienced with both (low and high) loading schemes is likely explained by the size principle (Henneman, 1957). According to the size principle, motor units are recruited in an orderly fashion to produce the force needed for a given task (Henneman, 1957). In general, smaller (low-threshold) motor units innervate type I muscle fibres and larger (high-threshold) motor units innervate type II muscle fibres (Burke, 1981). For most muscle groups, the upper limit of motor unit recruitment occurs when exercising with ~85% of maximum force (Duchateau et al., 2006). In other words, when exercising with high-loads (e.g., 80–90% of 1RM), all the available motor units are recruited at the onset of the exercise (Duchateau et al., 2006).

When exercising with low-loads, muscle fibres 'take turns' at producing force. At the beginning of a set with a low-load (e.g., 30% of 1RM), lower threshold motor units associated with type I muscle fibres are initially recruited to lift the load. As the set progresses, type I fibres fatigue, necessitating the recruitment of higher threshold motor units associated with type II muscle fibres to maintain force production. If the set is performed to repetition failure, there should be a recruitment of the entire motor unit pool (i.e., low and high threshold motor units). High levels of motor unit recruitment, coupled with the mechanical loading experienced by the muscle fibres, are likely the primary reasons for the similar effects of low-load and high-load RT on muscle hypertrophy (Schoenfeld et al., 2017a).

Studies also report comparable increases in MPS and anabolic signaling when exercising with 30% or 80–90% of 1RM— provided the sets are performed near to repetition failure (Burd et al., 2010; Morton et al., 2019). In summary, low-load and high-load RT performed near to repetition failure may produce similar increases in muscle size because of their comparable effects on motor unit recruitment, and subsequently, on MPS and anabolic signaling.

---

should not be dissuaded from RT as, with the correct programme design, it is possible to increase strength without significant hypertrophy.

Muscle fibre types

Skeletal muscle is composed of varied fibre types that have different contractile and metabolic properties. Several types of muscle fibres have been identified, but for simplicity fibres are usually categorised into two types (type I and II fibres). Type I fibres (slow oxidative) have high concentrations of mitochondria and aerobic enzymes; consequently, they are resistant to fatigue and are used extensively during endurance-type activities, such as long-distance running. Conversely, type II fibres (IIA fast-oxidative glycolytic; IIX fast glycolytic) have faster shortening and relaxation speeds, and anaerobic properties (Scott et al., 2001). Therefore, type II fibres can produce higher levels of force and are involved in high-intensity activities (e.g., sprinting). Type II fibres are thought to have a greater capacity for growth compared to type I fibres following RT (Adams & Bamman, 2012). The combination of muscle fibre types varies between muscles and between individuals, which partly explains why some people are more suited to and successful at certain sports (Costill et al., 1976). For example, athletes competing in strength/power sports tend to have a higher proportion of type II fibres (Fry, 2004).

Why do some individuals experience greater improvements in strength and hypertrophy than others?

Both environmental and genetic factors influence the adaptations to training. Hence, the adaptations and outcomes from RT are highly variable between individuals (Ogasawara et al., 2016; Trezise & Blazevich, 2019). For instance, the variance in maximal strength (1RM) gains have been shown to range from 0% to 250% between individuals following the same RT programme (Hubal et al., 2005). Unlike manageable factors (e.g., programme design, nutrition, sleep) that can be quantified and controlled, genetic factors cannot. For example, genotype and muscle fibre composition are hereditary. Moreover, epigenetic (i.e., genetic control by factors other than a person's DNA) responses to an identical RT programme are also different between individuals (Bagley et al., 2020).

A client's muscle morphology partly dictates improvements in strength and muscle mass following RT. For example, clients with a higher proportion of type II muscle fibres might experience greater improvements in strength and hypertrophy than clients dominant in type I fibres, despite following an identical RT programme (Fry, 2004). The composition of muscle fibres is hereditary, but the characteristics of muscle fibres can be modified through training (e.g., type IIX can become more like type IIA fibres), which is known as fibre type shifting (Eftestøl et al., 2016; Methenitis et al., 2020). The magnitude by which muscle fibre types can shift with training is debated by researchers (Wilson et al., 2012); nevertheless, training programmes designed to enhance performance should adhere to the principle of specificity (see Chapter 6). For example, athletes who compete in sports requiring maximal levels of strength and power benefit from training type II fibres using high-intensity and explosive training methods (Methenitis et al., 2020).

Adaptations summary

- Resistance training induces physiological and anatomical adaptations that improve muscular strength and size, which is beneficial for health and performance.
- Muscle growth occurs following regular RT, provided the muscle fibres are exposed to sufficient mechanical tension.
- Muscle growth can be achieved using both heavy and light loads, provided sets with light loads are performed near to repetition failure.
- Skeletal muscle is composed of different types of fibres, which are often categorised into two types. Type I fibres have endurance-oriented properties, whereas type II fibres have faster shortening and relaxation speeds and anaerobic properties.
- The composition of muscle fibres varies within (between muscles) and between individuals, partly explaining why the magnitude of responses to RT (e.g., strength, power, and hypertrophy) differs between individuals.

Resistance training terminology

The load/resistance used during RT influences the acute and chronic physiological adaptations (see Table 13.1). Training loads are usually selected relative to the client's level of strength, commonly assessed via one-repetition maximum (1RM) or repetition maximum (RM) testing (see Chapter 7). Training load zones are broadly defined within the RT literature as low (light), moderate or heavy. For clarity, the definitions used within this chapter are summarised in Figure 13.1.

Micro-resistance training

A RT session usually consists of a warm-up and a series of exercises within a set period (e.g., 5–6 exercises within a 45-minute session). Most RT programmes adopted within the scientific literature consist of one session within a day performed on 2–6 days/week. Although this approach is effective for improving health, strength and hypertrophy outcomes, it can lead to missed or incomplete training sessions when training time is limited due to work, family or other obligations. Micro-RT is an alternative approach where exercises are spread across a day. For example, completing a set of push-ups, dumbbell squats and inverted rows every three hours (i.e., a total of nine sets across the day). This structure enables individuals who cannot complete a regular RT session to perform some RT as opposed to nothing.

Micro-RT allows long recovery periods between exercises, which could reduce fatigue and improve exercise technique. Indeed, athletes often perform two daily sessions, instead of one, to minimise fatigue and maximise performance (Hartman et al., 2007). Nevertheless, there are potential

Training status

The time the client has been consistently (≥2 sessions per week) training for

Novice (untrained)	Intermediate	Advanced
<6 months	6 – 12 months	>12 months

Intensity of load

The percentage of one repetition maximum (1RM) used during an exercise

Intensity of effort

The perceived effort exerted during an exercise, generally assessed using a subjective scale or the proximity to repetition failure

Repetition failure (RF)

The point during an exercise where the muscles cannot produce enough concentric force to complete a full repetition, despite the lifter exerting maximal effort

Technical failure

The point during an exercise where the lifter's technique deteriorates due to fatigue

Proximity to failure

The point where the lifter ends the set before repetition failure (i.e., closeness to RF)

Repetition maximum (RM)

The maximum load lifted for a specified number of repetitions

Loading zones

Low Load	Moderate Load	Heavy Load
<65% 1RM	65 - 85% 1RM	≥85% 1RM
≥12RM	12 - 6RM	≤6RM

Repetition volume

Total number of repetitions completed during a RT session (sets x reps)

Volume-load

Combination of the load and repetition volume (sets x repetitions x load)

Hard set

A set performed with a high degree of perceived effort, at (or near) repetition failure

Set volume

The number of hard sets performed per muscle group over a defined period (e.g., one session or one week)

Inter-set rest interval duration

Time elapsed between consecutive sets of the same exercise

Short	Moderate	Long
<1 minute	1 – 2 minutes	>2-5 minutes

Figure 13.1 Resistance training terminology.

disadvantages with micro-RT. For example, the method is usually performed away from a gym (e.g., at home or work) where less equipment is available. The time-efficiency benefits are also reduced when an extended warm-up period is required before performing exercises with heavy loads.

Some high-intensity interval training (HIIT) research indicates that micro doses of HIIT spread across a day (aka high-intensity snacks) can improve health and fitness outcomes (see Chapter 11). However, the efficacy of micro-RT for improving health, strength and hypertrophy requires scientific investigation.

Exercise sequencing methods

The straight-set method involves performing a defined number of repetitions (a set) followed by a rest period before initiating the next set. Numerous set schemes can be employed, whereby the load/repetitions can remain constant or vary between sets (e.g., pyramids and wave-loading). The prescribed load will vary depending on the RT goals (see Chapter 7). A typical RT session includes a series of exercises performed for a target number of sets. For example, three sets of squats followed by three sets of bench press. Alternative exercise sequencing methods and techniques, often known as advanced methods (see Table 13.2), can be programmed to increase one or more training variables. However, advanced methods should be programmed carefully based on the client's readiness to train and the goal of the session.

When is it appropriate to increase the load or repetitions?

Several load progression models can be used to determine when it is appropriate to increase the training load. As progression is not linear (see Box 13.1), progression models should be used periodically. Relative intensity monitoring methods, such as repetitions in reserve (RIR), can be used during every training session to indicate when an increase in load is appropriate (see Chapter 7). For example, assuming a client did 12 repetitions on the bench press with 40 kg with an RIR rating of three, all things being equal (exercise, load, repetitions), an increase in load could be appropriate if the client provided an RIR of four during two consecutive sessions.

The 'two for two' method

In the 'two for two' method, the load or repetition prescription is increased when the client can perform two or more repetitions above the prescribed number of repetitions for two consecutive training sessions (without compromising technique). For example, if a client was prescribed 3 × 10 repetitions and he was able to perform 3 × 12 for two consecutive training sessions, an increase in load or another variable (see Table 13.3) could be indicated. A general recommendation is to apply a 2–10% increase in load (American College of Sports Medicine [ACSM], 2009). However, the load increment will vary depending on the exercise, the client's training status,

Table 13.2 Alternative exercise sequencing methods and techniques

Method	Description	Main purpose
Agonist-antagonist paired sets (super-sets)	Two exercises for opposing muscle groups performed in succession with minimal rest (e.g., bench press and barbell row)	↑ Volume (sets) ↑ Density (more work within a set time)
Compound sets	Two exercises for the same muscle group performed in succession with minimal rest (e.g., bench press and dumbbell flyes)	↑ Volume (sets) ↑ Density (more work within a set time)
Tri-sets	Three exercises for the same muscle group performed in succession with minimal rest	↑ Volume (sets) ↑ Density (more work within a set time)
Giant sets	More than three exercises for the same muscle group performed in succession with minimal rest	↑ Volume (sets) ↑ Density (more work within a set time)
Circuits	A sequence of consecutive RT exercises performed for a defined number of repetitions or set amount of time.	↑ Volume (sets) ↑ Density (more work within a set time)
Forced/assisted repetitions	A spotter provides the lifter with enough assistance to overcome the sticking point in the repetition	↑ Volume (repetitions) ↑ Intensity of effort
Partial Repetitions	Repetitions performed within a lesser range of motion than typically performed (e.g., achieving 70° knee flexion instead of 90° during the squat)	↑ Intensity of load ↑ Volume (repetitions)
Cheating	Modifying technique to continue to perform more repetitions	↑ Intensity of effort ↑ Volume (repetitions)
Drop sets/strip sets	Decreasing the resistance used immediately after reaching repetition failure to allow additional repetitions to be performed	↑ Volume
Eccentric training/heavy negatives	Focussing on the eccentric component of an exercise using a load greater than can be lifted concentrically (i.e., >1RM)*	↑ Intensity of load

Usually requires a spotter

and equipment. For example, larger increments of 2.5–5 kg (~5–10 lbs) are usually possible in compound exercises, such as a deadlift, although exercises involving fewer muscle groups require smaller increments (e.g., 1.25–2.5 kg). As a client accrues RT experience and less trainability (see Chapter 6), the load progression typically becomes smaller. Novice clients could increase load by 5–10%, whereas 2–5% increments are more appropriate and realistic for advanced clients.

BOX 13.2

Applying progressive overload in resistance training

Bret Contreras

It is important to recognise that the body adapts to a stressor, not a specific load or number of repetitions. Most RT programmes are based on providing an overload quantitatively (i.e., more load and/or repetitions). However, several other methods can be applied to increase physiological stress. In simple terms, progressive overload (PO) means doing more over time (see Chapter 6). While the art of PO would require an entire chapter to discuss, the fundamental premise is that regularly setting personal records (PRs) and gaining strength in various repetition ranges and modalities increases the tension applied to muscles over time. This leads to favourable neuromuscular adaptations (Trezise & Blazevich, 2019) and increases mechanical tension; the primary driver of hypertrophy (Burkholder, 2007). Novices often, mistakenly, believe that PO only involves increasing load (lifting heavier weights), but there are several ways to apply PO. Ten of the most common methods are listed in Table 13.3. These include abbreviations to assist in recording the type of PRs within a training log.

Applying progressive overload in practice

Clients should not be expected to set PRs every workout or even every week, particularly as they become more experienced with RT. If a client increased load on the bench press by 5 lbs/week, she would be bench pressing 260 more pounds for the same number of repetitions in one year, which obviously will not happen. Furthermore, even a monthly increase of 5 lbs on the bench press is unlikely on a consistent basis; otherwise, the client would be lifting 60 lbs more every year for the same number of repetitions. Using repetitions as an example, if a client performed one additional repetition a month on the chin up, she would, theoretically, achieve 12 additional repetitions in a year. This would mean 60+ consecutive chin-ups in five years. Again, it should be evident to most trainers that this linear progression does not happen in practice. PO is a slow and non-linear process. However, every six months clients should be noticeably stronger at some exercises in specific repetition ranges, and trainers should always strive to increase the challenge to the muscles over time, using a combination of the approaches described in Table 13.3.

Tempo

The duration of a repetition and set is determined by the tempo used during the exercise. The tempo of a dynamic exercise is often conveyed as a three-number sequence, where each number represents time in seconds (e.g., 1-1-3). The first number is the time to complete the concentric action (e.g., lifting the weight); the second number is the transition (isometric) phase between the concentric and eccentric actions (e.g., the bottom of a

Table 13.3 Examples of progressive overload methods (Contreras, 2021)

Method	Description	Example
Intensity of load	More load for same number of reps	Bench pressing 100 kg for 6 reps to 110 kg for 6 reps.
Intensity of effort	Same load × reps with lower rating of perceived exertion (RPE)	Bodyweight chin ups for 3 × 6 reps to 3 × 6 reps with a lower RPE.
Volume (repetitions)	More reps with same load	Back extensions with 30 kg for 10 reps to 30 kg for 11 reps.
Volume (sets)	More sets with same load × reps	Bent over row 80 lbs for 3 × 10 reps to 80 lbs for 4 × 10 reps.
Range of motion (ROM)	Increased ROM with same load × reps	Squatting 205 lbs × 5 reps to parallel to 205 lbs × 5 reps 2 inches below parallel.
Form	Improved technique with the same load × reps	Deadlifting 180 kg × 3 reps to 180 kg × 3 reps without rounding the back.
Mind-muscle connection (MMC)	Increasing muscle squeeze with same load × reps	Hip thrusting 100 kg × 12 reps to 100 kg × 12 reps while feeling the contraction more in the gluteals.
Time	Same volume-load in less time	Military pressing 50 kg for 3 × 8 reps with 3 minutes rest between sets to 50 kg for 3 × 8 reps with 2 minutes rest between sets.
Bodyweight	Same load × reps with a change in bodyweight	Doing 16 push-ups while weighing 75 kg to doing 16 reps while weighing 80 kg (weighing more with BW exercises), or 50 kg lunges × 8 reps while weighing 80 kg to 50 kg lunges × 8 reps while weighing 75 kg (weighing less with free weight exercises).
Advanced methods	Increasing volume, intensity or density	See Table 13.2

BW = Bodyweight; Reps = Repetitions; RPE = Rating of perceived exertion

squat); the third number is the duration of the eccentric action. The load used for an exercise usually dictates the tempo because the muscle fibres require more time to produce force as the load increases. The tempo is also affected by set volume, as the repetition duration usually decreases towards the end of a set due to fatigue. Although the tempo is mostly a function of an exercise's load and volume, it can be manipulated by intentionally performing exercises at a faster or slower cadence.

Is there an optimal tempo for resistance training exercises?

During the concentric action of most exercises the goal should be to exert force as quickly as possible, particularly when training to improve power

(Methenitis et al., 2020). Intentionally performing the concentric portion of the lift very slowly can reduce muscle activation and result in sub-optimal adaptations (Schuenke et al., 2012). However, when using very light loads (<50% 1RM) a slightly slower (~2 seconds), concentric action can be used to maintain attentional focus and ensure the load is lifted under control. A one second isometric pause at the end of the concentric action facilitates maintaining proper exercise form and minimises the stretch-shortening cycle (SSC). The SSC is a neuromuscular spring-like mechanism that can be exploited during plyometric exercises.

Deliberately slowing the eccentric action of an exercise could result in greater improvements in strength (Westcott et al., 2001) and hypertrophy (Shibata et al., 2018). However, adopting a very slow tempo could decrease the recruitment of type II muscle fibres, which are more responsive to growth (Schuenke et al., 2012). There is likely a repetition duration threshold, where very slow repetitions necessitate a reduction in intensity or repetitions/set, which is sub-optimal for strength and hypertrophy outcomes. Repetitions lasting 0.5–8 seconds seem to produce similar hypertrophy when sets are performed to repetition failure; however, extending the duration of repetitions to ≥10 seconds could reduce the hypertrophic effect (Schoenfeld et al., 2015).

Performing exercises at a deliberately slow tempo (particularly eccentric actions) can increase muscle damage and soreness (Fridén & Lieber, 1992), which could increase discomfort and extend the recovery time required between training sessions. Conversely, rapid eccentric actions (e.g., dropping into the bottom of a squat) can decrease muscle activation, resulting in sub-optimal technique and potential injury. Therefore, performing the eccentric action of most RT exercises at a measured speed (1–3 seconds) encourages the exercise to be performed under control with high attentional focus (Calatayud et al., 2016). In summary, a tempo of 1-1-2 or 1-1-3 is recommended for most exercises.

Exercise technique

Exercise technique and the range of motion (ROM) used during an exercise affects muscle activation patterns, the torques (turning forces) at each joint and the points in the movement where peak forces occur (Chiu et al., 2017; Slater & Hart, 2017). Consequently, changes in technique during an exercise can affect how the tissues (e.g., bone, muscle and tendon) are loaded. Therefore, each repetition during a set should be performed with a consistent technique to reduce injury risk and optimise technique.

Is there an optimal range of motion for an exercise?

Strength is ROM-specific meaning that strength improvements occur in the movements, joint angles and muscle lengths used during the exercise

(Pedrosa et al., 2021). Altering ROM during a set can make it difficult to quantify progressive overload between sessions. For example, reducing the ROM towards the end of a set of squats (less depth) could allow more repetitions to be completed. However, an apparent improvement in strength (more repetitions) could be due to the decrease in ROM rather than an improvement in neuromuscular adaptations. Furthermore, significant changes in ROM during an exercise could shift loading and recruitment patterns between muscle groups and may result in suboptimal hypertrophy of the target muscle group.

The ROM used for an exercise will vary between clients based on their anthropometry, strength and mobility. Performing exercises through a full ROM and training muscles at long (stretched) lengths, can promote hypertrophy of the lower-body musculature, at least in certain muscles (Maeo et al., 2021; Schoenfeld & Grgic, 2020) Similarly, superior neuromuscular adaptations were reported in participants performing a full ROM bench-press compared to partial ROM variations during a 10-week training programme (Martínez-Cava et al., 2019). Therefore, clients should be encouraged perform exercises using their full ROM.

Should training through a partial range of motion be avoided?

Performing exercises through a full ROM can produce greater strength and hypertrophy outcomes, but this does not mean exercises performed with a partial ROM should be avoided altogether. Using a partial ROM enables heavier loads to be used, which could improve strength in the full ROM version of the exercise (Bazyler et al., 2014). Furthermore, the passive mechanical tension generated when a muscle is stretched during a RT exercise could provide an added hypertrophic stimulus (Simpson et al., 2017; Tatsumi, 2010). Therefore, performing a specific exercise with a partial ROM, focussing on the position where the target muscle is maximally stretched, could be a viable technique to promote hypertrophy of certain muscles (Pedrosa et al., 2021).

Resistance training for health
Paul Hough

Exercise recommendations for improving health have traditionally focused on endurance (cardiorespiratory) exercise. However, RT is also beneficial for the general population (Wescott, 2012; WHO, 2020). Alongside improving strength, regular RT is associated with reduced risk of cardiovascular disease, type II diabetes, certain cancers and other chronic diseases (Saeidifard et al., 2019; Stamatakis et al., 2018). Furthermore, RT is particularly beneficial for older adults (see Chapter 16). The improvements in neuromuscular adaptations following RT (see Table 13.1) are well-documented. Over the past 20 years, numerous other physiological benefits from RT that contribute to improved health outcomes have been identified; these are briefly summarised below.

Physiological benefits of resistance training

Systemic benefits

During RT, skeletal muscle releases cytokines and other muscle fibre-derived peptides, collectively termed 'myokines'. The release of myokines, such as IL-15, and brain-derived neurotrophic factor (BDNF), seem to positively affect other tissues and organs, such as the liver and brain (Lee & Jun, 2019; Pedersen et al., 2007). Furthermore, myokines could provide beneficial health effects by regulating skeletal muscle regeneration, and improving glucose uptake and fat oxidation (Leal et al., 2018; Pedersen et al., 2007). Indeed, a promising metabolic effect of RT is improving glucose and insulin metabolism (Thyfault & Bergouignan, 2020).

Insulin sensitivity

Insulin is a hormone that enables cells throughout the body to absorb glucose from the blood. When the cells do not respond adequately to insulin (insulin resistance), this causes hyperglycemia (high blood glucose), the predominant symptom of diabetes mellitus. Muscle tissue is the largest disposal site for ingested glucose and plays a vital role in glucose metabolism (Holloszy, 2005). Thus, increasing muscle mass, through progressive RT can improve glucose metabolism. The improvement in glucose metabolism following RT is not purely a consequence of an increase in muscle size. Regular RT also induces favourable metabolic changes within skeletal muscle, such as enhanced insulin action (Ishii et al., 1998) and increased GLUT-4 (glucose transporter protein) translocation (Strasser & Pesta, 2013).

Cardiovascular disease risk factors

Emerging research indicates regular RT can improve several markers of cardiovascular health, such as lowering blood pressure (MacDonald et al., 2016), reducing visceral fat (Dutheil et al., 2013), and improving endothelial function (Boeno et al., 2019).

Resting metabolic rate

Muscle is a metabolically active tissue that contributes to the resting metabolic rate (RMR), which is the energy required by the body at rest. Skeletal muscle mass and RMR decline with age; however, regular RT can reduce muscle loss, improving metabolic function and reducing the increase in body fat that occurs with ageing (Tresierras & Balady, 2009). An increase in muscle mass following regular RT can also increase RMR by approximately 100 kcal/day, which could have a meaningful effect on bodyweight management over time (MacKenzie-Shalders et al., 2020). The magnitude of the increase in RMR varies between individuals due to factors, such as sex and the volume of muscle gained (Aristizabal et al., 2015).

Bone and connective tissue health

Regular RT, combined with high-impact exercises (e.g., running, hopping and jumping), can help to maintain or improve bone mineral density and reduce the risk of fractures (Cauley & Giangregorio, 2020). Additionally, RT is a proven therapeutic strategy to treat and manage musculoskeletal conditions, such as osteosarcopenia (Hong & Kim, 2018). Less research has been conducted into how connective tissues respond to long-term RT. However, RT can increase tendon stiffness, which could improve the force-generating capacity of muscles (Kubo et al., 2002). Additionally, RT could also reduce the age-related deterioration of tendons (Guzzoni et al., 2018).

The brain and cognitive function

The structure and function of the brain are negatively affected with ageing, resulting in a decline in cognitive function, such as memory and processing speed (Buckner, 2004; Raz et al., 2010). Encouragingly, several studies show that RT can induce structural changes in the brain associated with improvements in cognitive function (Landrigan et al., 2020; Wilke et al., 2019). Improved cognitive function following RT could partly be attributed to an increase in certain neurochemicals (e.g., IGF-1 and BDNF) that activate complex neurobiological processes and evoke functional and/or structural adaptations in the brain (Cotman et al., 2007; Hötting & Röder, 2013). For example, one study reported a strong relationship between increased levels of IGF-1 and improvements in executive functions (e.g., reaction time) after a year of RT in older adults (Tsai et al., 2015).

Resistance training for health recommendations

Exercise selection for health

Exercises should be selected based on the client's fitness, training experience and goals (see Chapter 7). Compound (multiple-joint) exercises that target the major muscle groups should be prioritised after the warm-up when the objective is to improve maximal strength; however, exercise order is less important for hypertrophy outcomes (Nunes et al., 2020). Novice clients may benefit from using resistance machines at the start of a training programme to build strength and condition the joints. Free-weight exercises can be introduced as the client's strength and exercise competency improves. Isolation (single-joint) exercises can be included after compound exercises to target the smaller muscle groups and address weaknesses or asymmetries (see Chapters 5 and 7).

Intensity of load for improving health outcomes

The strength-endurance continuum (aka the repetition maximum continuum) has historically been used to prescribe load based on the goal of the RT programme, where heavy (~≥85% 1RM) loads are recommended for improving strength, moderate (~67–85% 1RM) loads for hypertrophy, and light (≤67% 1RM) loads for local muscular endurance (Garber et al., 2011; Haff & Triplett, 2016). Research supports the concept of a strength-endurance continuum for improving maximal strength (see page 248). However, the prescription of near-maximal (≥85% 1RM) loads is not required to improve strength amongst novice or intermediate clients. Indeed, using near-maximal loads can increase the difficulty of developing the correct exercise technique, particularly with free-weight exercises.

Using loads between 30–85% 1RM has been shown to improve various health outcomes (see Figure 13.3). However, optimal loading ranges to improve specific health outcomes are uncertain due to differences in training protocols (e.g., intensity, proximity to failure, rest periods) between studies. The optimal intensity likely varies depending on the desired adaptation and the client's health status. For example, a higher (>75% 1RM vs. <75% 1RM) intensity RT programme was more effective in reducing glycated haemoglobin and insulin in patients with type II diabetes (Liu et al., 2019). Additionally, training with heavier loads may produce greater improvements in bone mineral density (Vincent & Braith, 2002). An optimal RT prescription for enhancing brain health and cognitive function has not been identified, as the neurobiological mechanisms of how RT can induce functional brain changes are currently under investigation.

Strength

Training with heavier loads (>60% of 1RM) tends to produce greater gains in dynamic strength than training with lighter (≤60% of 1RM) loads (Schoenfeld et al., 2017a). However, novice clients can benefit from using lighter (40–60% 1RM) loads to develop proficient technique and gradually increase the load as exercise proficiency improves. Conversely, trained clients may need to strategically lift heavier (≥80% 1RM) loads (see page 248).

Hypertrophy

Training with moderate loads (~67–85% 1RM), corresponding to a medium (6–12 RM) repetition range, provides a combination of mechanical tension and metabolic stress. Therefore, the 6–12 repetition range has historically been recommended for hypertrophy (Haff & Triplett, 2016; Kraemer & Ratamess, 2004). However, as discussed in Box 13.1, training with lighter loads produces similar hypertrophy compared to heavier (>70% 1RM) loads when exercises are performed to (or near to) repetition failure or when using blood flow restriction methods (see Box 13.3). In short, a broad range of loads can be used if hypertrophy is sought alongside other health outcomes (see Figure 13.3).

In summary, trainers should modify the training load based on the client's experience, health/fitness status and desired adaptations. Using loads between 50–80% 1RM is an appropriate general guideline for health-focused RT programmes, and near-maximal loads (≥85% 1RM) should be used with caution.

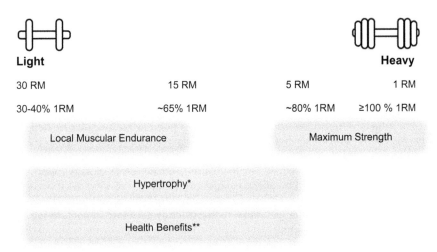

RM = Repetition maximum; 1RM = One repetition maximum; *Based on performing sets near repetition failure; **Some health outcomes may require loads towards the heavier end of the zone.

Figure 13.2 Intensity of load recommendations for different training goals.

Training to failure

Failure to complete a repetition at the end of a set occurs due to numerous physiological and psychological factors (e.g., neuromuscular fatigue, cardiovascular strain, and perception of fatigue and pain). Training to failure (TTF) describes lifting a load to the point where the muscles fail to produce enough concentric force to complete a full repetition, despite the lifter exerting maximal effort. As shown in Figure 13.4, the proximity to failure decreases as load increases due to the inverse relationship between the intensity of load and (repetition) volume.

BOX 13.3

Blood flow restriction: applications from the laboratory

Zachary Bell and Jeremy Loenneke

Blood flow restriction (BFR) is a training method whereby blood flow is reduced into the muscle of interest by the application of a cuff or wrap. BFR by itself, or in combination with low intensity/load exercise, has been shown to produce beneficial muscle adaptations (Patterson et al., 2019). Most of the research has focused on low load (20–30% maximum) resistance exercise in combination with BFR, which results in changes in muscle size and strength greater than performing the same exercise without BFR (Loenneke et al., 2012). The changes in muscle mass are comparable to that observed with high load exercise, but the changes in strength are typically less. Available evidence indicates that BFR is relatively safe, assuming the pressure is applied appropriately. For example, the pressure should be applied so that blood flow into the limb is only partially reduced (i.e., not arterial occlusion). BFR is primarily induced through the application of a cuff or wrap (see Figure 13.3), placed at the top of the arm or leg (Mattocks et al., 2018). BFR can also be applied practically via an elastic wrap, but this coincides with the inability to quantify the pressure being applied. The use of a subjective tightness scale ('7' out of 10) is popular but unreliable (Bell et al., 2019). Alternative methods include using a percentage of wrap length (Abe et al., 2019) or estimating the degree of restriction based on the number repetitions completed. If low loads are used (20–30% of maximum), then individuals should be able to achieve the majority of the goal repetitions across 4 sets of an exercise (75 total reps, 30-15-15-15, rest intervals of 30–60 s). If an individual is unable to consistently get close to completing that number of repetitions, then either the load is too high or the wraps are too tight. This technique has been effectively used in a variety of populations including those who are healthy as well as those rehabilitating from injury (Patterson et al., 2019).

- The benefit of BFR is that it allows an individual to train with low loads (20–30% maximum) and increase muscle size and strength over repetition matched exercise without restriction. Combining BFR with high loads (70% maximum) does not provide additional benefit over high loads without restriction.
- For changes in muscle size and strength, moderate pressures are as effective as high pressures (40–50% of pressure needed to cease blood flow). Applying practical BFR along with goal repetitions is a pragmatic way to monitor the level of restriction.
- BFR can be applied with a variety of exercises (e.g. squat, bench press, leg press, leg extension/flexion, bicep curls) but the cuffs/wraps should be placed only at the top of the arms or the top of the legs.

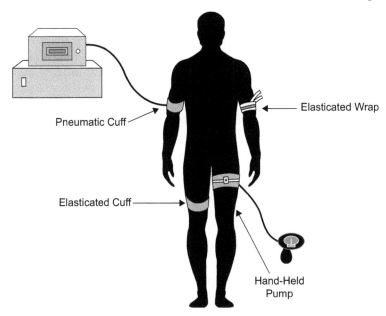

Figure 13.3 Blood flow restriction schematic.

Is training to failure necessary to improve health outcomes?

Novice clients have a high degree of trainability and require less training to elicit adaptations than intermediate and advanced counterparts (see Chapter 6). Adding more training stimulus, such as TTF, does not necessarily yield more benefits (Martorelli et al., 2017). Indeed, TTF is not essential to maximise MU recruitment (Sundstrup et al., 2012), does not necessarily produce superior improvements in strength (Davies et al., 2016), and could produce inferior muscle fibre adaptations than non-failure training (Carroll et al., 2019). Therefore, regular TTF is not obligatory, provided clients perform exercises within reasonable proximity to failure (e.g., 1–3 RIR). However, TTF is necessary and beneficial in certain circumstances, discussed next.

When determining a repetition maximum (RM) for an exercise (see Chapter 7), repetition failure will occur after the RM has been achieved (i.e., the RM will be the number of *complete* repetitions executed before failure). Periodically TTF allows clients to appreciate what it feels like to reach repetition failure, enabling proximity to failure (i.e., RIR) to be calibrated. Additionally, training close to failure with a high intensity of effort is indicated within low volume (e.g., 2–3 sets/week) training programmes (Androulakis-Korakakis et al., 2020) and when training for hypertrophy using light loads (see Box 13.1).

Issues with training to failure

Regular TTF, particularly when combined with short rest periods, could decrease the repetitions in proceeding sets and total training volume due to accumulative fatigue (Willardson, 2007; Willardson & Burkett, 2006). A reduction in volume with the target load could have a negative long-term effect on strength and hypertrophy outcomes. Moreover, TTF appears to prolong post-training neuromuscular fatigue compared to training short of failure (Morán-Navarro et al., 2017; Pareja-Blanco et al., 2020). Following a single-limb exercise performed to failure, the untrained limb demonstrates a reduction in strength 48-hours after training, indicating central nervous system (CNS) fatigue (Farrow et al., 2020). Interestingly, TTF with a lighter load has been reported to cause greater CNS fatigue in both the exercised and non-exercised limb compared to TTF with a heavier load (Farrow et al., 2020). Therefore, an extended recovery period between training sessions might be required after TTF with light loads (Izquierdo-Gabarren et al., 2010).

The acute physiological and psychological responses between TTF with light and heavy loads are different. As the load is decreased the set becomes longer (see Figure 13.4), and the accumulation of metabolites and cardiovascular strain increases (Gjovaag et al., 2016); these factors are associated with increased perception of discomfort during and after the exercise (Krieger, 2009; Ralston et al., 2017). Some clients may be deterred from TTF with light loads, although further research is needed to establish if the discomfort associated with high repetition training decreases with training experience. Finally, the perception

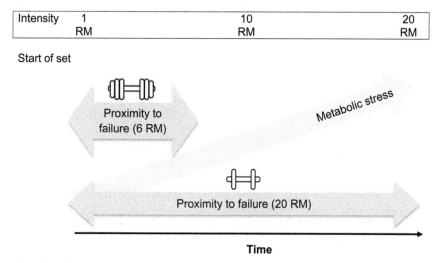

RM = Repetition maximum.

Figure 13.4 Training to failure.

of effort and discomfort is influenced by the type of exercise, particularly when TTF. Compound exercises, performed with moderate-heavy loads, are more technically demanding, require higher levels of stability/coordination, and induce more physiological strain than isolation exercises. Thus, TTF on technically demanding exercises with moderate-heavy loads should generally be avoided. In instances where TTF is deemed necessary, training to technical failure (see Figure 13.1) is more appropriate.

Volume for health RT programmes

Sets per session

Performing one set/exercise can produce meaningful improvements in strength amongst untrained men and women (Humburg et al., 2007; Radaelli et al., 2015). However, performing more than one set/exercise produces greater gains in strength and hypertrophy in both trained and untrained individuals (Krieger, 2009; Ralston et al., 2017). Performing three sets/exercise could also be more effective in reducing cardiovascular disease risk factors than one set/exercise (Correa et al., 2015).

Is there an upper limit of sets within a session?

The dose-response to training is not infinite (i.e., more training is not always better) as the body's adaptive capacity is limited (see Chapters 6 and 7). For example, one study showed that moderate volume (~9 sets/muscle group) training resulted in better strength and hypertrophy outcomes than high volume (~14 sets/muscle group) training during a six-week programme (Amirthalingam et al., 2017). Increasing training volume beyond an individual's adaptation threshold (see Chapter 6) does not stimulate a greater adaptive response and merely increases neuromuscular fatigue and possibly muscle damage (Boyas & Guével, 2011). Collectively, the RT literature indicates that the upper limit of productive training volume is ~9–13 hard sets/muscle group/session, although this varies between individuals. For instance, performing 3–5 sets/muscle group/session (possibly less) can produce beneficial outcomes for novice clients (Humburg et al., 2007; Radaelli et al., 2015).

Is single set training effective for trained clients?

Even clients with RT experience can improve strength by performing one set (2–3 sessions per week) using a load of ~70–85% 1RM, provided each set is performed close to failure (Androulakis-Korakakis et al., 2020).

However, most studies (e.g., Krieger et al., 2010) indicate that single set training is not optimal for improving strength or hypertrophy.

Sets per week

Increasing the number of sets/muscle-group/week tends to produce greater improvements in strength and hypertrophy, up to a point (Ralston et al., 2017; Schoenfeld et al., 2019a). However, an optimal weekly set volume has not been identified. Some studies have indicated that exceeding a particular training volume does not yield further benefits. For example, exceeding 20 sets/muscle-group/week does not seem to enhance the hypertrophic response (Haun et al., 2018). A study comparing the effects of training volume on strength and hypertrophy of the biceps reported a trend for greater strength and hypertrophy improvements with a moderate (18 sets/week) compared to a low (9) and high (27) number of weekly sets (Heaselgrave et al., 2019). There is a large interindividual response to volume and no universal optimal weekly set prescription. A broad recommendation is to perform 10–20 sets/muscle-group/week. Where practical, the weekly set volume can gradually increase as clients accrue training experience until an upper limit of productive weekly volume is reached.

Why is the weekly volume threshold unclear?

The lack of consensus regarding a weekly volume threshold (or optimal dose) is due to the numerous factors that affect how an individual will respond to an increase in volume (e.g., genetics, nutrition, sleep). For example, a study that compared the effects of a low and moderate volume programme on strength and hypertrophy outcomes reported that 13 out of 34 participants displayed enhanced molecular adaptations from the moderate (3 sets/exercise) compared to the low (1 set/exercise) volume training (Hammarström et al., 2020). However, there was a variable response to training volume between participants, as some did not experience enhanced hypertrophy and strength when training volume was increased (Hammarström et al., 2020).

Volume summary

Performing more than ten hard sets/muscle group within a training session results in diminishing returns. A weekly training volume of 10–20 sets/muscle-group/week can produce significant improvements in strength and hypertrophy. However, the weekly set volume should be adjusted based on the client's goals and training history. Training programmes focused on improving general health outcomes can adopt a low weekly volume prescription and adjust based on the client's responses (Gomes et al., 2019). Finally, the range of effective training volumes reported within the literature could be due to differences in inter-set rest intervals and training frequencies between studies. For instance, studies indicating higher volume programmes produce better outcomes tend to have distributed training volume across the week (Hammarström et al., 2020; Schoenfeld et al., 2019b), rather than condensing the volume within fewer sessions (Aube et al., 2020). Therefore, training frequency and inter-set rest periods should be considered when prescribing training volume.

Training frequency for health RT programmes

Training frequency refers to the number of sessions performed within a defined period (usually one week). In general, a minimum of two RT sessions/week are recommended to improve health and hypertrophy outcomes (Garber et al., 2011; Schoenfeld et al., 2016b). The optimal training frequency varies between clients due to individual factors. For instance, a variation in the training stimulus (e.g., exercise type, intensity, volume) will affect the magnitude of fatigue the client experiences and could necessitate a longer recovery period between training sessions. For novice clients and older adults, a period of 48 hours between sessions is recommended to facilitate recovery before training the same muscle-groups. After considering recovery between sessions, training frequency is dictated by the client's availability, preferences, training history, and goals (see Case Study 13.1).

When should frequency be increased?

Most health benefits can be achieved with 2–3 non-consecutive RT sessions/week (ACSM, 2009). Training frequency should be evaluated as the client's goals, fitness, and circumstances change. It can be impractical (due to time constraints) or ineffective (due to fatigue, motivation and diminishing returns) to increase the number of sets or exercises performed in a session. Therefore, increasing training frequency can be an effective strategy to increase training volume and manage fatigue (see Case Study 13.1).

CASE STUDY 13.1

John has been performing three RT sessions/week for a year, and he is no longer gaining muscle. John wishes to increase muscle mass, which can be facilitated by increasing training volume (Schoenfeld et al., 2019a). However, John trains in his lunch hour and (after travel, changing and showering) he only has 40 minutes to train. John could increase volume by using advanced methods (see Table 13.2). Alternatively, John could increase his training frequency to four days/week, distributing the increased volume across the week.

Does training less frequency reduce strength and hypertrophy?

There are times when clients cannot maintain their training frequency (e.g., during holidays), which could potentially lead to detraining effects, such as decreases in muscle mass and strength. However, several studies have demonstrated that muscle size and strength can be maintained with a lower training frequency and total volume. For example, participants who reduced their training frequency from three to one session/week for eight weeks experienced no significant changes in strength (1RM half squat) or muscle (quadriceps) mass, despite decreasing volume-load by approximately 50% (Tavares et al., 2017).

Frequency summary

Training frequency should be individualised according to the client's fitness, preferences and goals. Health outcomes can be improved by performing two RT sessions/week, allowing 48 hours of recovery between sessions. Intermediate and advanced clients, requiring higher training volumes, may benefit from increasing frequency to distribute volume and manage fatigue. The current literature indicates that training 2–4 days/week is optimal for health outcomes.

Inter-set rest periods for health RT programmes

In general, novice and intermediate clients are advised to rest for 1–2 minutes between hard sets (Garber et al., 2011). However, the inter-set rest period should be modified based on the previous and current type of RT exercise, and the intensity of effort used in the previous set. Even the client's sex should be considered, as females appear to demonstrate better inter-set recovery than males (Celes et al., 2010). Compound exercises, particularly free-weight, are more physiologically and psychologically demanding than isolation exercises and necessitate a longer recovery period (Senna et al., 2016). After a set performed close to failure, some degree of residual neuromuscular fatigue is likely. Thus, a 2–3 minute inter-set rest period may be required to enable the client to maintain proper technique and achieve the required intensity on the next set.

Do shorter inter-set rest periods produce better outcomes?

Some clients may intuitively believe they are saving time or 'working harder' by taking short rest periods. However, the physiological consequences of insufficient rest periods can reduce training efficacy. For example, a shorter (1 vs. 5 minute) rest period between four sets of leg press and leg extension exercises was shown to increase lactate accumulation and reduce muscle protein synthesis (McKendry et al., 2016). Additionally, as observed in TTF studies, higher levels of metabolites following short rest periods could increase perceived effort and discomfort during training. Taking very short (<1 minute) rest periods between consecutive sets should generally be avoided as neuromuscular fatigue is likely to be high at the start of the next set. The inadequate recovery could result in fewer repetitions being achieved on subsequent sets (i.e., reduced training volume).

What is the optimal inter-set rest period?

There is a trade-off between optimal and practical when selecting rest periods. Although longer (3 vs. 1 minute) rest periods produce better hypertrophy and strength outcomes (Schoenfeld et al., 2016c), the additional time resting between sets can increase the duration of a session. Adopting advanced techniques (see Table 13.2) can enable the same number of hard sets to be completed, with 2–3-minute rest periods between sets, without significantly increasing the session duration. However, advanced techniques are not always appropriate, particularly with novice clients. Thus, a rest period of 1–2 minutes is logical for health programmes, prioritising two minutes rest between compound exercises.

Resistance training for muscle hypertrophy
Michael Israetel

Basic mechanisms of hypertrophy

The fundamental training stimulus of hypertrophy is the generation of tension within working muscle fibres (Burkholder, 2007; Wackerhage et al., 2019). Muscle fibres that contract against a resistance and generate tension will experience the activation of some hypertrophic pathways, regardless of whether the amount of stimulus rises above the level needed to gain *net* muscle tissue. Hypertrophy via the direct imposition of contractile tension has been well documented, and numerous candidate mechanisms have been both proposed and observed (Sartori et al., 2021; Wackerhage et al., 2019). However, a direct 'molecule by molecule' cascade of how muscle fibres detect tension and translate it into a growth signal is currently undocumented (Burkholder, 2007; Glass, 2005).

The generation of tension within muscle fibres might not have to come from the fibre itself, as extreme stretching and compression via forces external to the fibre's contractile machinery can also stimulate growth, albeit less robustly than internally generated forces (Nunes et al., 2020; Simpson et al., 2017). When forces are internally generated, they can stimulate growth regardless of the contraction type, as concentric, isometric, and eccentric actions all incite a growth stimulus, perhaps via somewhat independent mechanisms. Therefore, it is prudent to perform all three muscle actions when the goal is to maximise hypertrophy (Oranchuk et al., 2019; Schoenfeld et al., 2017b).

Table 13.4 Resistance training guidelines for improving health outcomes

	Recommendation	Further details
Exercise sequencing method	Performing a set followed by a rest period before the subsequent set (i.e., the straight set method). Alternative exercise sequencing methods and techniques (see Table 13.2) can be programmed to increase the training volume, intensity and density	Alternative sequencing methods should be programmed carefully.
Progression	Load or repetitions can be increased using subjective (e.g., RIR) and objective systems (e.g., 'two for two' method).	Weekly progression should not be expected (see Box 13.3).
Tempo	Concentric (as fast as possible*) Isometric: 1 second Eccentric: 2–3 seconds * When using light loads (<50% 1RM) a 1–2 second concentric action can facilitate attentional focus and technique.	Slowing the eccentric action of an exercise (>3 seconds) could result in greater improvements in strength and hypertrophy outcomes. However, slow eccentrics can increase muscle damage and soreness.
Technique	Each repetition should be performed through the client's full ROM*. *ROM is specific to the client's characteristics (anthropometry, strength, mobility etc.).	The strategic use of a partial ROM exercises with heavier loads could facilitate hypertrophy and strength gains.
Exercise selection	Compound exercises, targeting the major muscle groups. Isolation exercises can be included to target the smaller muscle groups.	Novice clients may benefit from using resistance machines initially and free-weight exercises can be introduced as strength and exercise competency improves.
Intensity of load	60–80% 1RM to improve strength and achieve health benefits. 30–50 % 1RM effective for hypertrophy, provided exercises are performed to (or near to) repetition failure.	The optimal intensity of load for different health targets is uncertain. Advanced clients may need to strategically use heavier (≥80% 1RM) loads to improve maximal strength.

(Continued)

Table 13.4 Resistance training guidelines for improving health outcomes (Continued)

	Recommendation	Further details
Training to failure (TTF)	TTF is not required to achieve improvements in health and strength outcomes. Training near to failure (0–3 **RIR**) is necessary when using light (30–50% 1 RM) loads and hypertrophy is sought. Occasional TTF could help clients to calibrate their **RIR** ratings.	Regularly TTF should be avoided as it can increase cardiovascular strain, discomfort and post-training fatigue. The negative effects of TTF could compromise training volume and the quality of other exercises.
Session volume (hard sets)	1–3 sets/exercise (3 sets produce better gains in strength and hypertrophy) No more than 10 sets/muscle group within a session.	Session volume should be individualised based on the client's training status. Novice clients will likely experience benefits with 3–5 sets/muscle group/session.
Weekly volume (hard sets)	10–20 sets/muscle group.	Novice clients will likely experience benefits with less than 10 sets/muscle group/week.
Frequency (sessions/week)	2–4 sessions/week. Allow 48 hours recovery between sessions when training the same muscle group.	Frequency should be individualised according to the client's circumstances.
Inter-set rest periods	2 minutes between compound exercises. 1–2 minutes between isolation exercises.	Advanced techniques (see Table 13.2) can increase session volume without reducing inter-set rest periods. Advanced techniques are not always appropriate or practical with novice clients.

RIR = Repetitions in reserve; RM = Repetition maximum; ROM = Range of motion.

In addition to tension, at least two other factors have potential hypertrophic mechanisms; cell swelling and metabolic stress (Sartori et al., 2021; Wackerhage et al., 2019). Muscle damage has been proposed as another hypertrophy mechanism but is of secondary importance for at least two reasons. First, there is a lack of direct evidence that muscle damage promotes hypertrophy. Second, damage almost certainly occurs via the imposition of tension, metabolic stress, and cell swelling, making its inclusion as an independent hypertrophic factor erroneous. Cell swelling, as observed when a 'muscle pump' is experienced during bodybuilding-style training, has been demonstrated in vitro to increase protein synthesis and reduce proteolysis (breakdown)—primary factors in long-term muscle growth (Grant et al., 2000; Millar et al., 1997). Metabolites (e.g., lactate and inorganic phosphate) have been shown to initiate muscle growth when introduced into cells (Li et al., 2014; Oishi et al., 2015) and are generated in large concentrations in the muscles generating peak tension continuously during intense bouts of hypertrophy-oriented training (Lagally et al., 2002).

Fortunately, producing high degrees of concentric, isometric, and eccentric tension for continual periods (e.g., during a set of biceps curls) also generates high concentrations of metabolites and initiates cell swelling (Grant et al., 2000; Schoenfeld et al., 2014). Thus, performing straight sets of intensive resistance exercises can stimulate the fundamental mechanisms (i.e., tension, cell swelling and metabolite sequestration) required for muscle growth, provided a sufficient intensity of effort is applied (Fischer, 2014).

Intensity for hypertrophy

In RT, there are two primary approaches to determine the difficulty of any given unit of training time: how much load is being lifted (intensity of load), and how close to muscular failure the load is being lifted (relative intensity).

Intensity of load

Research on hypertrophy training loading over the past decade has provided clearer recommendations than ever before. Training with loads as light as 20% 1RM can elicit robust hypertrophy if the sets are performed close to failure (Lasevicius et al., 2018). Loads of 30–40% 1RM generate a more significant hypertrophic stimulus than sets of 20% 1RM, but loads of 40–50% 1RM do not generate significantly more hypertrophy than loads of 30–40% 1RM (Lasevicius et al., 2018; Schoenfeld et al., 2017a). Thus, the current best estimate of the lowest intensity to provoke a significant hypertrophy stimulus is around 30% 1RM. Using loads <30% 1RM can stimulate muscle growth, but considerably less than heavier loads (Lasevicius et al., 2018).

At the heavier end of the load spectrum, loads of 100% (or more) of 1RM stimulate hypertrophy very robustly per-repetition. However, the magnitude of hypertrophy stimulus for sets using 100% 1RM is lower compared to slightly lighter (e.g., 85% 1RM) loads due to the low total number of repetitions/set. For example, a 100% 1RM load might stimulate 25% more muscle growth than an 85% 1RM load *per repetition*, but if a client can perform five complete repetitions at 85% 1RM, the single 100% of 1RM repetition dose cannot make up that much difference in hypertrophic stimulus. Consistent with this hypertrophic shortcoming with using very heavy loads, research indicates that sets of ~3 repetitions do not stimulate as much growth *per set* than sets of ~10 repetitions (Schoenfeld et al., 2016a). Although the stimulatory effects of loading exist on a continuum, it can be speculated that a top-end 'optimal' loading cut-off for hypertrophy is achieved at around 85% 1RM (see Figure 13.3).

In summary, short-term studies indicate that training anywhere between 30% 1RM (sets of ~30 repetitions close to failure) to 85% 1RM (sets of around five repetitions close to failure) is likely best practice for the stimulation of maximum muscle growth.

Relative intensity (intensity of effort)

The listed repetition ranges discussed above correspond to sets performed close to muscular failure. Thus, training to failure (TTF) is pertinent to the discussion on stimulating hypertrophy. Though there does not seem to be any unique mechanism by which failure itself stimulates muscle growth, the path to failure confers certain advantages (see Box 13.1). When TTF on higher repetition sets (e.g., 15–30 repetition range) the faster twitch fibres seem to experience excitation-contraction uncoupling from fatigue and metabolite accumulation more profoundly and earlier than slower-twitch fibres (Fryer & Stephenson, 1996; Lamb, 2002). Therefore, going close to failure on higher (15–30) repetition sets may not maximally activate the faster twitch fibres as much as a lower repetition set. However, the increase in metabolite levels and greater cell swelling effects from higher repetition training makes it a viable alternative strategy to maximise muscle growth.

Is training to failure always necessary?

Training close to failure on working sets in the 5–30 repetition range maximises hypertrophy, but it is not exactly clear *how close* to failure sets need to be to maximise the hypertrophic effect. In TTF studies the researchers have difficultly discriminating the hypertrophic effects of going to all-out failure versus stopping three repetitions short of failure. Most of the TTF research is in beginners, who often underestimate their true failure point, often by five repetitions per set or more (Barbosa-Netto et al., 2017). Therefore, performing sets at three or fewer RIR should ensure maximal hypertrophic effects. Individuals with resistance training experience may experience an additional growth stimulus from TTF; however, this approach can cause a disproportionate rise in fatigue accumulation (see Chapter 6), which could decrease training sustainability and productivity (Morán-Navarro et al., 2017; Willardson, 2007).

In summary, training should consist of hard sets (see Chapter 7), where each set is performed to three or fewer RIR. Exactly how many RIR below three is of little consequence on hypertrophy (Baz-Valle et al., 2018). The discussion will now focus on how much training volume is required for hypertrophy.

Volume for hypertrophy

Sets per session

When growth is measured for only the first month of training, one set/session stimulates approximately the same hypertrophy as three sets. Still, over several months, three sets/session stimulates more growth than one set/session (Rønnestad et al., 2007). For clients training for several months (and those with years of training history), it seems that the optimum number of sets/session for muscle growth is within the range of 5–10, with an average of around eight sets (Krieger, 2010; Schoenfeld et al., 2017b). However, there is undoubtedly considerable individual variance, with some individuals optimising hypertrophy at around three sets/muscle/session, and others at 12 or more (Scarpelli et al., 2020).

Novice clients should begin with 1–2 hard sets/muscle/session, perhaps taking more warm-up (easy) sets to learn and improve technique. When the client is comfortably recovering from two sets per session, additional sets can be added, and recovery re-assessed several sessions later. When starting a new training cycle (with new exercises and repetition ranges), it is wise to begin at the lower end (3–6 sets/muscle/session) of the client's simulative range from an injury prevention perspective. Hard sets can be slowly added as recovery allows (and no faster) during the following training weeks (Gabbett, 2016; Israetel et al., 2019). When a client cannot recover from the workload every week (e.g., he/she cannot lift the same weight for the same repetitions) a reduction in volume (and relative effort) for a week or so can be programmed. A recovery (or de-load) phase reduces accumulated fatigue and promotes recovery before the next productive training cycle, which should begin at the lower end (~3 sets/muscle/session) of volume ranges (Israetel et al., 2019).

Sets per week

Every training session of a given muscle group stimulates growth, but also creates fatigue (Miranda et al., 2018; West et al., 2009). An optimal weekly set volume for hypertrophy has not been identified as this depends on the client's training experience and ability to recover between sessions, which is influenced by the volume completed in the last session (McLester et al., 2003; Morán-Navarro et al., 2017). Therefore, there is an interaction between the number of sets performed within a session and the total sets completed in a week. For instance, performing more than ten sets/muscle in one session would create extensive tissue damage, thereby extending the required recovery period before more sets for the same muscle groups could be executed (Damas et al., 2016; Schoenfeld, 2012). The target muscle groups being trained should be recovered from previous training; this can be gauged by assessing if the target muscle groups can perform at or above prior levels (e.g., the same number of repetitions/set with a given load and RIR). Subjective recovery markers can also be used; for instance, any perceived muscle soreness should have dissipated (Ferreira et al., 2017).

Training frequency for hypertrophy

If a client performed two hard sets on Monday, he might be able to train the same muscle group hard again on Tuesday (Yang et al., 2018). However, if he did six hard sets on Monday, he might not be recovered until Wednesday or Thursday. As long as the client modulates per-session volume, several training frequencies seem to be roughly equivalent for hypertrophy, provided the training programme is sufficiently hard, allows adequate recovery, and training is scheduled again reasonably soon after recovery (Schoenfeld et al., 2016b). In general, 2–6 weekly sessions typically allow hard-yet-recovered training with per-session volumes of 5–10 sets/muscle group.

The weekly training frequency will vary between clients depending on personal circumstances (e.g., work/family commitments), the number of sets performed in previous sessions, and the recovery capacity of different muscle groups (McLester et al., 2003; Morán-Navarro et al., 2017). For example, a client may only train his hamstrings twice a week because the muscle group recovers more slowly than others. Conversely, the same client might be able to comfortably train his lateral deltoids five times a week, even at the higher per-session volumes.

Inter-set rest periods for hypertrophy

Type II (fast) muscle fibres display greater growth than type I (slower) fibres but also fatigue more quickly (Fryer & Stephenson, 1996; Lamb, 2002). Trying to perform all sets with minimal rest results in accumulating fatigue without the corresponding hypertrophic stimulus (Henselmans & Schoenfeld, 2014). Therefore, taking adequate rest between sets is important for hypertrophy. By performing sets of 5–30 total repetitions followed by sufficient rest periods (discussed below), it is possible to yield more type II fibre (and total) growth from each successive set. Inter-set rest periods can be established using four conditions. A client can consider performing another set when:

1   at least five repetitions could be performed in the next set, ensuring the stimulus is sufficient to justify doing the set.
2   Physiological systems (e.g., neuromuscular and cardiovascular) are sufficiently recovered to allow for a near-maximal effort in the upcoming set. If the client feels like he/she will not be able to achieve the target intensity, a longer rest period would be beneficial.
3   The cardiovascular system should be sufficiently recovered to not be a limiting factor on the next set; this ensures that the target muscle can reach near-failure. A significantly elevated breathing rate indicates more rest is required.
4   All supporting muscles must be *more recovered* than the target muscle, so that they do not fail before the target muscle(s) and become the limiting factor. For example, a client's quadriceps might be capable of generating enough force to complete 12 repetitions of the squat with a given load; however, fatigue in the lower back might limit the set to eight repetitions. In this case, the client needs to rest longer until his/her lower back can tolerate *at least* 12 repetitions.

The above rest factors imply that the client needs to rest as long it takes to be recovered enough to do another hard set (5–30 repetitions; ≤3 RIR) *in which the target muscle is the limiting factor.* The precise amount of time this takes can vary greatly depending on several factors, including the number of joints involved, the demands placed on stabiliser muscle groups, what muscle groups are being targeted and their respective sizes. In short, if a client performs at least five repetitions, and she stops because the target muscle was trained as close to failure (as planned), then the rest period was sufficient. However, if she achieved fewer than five repetitions or stopped the set for any reason other than impending target muscle failure, the rest period was likely insufficient.

Training to develop maximal strength
Greg Nuckols

Developing muscular strength is a primary goal of many RT programmes, particularly for athletes involved in strength and power sports. This section will focus on two definitions of strength and applications: (1) the capacity of skeletal muscles to generate contractile force and (2) the capacity of individuals to move or resist external loads. The sheer capacity of skeletal muscles to generate contractile force is generally measured with single-joint isometric strength assessments, and the ability to move external loads is most commonly measured using one repetition maximum (1RM) tests, though isokinetic strength tests are also used in research settings.

Table 13.5 Resistance training guidelines for maximising muscle hypertrophy

	Recommendation	Further details
Exercise sequencing method	Use the straight set method supplemented with alternative exercise sequencing methods and techniques (see Table 13.2).	Alternative sequencing methods should be programmed carefully.
Progression	When the client is comfortably recovering from 1–2 sets/session, 1–2 sets can be added, and recovery re-assessed several sessions later.	Weekly load progression should not be expected (see Box 13.3).
Exercise selection	Select exercises involving concentric, isometric and eccentric actions. Include a variety of exercises that target the muscles intended to be grown.	The target muscle group should be the limiting factor during a set.
Intensity of load	Select loads in the 5–30 repetition (~40–85% 1RM) range.	A range of loads can be used provided exercises are performed close to repetition failure.
Training to failure (TTF)	Perform all hard sets at an RIR of ≤3, and closer to failure on occasions (i.e., 0 RIR). TTF on every set is not required.	TTF on every session should be avoided as it could increase recovery time and compromise total training volume.
Session volume (hard sets)	3–12 hard sets per muscle/session, starting at the lower range.	Slowly increase volume as recovery allows.
Weekly volume (hard sets)	10–20 sets/muscle group.	Novice clients will likely experience benefits with less than 10 sets/muscle group/week.
Frequency (sessions/week)	2–6 sessions/week starting at the lower range. Only add sessions if recovery between sessions is sufficient.	Match the per-session volume to the session number.
Inter-set rest periods	Rest long enough between sets so that the target muscle is the limiting factor and at least five repetitions can be completed.	A significantly elevated breathing rate indicates more rest is required.

RIR = Repetitions in reserve; RM = Repetition maximum; ROM = Range of motion;

Factors that contribute to maximal strength

Alongside neural factors and hypertrophy, other structural factors contribute to torque production at joints and facilitate improvements in strength. The three most important (non-hypertrophic) structural factors seem to be pennation angle (for pennate muscles), internal moment arms created by the muscle, and connective tissue adaptations that affect the ability of muscle fibres to transmit force laterally to the surrounding connective tissue matrix.

Pennation angles simultaneously influence the number of sarcomeres in parallel for a muscle (a larger pennation angle allows for more sarcomeres in parallel), and the efficiency that muscle fibre contractions contribute to the contractile force of the entire muscle (a smaller pennation angle yields more efficient force transmission). Thus, both increases and decreases in pennation angles could come with significant tradeoffs; however, in theory, pennation angles of approximately 45° should be optimal for maximizing whole-muscle contractile force (Aagaard et al., 2001). Most muscles have pennation angles of <30°, so increasing pennation angles is generally beneficial for force production (Lieber & Fridén, 2000). Internal moment arms directly impact the degree to which muscle contractile forces are capable of generating torque at the joint(s) those muscles cross. Longer internal moment arms allow for the generation of greater joint torques per unit of muscle contractile force. While the length of an internal moment arm is primarily defined by the location of the muscles attachment point(s) relative to the centre of the joint(s) it moves, internal moment arms for some muscles may be longer if the muscle is larger (Vigotsky et al., 2015). Finally, connective tissue adaptations – an increased density of focal adhesions between muscle fibres and the surrounding connective tissue matrix – are thought to enhance the efficiency with which contractile force generated by muscle fibres is transferred to the muscle's tendons (Jones et al., 1989).

The pennation angles in pennate muscles and internal moment arms lengths tend to increase with hypertrophy (Ema et al., 2016; Vigotsky et al., 2015). Little is known about connective tissue adaptations to know what training variables influence them, beyond stating that they likely occur with resistance exercise *per se* (Erskine et al., 2011). Finally, for isometric strength production, the impact of coordination and technique is minimal, and healthy individuals seem to be capable of voluntarily recruiting virtually all of their motor units, even without training (Noorkõiv et al., 2014). Thus, if a client wishes to simply increase the capacity of a muscle to produce contractile force or increase isometric joint moments, training for strength seems to be virtually synonymous with training for hypertrophy. Further improvements due to specific maximal isometric training are also likely (Jones & Rutherford, 1987).

Is a bigger muscle a stronger muscle?

Muscle size – specifically the number of sarcomeres in parallel – contributes to muscular strength because the actin and myosin proteins within sarcomeres are the basic contractile unit within skeletal muscle tissue. The ability of a muscle to generate active contractile force is constrained by the number of sarcomeres it possesses. In general, training to increase the muscle's ability to generate contractile force seems to be virtually synonymous with hypertrophy training. As muscles grow following RT, functional adaptations of muscle fibres suggest that the density of contractile proteins increases or remain stable. Sarcoplasmic hypertrophy, a disproportionate increase in non-contractile elements of muscle fibres, may exist, but it seems to be the exception rather than the rule, and it is unknown what training variables may encourage it (Dankel et al., 2018). Muscle size is also strongly associated with maximal isometric force production (Trezise et al., 2016).

As with isometric strength, dynamic strength is likely constrained by muscle size. In trained athletes, increases in fat-free mass and increases in maximal dynamic strength seem to be closely associated (Appleby et al., 2012; Baker et al., 1994) and maximal dynamic strength seems to correlate almost perfectly with fat free mass or the thickness of agonist muscles amongst elite athletes (Brechue & Abe, 2002; Siahkouhian & Hedayatneja, 2010). However, hypertrophy may not acutely result in increases in dynamic strength, especially if the hypertrophy is accomplished using non-specific means (exercises other than those used to assess maximal dynamic strength) or low loads, due to the skill component of maximal dynamic strength expression.

Training recommendations for maximal strength development

Although muscle size influences dynamic strength, merely training to maximise hypertrophy is insufficient for maximising dynamic strength development. The rest of this section will focus on the development of dynamic strength – primarily 1RM strength.

Movement specificity

Coordination and technique are important for strength development; hence, strength increases to a greater degree in specific movements that are regularly performed. For example, a RT program that includes barbell squats is more likely to increase a client's 1RM squat to a greater extent than a programme that excludes the barbell squat but includes other exercises that train all the muscles associated with squat 1RM strength (e.g., leg press, leg extension) (Paoli et al., 2017).

Muscle action

Strength gains seem to be specific to the muscle action being trained. For instance, specific eccentric-only training at relatively high intensities is necessary to maximise eccentric strength gains (Roig et al., 2009), and relatively high-intensity concentric-only training is necessary to maximise concentric strength.

Intensity for maximal strength development

In general, training at a higher intensity (% 1RM) leads to larger dynamic strength increases than training at a lower intensity (% 1RM), likely because training at a higher intensity is necessary for improving inter- and intra-muscular coordination with heavy loads, and improving the lifter's skill at maintaining technique under heavy loads during 1RM testing (Schoenfeld et al., 2017a). Training intensities of ≥80% of 1RM are often recommended for maximizing dynamic strength increases. Training with lower loads (<80% 1RM) can increase dynamic strength – albeit to a lesser degree.

It is unclear how often high-intensity loading is required for maximising strength gains. For example, training with 80% 1RM would be expected to produce greater strength gains than training with 50% 1RM. However, a study that compared a high (80% 1RM) versus low (50% 1RM) intensity training programme reported similar strength gains between groups when monthly 1RM tests were performed (Morton et al., 2016). Thus, high-intensity loading may not be necessary on a weekly basis. High-intensity training every 2–4 weeks, interspersed with lower-intensity training, may be sufficient to improve strength; however, more research is needed in this area.

Proximity to failure

A 2016 meta-analysis found that training to failure (TTF) and non-failure training led to similar increases in dynamic strength (Davies et al., 2016). Since then, several studies have compared the effects of training with different degrees of velocity loss per set (i.e., training closer to or further from failure). Most of these studies suggest that, over the short-to-moderate term, proximity to failure, ranging from 0–10 repetitions in reserve, has little impact on strength gains, as long as intensity is adequate (>70% of 1RM) (Galiano et al., 2020; Carroll et al., 2018; Sánchez-Moreno et al., 2020). However, constantly training too far away from failure may lead to less hypertrophy (see previous section), which could indirectly limit long-term strength development. As discussed previously, TTF or very close to failure causes greater acute fatigue and is associated with longer recovery times after a training session. Thus, training close to failure is not recommended during the week before a 1RM assessment.

In summary, proximity to failure during a training program should depend on the clients' goals (are they trying to develop muscle hypertrophy?), their training frequency per lift (failure and near-failure training impose fewer constraints on lower-frequency programs), and their proximity to a 1RM assessment.

Autoregulation

Autoregulation refers to strategies used to adapt training variables to an athlete's momentary capabilities (see Chapter 7). Autoregulation differs from 'training by feel' as it incorporates quantitative feedback, such as repetition velocity and rating of perceived exertion (RPE), instead of relying on mere intuition.

Several methods can be used to autoregulate RT. The two common methods of autoregulation were discussed in Chapter 7: repetitions in reserve (RIR) and RPE. Over the past decade, velocity-based RT has become popular (Galiano et al., 2020; Sánchez-Moreno et al., 2020). The three most common training variables that are autoregulated are load selection, repetitions per set, and sets per exercise.

The theoretical basis of prescribing training using autoregulation is that clients' performance and readiness to train can fluctuate over time (see Case Study 13.2). Autoregulated training can better accommodate acute increases and decreases in performance than rigid prescriptions (e.g., % 1RM). If a client is feeling and performing better than normal, autoregulation enables them to increase training intensity or volume to take advantage of the acute improvement in performance. Conversely, if a client is feeling fatigued, training loads and/or volume can be reduced (see Table 13.6). Autoregulated training also requires less frequent strength testing. For example, if training is prescribed based on a 1RM lift performed three months ago, this may no longer be very informative when attempting to assign training loads. Alternatively, quantitative feedback regarding load and/or volume selection using autoregulation is updated on a set-by-set basis.

Research comparing autoregulated vs. static training prescriptions have largely found that employing autoregulation has a neutral (Orange et al., 2019) or positive (Dorrell et al., 2020; Helms et al., 2018) impact on strength adaptations. Thus, autoregulating training does not seem to have any clear drawbacks (other than the cost of a velocity device, if using velocity-based training), but may improve strength results, especially for clients with larger-than-average fluctuations in daily performance.

CASE STUDY 13.2

Autoregulation

Oswald is a policeman who usually trains after work. Due to his unpredictable work schedule, his readiness to train and his strength can fluctuate considerably during a hectic week. However, he likes knowing what weights he is going to lift before each training session, and dislikes using lower loads than he has lifted before. Some weeks he has to work considerably longer hours and he often recovers poorly when he trains to failure.

In Oswald's case it would be appropriate to assign his loads using percentages of his last tested 1RM, but allow the repetitions/set to be dictated using RIR. For instance, the prescription could be 75% 1RM for five sets, but he could use an RIR of two to determine the number of repetitions performed (75% x5 @ RIR 2). On days when he is feeling good, he could perform 8–10 repetitions (@2 RIR). On days when he is fatigued, he may only complete 5–7 repetitions per set with the same (2) RIR.

Table 13.6 Advantages and disadvantages of using the rating of perceived exertion (RPE) scale measuring repetitions in reserve (RIR)

Advantages	Disadvantages
Simple to explain and administer.	Some individuals find it difficult to accurately rate their RIR.
Does not require purchasing or learning how to use additional equipment.	Some individuals who rate their RIR accurately still lack confidence in their ratings, which can cause stress and distraction during training.
Does not require ongoing testing for RIR ratings to maintain utility.	The accuracy of RIR ratings are lower for individuals with limited training experience than trained individuals.
	Reduced accuracy when training with more than 3–4 RIR. Therefore, RIR is only useful when lifters are training reasonably close to failure.

Volume for maximum strength development

Research suggests that a moderate-to-high volume of sets per exercise per week (5–10+) leads to larger strength gains than a low (<5 sets per week) set volume (Ralston et al., 2017). Larger strength gains resulting from higher training volumes may be due to increased opportunities to practice exercise technique under load, or to higher training volumes typically being associated with greater hypertrophy. However, training volume can become excessive, with very high training volumes potentially producing smaller strength gains than moderate volumes (Aube et al., 2020; González-Badillo et al., 2005). More research is needed to establish the full dose-response relationship between training volume and strength gains; however, as with hypertrophy, training volume depends on individual characteristics of the client, training status, the exercise being trained, intensity, and the typical proximity to failure (see Figure 13.3).

Frequency for maximum strength development

Previous research suggested that higher training frequencies on a per-exercise basis may lead to larger strength gains, possibly due to increased opportunities for skill development and acquisition (Hunter, 1985). However, a recent meta-analysis found that higher training frequencies were associated with greater strength gains, but not in studies when weekly training volume was equated (Grgic et al., 2018). In other words, when higher frequencies were associated with higher volume (i.e., more total sets) higher frequency training led to larger strength gains. In studies where weekly volume was the same in all conditions, higher frequency training did not lead to greater strength gains. Thus, increases in strength associated with increases in training frequency may be attributable to difference in training volume, rather than frequency. In practice, higher training frequencies may allow for higher volumes to be productive and tolerable (see Case Study 13.1).

Inter-set rest intervals for maximum strength development

Taking longer rest intervals has been associated with greater strength development in some (Hill-Haas et al., 2007; Schoenfeld et al., 2016c), but not all studies (Buresh et al., 2009; Willardson & Burkett, 2008). The discrepancy within the literature could relate to the training status of the participants, the duration of the studies, or the types of exercises tested. In general, compound (particularly lower body) exercises performed for more repetitions with higher absolute loads will cause more acute metabolic stress, and will likely require longer rest intervals for the lifter to adequately recover for the next set. However, the body of research suggests that performance does not need to be fully maintained set-to-set to maximise strength adaptations. In general, rest intervals of 1–2 minutes should be sufficient for most single-joint exercises, while rest intervals of 2–5+ minutes may be more prudent for compound exercises, particularly lower-body exercises.

Periodisation for maximum strength development

Periodised RT (see Chapter 8) has been reported to promote larger gains in dynamic strength than non-periodised RT (Williams et al., 2017), and linear and undulating periodisation models seem to have similar effects on strength development (Harries et al., 2015). However, the research comparing periodised and non-periodised training has generally allowed participants to train at higher peak intensities than the non-periodised programs they are compared against (e.g., Willoughby, 1993). Consequently, some studies could, inadvertently, have assessed the impact of peak training intensity on strength gains, rather than the independent effect of periodisation *per se*. The minority of studies that equated peak intensity between periodised and non-periodised programmes did not seem to result in greater strength gains in the periodised group (Antretter et al., 2017; Antretter et al., 2019). Thus, periodising programs designed for strength development is likely to have a neutral-to-positive effect on strength gains, but more research is needed in this area.

Table 13.7 Resistance training guidelines for maximising maximal dynamic strength

	Recommendation	Further details
Exercise selection	Select exercises in which improvements in strength are sought. Use the ROM relevant to the desired goal.	Strength gains are partially specific to the muscle action being trained. Most exercises are constrained by concentric strength. If a lifter wants to maximise isometric and eccentric strength, dedicated isometric and/or eccentric training is necessary.
Intensity of load	In the short-to-moderate term, intensities at or above 80% 1RM are recommended.	Occasionally lifting very heavy loads (90–95% 1RM) enables clients to feel comfortable with these loads for testing maximal strength. Training with 90–95% 1RM is not necessary in every training session.
Training to failure (TTF)	In the short-to-moderate term, TTF does not seem very important for strength development.	In the long term, a proportion of training needs to be performed reasonably close to failure to facilitate hypertrophy to maximise strength development.
Session volume (hard sets)	In general, 3–5 sets per exercise is a decent starting point. Set volume primarily depends on proximity to failure, prior experience, and training frequency.	1–2 sets per exercise/session may be sufficient for untrained clients, training near failure, with relatively high training frequency (3+ times per muscle group per week). Up to 10+ sets may be advisable for well-trained lifters, training with lower frequency or more RIR.
Weekly volume (hard sets)	Set volume depends partially on proximity to failure. If training to failure or very close to failure, 5–20 sets per primary exercise per week is advisable.	If regularly training 3–4+ reps from failure, higher weekly set volumes may be advisable.
Frequency (sessions/ week)	Training each muscle group/ exercise 2–3 times per week seems to be a good starting point for most applications.	Weekly training frequency for each primary exercise largely depends on per-session volume. With high per-session volumes (8–10+ working sets for primary exercises), frequencies of once or twice per week are advisable. With low-to-moderate per session volumes (<8 working sets for primary exercises), higher frequencies (3+) are possible and potentially advisable.

(Continued)

Table 13.7 (Continued)

	Recommendation	Further details
Inter-set rest periods	Rest intervals of 1–2 minutes for single-joint and 2–5+ minutes for multi-joint exercises. Longer rest intervals are usually needed for lower-body multi-joint exercises than upper-body exercises.	Rest intervals do not always need to be timed. Experienced lifters typically self-determine appropriate rest intervals.
Periodisation	In general, research suggests that training for strength development should be periodised.	Periodising training has a neutral-to-positive impact on strength development. Linear and undulating periodization models seem to be similarly effective.

RIR: Repetitions in reserve; ROM: range of motion; MJ: multiple-joint; SJ: single-joint; RM: repetition maximum.

References

Abe, T., Mouser, J., Dankel, S., et al. (2019). A method to standardize the blood flow restriction pressure by an elastic cuff. *Scandinavian Journal of Medicine & Science in Sports, 29*(3), 329–335.

Adams, G., & Bamman, M. (2012). Characterization and regulation of mechanical loading-induced compensatory muscle hypertrophy. *Comprehensive Physiology, 2*(4), 2829–2870.

Aagaard, P., Andersen, J., Dyhre-Poulsen, P., et al. (2001). A mechanism for increased contractile strength of human pennate muscle in response to strength training: changes in muscle architecture. *The Journal of Physiology, 534*(Pt 2), 613–623.

American College of Sports Medicine (2009). American College of Sports Medicine position stand. Progression models in resistance training for healthy adults. *Medicine and science in sports and exercise, 41*(3), 687–708.

Amirthalingam, T., Mavros, Y., Wilson, G., et al. (2017). Effects of a modified German volume training program on muscular hypertrophy and strength. *Journal of Strength and Conditioning Research, 31*(11), 3109–3119.

Androulakis-Korakakis, P., Fisher, J., & Steele, J. (2020). The minimum effective training dose required to increase 1RM strength in resistance-trained men: a systematic review and meta-analysis. *Sports Medicine, 50*(4), 751–765.

Appleby, B., Newton, R. U., & Cormie, P. (2012). Changes in strength over a 2-year period in professional Rugby Union players. *The Journal of Strength & Conditioning Research, 26*(9), 2538–2546.

Aristizabal, J., Freidenreich, D., Volk, B., et al. (2015). Effect of resistance training on resting metabolic rate and its estimation by a dual-energy X-ray absorptiometry metabolic map. *European Journal of Clinical Nutrition, 69*(7), 831–836.

Aube, D., Wadhi, T., Rauch, J., et al. (2020). Progressive resistance training volume: effects on muscle thickness, mass, and strength adaptations in resistance-trained individuals. *The Journal of Strength & Conditioning Research*. Publish Ahead of Print.

Bagley, J., Burghardt, K., McManus, R., et al. (2020). Epigenetic responses to acute resistance exercise in trained vs. Sedentary men. *The Journal of Strength & Conditioning Research, 34*(6), 1574–1580.

Baker, D., Wilson, G., & Carlyon, R. (1994). Periodization: the effect on strength of manipulating volume and intensity. *The Journal of Strength & Conditioning Research, 8*(4), 235–242.

Barbosa-Netto, S., d'Acelino-E-Porto, O., & Almeida, M. (2017). Self-selected resistance exercise load: implications for research and prescription. *Journal of Strength and Conditioning Research, 35*, S166-S172.

Bazyler, C., Sato, K., Wassinger, C., et al. (2014). The efficacy of incorporating partial squats in maximal strength training. *Journal of Strength and Conditioning Research, 28*(11), 3024–3032.

Baz-Valle, E., Fontes-Villalba, M., & Santos-Concejero, J. (2018). Total number of sets as a training volume quantification method for muscle hypertrophy. *Journal of Strength and Conditioning Research, 1*.

Bell, Z., Dankel, S., Spitz, R., et al. (2019). The perceived tightness scale does not provide reliable estimates of blood flow restriction pressure. *Journal of Sport Rehabilitation, 29*(4), 516–518.

Boeno, F., Farinha, J., Ramis, T., et al. (2019). Effects of a single session of high- and moderate-intensity resistance exercise on endothelial function of middle-aged sedentary men. *Frontiers in Physiology, 10*.

Boyas, S., & Guével, A. (2011). Neuromuscular fatigue in healthy muscle: underlying factors and adaptation mechanisms. *Annals of Physical and Rehabilitation Medicine, 54*(2), 88–108.

Brechue, W., & Abe, T. (2002). The role of FFM accumulation and skeletal muscle architecture in powerlifting performance. *European Journal of Applied Physiology, 86*(4), 327–336.

Buckner, R. (2004). Memory and executive function in aging and AD: multiple factors that cause decline and reserve factors that compensate. *Neuron, 44*(1), 195–208.

Buresh, R., Berg, K., & French, J. (2009). The effect of resistive exercise rest interval on hormonal response, strength, and hypertrophy with training. *Journal of Strength and Conditioning Research, 23*(1), 62–71.

Burd, N., West, D., Staples, A., et al. (2010). Low-load high volume resistance exercise stimulates muscle protein synthesis more than high-load low volume resistance exercise in young men. *PLoS ONE, 5*(8), e12033.

Burke, R. (1981). Motor units: anatomy, physiology, and functional organization. In *Comprehensive physiology* (pp. 345–422). American Cancer Society.

Burkholder, T. (2007). Mechanotransduction in skeletal muscle. *Frontiers in Bioscience: A Journal and Virtual Library, 12*, 174–191.

Calatayud, J., Vinstrup, J., Jakobsen, M., et al. (2016). Importance of mind-muscle connection during progressive resistance training. *European Journal of Applied Physiology, 116*(3), 527–533.

Carroll, K., Bernards, J., Bazyler, C., et al. (2018). Divergent performance outcomes following resistance training using repetition maximums or relative intensity. *International Journal of Sports Physiology and Performance, 1–28*.

Carroll, K., Bazyler, C., Bernards, J., et al. (2019). Skeletal muscle fiber adaptations following resistance training using repetition maximums or relative intensity. *Sports (Basel, Switzerland), 7*(7).

Cauley, J., & Giangregorio, L. (2020). Physical activity and skeletal health in adults. *The Lancet. Diabetes & Endocrinology, 8*(2), 150–162.

Celes, R., Brown, L., Pereira, M., et al. (2010). Gender muscle recovery during isokinetic exercise. *International Journal of Sports Medicine, 31*(12), 866–869.

Chiu, L., vonGaza, G., & Jean, L. (2017). Net joint moments and muscle activation in barbell squats without and with restricted anterior leg rotation. *Journal of Sports Sciences, 35*(1), 35–43.

Coffey, V., & Hawley, J. A. (2007). The molecular bases of training adaptation. *Sports Medicine, 37*(9), 737–763.

Correa, C., Teixeira, B., Cobos, R., et al. (2015). High-volume resistance training reduces postprandial lipaemia in postmenopausal women. *Journal of Sports Sciences, 33*(18), 1890–1901.

Costill, D., Fink, W., & Pollock, M. (1976). Muscle fiber composition and enzyme activities of elite distance runners. *Medicine and Science in Sports, 8*(2), 96–100.

Cotman, C., Berchtold, N., & Christie, L. (2007). Exercise builds brain health: key roles of growth factor cascades and inflammation. *Trends in Neurosciences, 30*(9), 464–472.

Damas, F., Phillips, S., Libardi, C., et al. (2016). Resistance training-induced changes in integrated myofibrillar protein synthesis are related to hypertrophy only after attenuation of muscle damage. *The Journal of Physiology, 594*(18), 5209–5222.

Dankel, S., Kang, M., Abe, T., et al. (2019). Resistance training induced changes in strength and specific force at the fiber and whole muscle level: A meta-analysis. *European Journal of Applied Physiology, 119*(1), 265–278.

Davies, T., Orr, R., Halaki, M., et al. (2016). Effect of training leading to repetition failure on muscular strength: a systematic review and meta-analysis. *Sports Medicine, 46*(4), 487–502.

Del Vecchio, A., Casolo, A., Negro, F., et al. (2019). The increase in muscle force after 4 weeks of strength training is mediated by adaptations in motor unit recruitment and rate coding. *The Journal of Physiology, 597*(7), 1873–1887.

Dorrell, H., Smith, M., & Gee, T. (2020). Comparison of velocity-based and traditional percentage-based loading methods on maximal strength and power adaptations. *Journal of Strength & Conditioning Research, 34*(1), 46–53.

Duchateau, J., Semmler, J., & Enoka, R. (2006). Training adaptations in the behavior of human motor units. *Journal of Applied Physiology (Bethesda, Md.: 1985), 101*(6), 1766–1775.

Dutheil, F., Lac, G., Lesourd, B., et al. (2013). Different modalities of exercise to reduce visceral fat mass and cardiovascular risk in metabolic syndrome: the RESOLVE randomized trial. *International Journal of Cardiology, 168*(4), 3634–3642.

Eftestøl, E., Egner, I., Lunde, I., et al. (2016). Increased hypertrophic response with increased mechanical load in skeletal muscles receiving identical activity patterns. *American Journal of Physiology. Cell Physiology, 311*(4), C616–C629.

Ema, R., Akagi, R., Wakahara, T., et al. (2016). Training-induced changes in architecture of human skeletal muscles: current evidence and unresolved issues. *The Journal of Physical Fitness and Sports Medicine, 5*(1), 37–46.

Erskine, R., Jones, D., Maffulli, N., et al. (2011). What causes in vivo muscle specific tension to increase following resistance training? *Experimental Physiology, 96*(2), 145–155.

Farrow, J., Steele, J., Behm, D., et al. (2020). Lighter-load exercise produces Greater acute- and prolonged-fatigue in exercised and Non-exercised limbs. *Research Quarterly for Exercise and Sport, 0*(0), 1–11.

Ferreira, D., Gentil, P., Ferreira-Junior, J., et al. (2017). Dissociated time course between peak torque and total work recovery following bench press training in resistance trained men. *Physiology and Behavior, 179,* 143–147.

Felici, F., Rosponi, A., Sbriccoli, P., et al. (2001). Linear and non-linear analysis of surface electromyograms in weightlifters. *European Journal of Applied Physiology, 84*(4), 337–342.

Fischer, J. (2014). The effects of load and effort-matched concentric and eccentric knee extension training in recreational females. *Human Movement, 15*(3), 147–151.

Folland, J., & Williams, A. G. (2007). The adaptations to strength training: morphological and neurological contributions to increased strength. *Sports Medicine, 37*(2), 145–168.

Fridén, J., & Lieber, R. (1992). Structural and mechanical basis of exercise-induced muscle injury. *Medicine and Science in Sports and Exercise, 24*(5), 521–530.

Fry, A. (2004). The role of resistance exercise intensity on muscle fibre adaptations. *Sports Medicine, 34*(10), 663–679.

Fryer, M., & Stephenson, D. (1996). Total and sarcoplasmic reticulum calcium contents of skinned fibres from rat skeletal muscle. *Journal of Physiology, 493,* 357–370.

Gabbett, T. (2016). The training-injury prevention paradox: should athletes be training smarter and harder? *British Journal of Sports Medicine, 50*(5), 273–280. BMJ Publishing Group.

Garber, C., Blissmer, B., Deschenes, M., et al. (2011). American College of Sports Medicine position stand. Quantity and quality of exercise for developing and maintaining cardiorespiratory, musculoskeletal, and neuromotor fitness in apparently healthy adults: guidance for prescribing exercise. *Medicine and Science in Sports and Exercise, 43*(7), 1334–1359.

Galiano, C., Pareja-Blanco, F., Hidalgo de Mora, J., et al. (2020). Low-velocity loss induces similar strength gains to moderate-velocity loss during resistance training. *Journal of strength and Conditioning Research,* 10.

Gjovaag, T., Hjelmeland, A., Oygard, J., et al. (2016). Acute hemodynamic and cardiovascular responses following resistance exercise to voluntary exhaustion. Effects of different loadings and exercise durations. *The Journal of Sports Medicine and Physical Fitness, 56*(5), 616–623.

Glass, D. (2005). Skeletal muscle hypertrophy and atrophy signaling pathways. *The International Journal of Biochemistry & Cell Biology, 37*(10), 1974–1984.

Glover, I., & Baker, S. (2020). Cortical, corticospinal and reticulospinal contributions to strength training. *The Journal of Neuroscience, 40*(30), 5820–5832.

Gomes, G., Franco, C., Nunes, P., et al. (2019). High-frequency resistance training is not more effective than low-frequency resistance training in increasing muscle mass and strength in well-trained men. *Journal of Strength and Conditioning Research, 33*(1), S130–S139.

González-Badillo, J., Gorostiaga, E., Arellano, R., et al. (2005). Moderate resistance training volume produces more favorable strength gains than high or low volumes during a short-term training cycle. *Journal of Strength and Conditioning Research, 19*(3), 689–697.

Grant, A., Gow, I., Zammit, V., et al. (2000). Regulation of protein synthesis in lactating rat mammary tissue by cell volume. *Biochimica et Biophysica Acta, 1475*(1), 39–46.

Grgic, J., Schoenfeld, B., Davies, T., et al., (2018). Effect of resistance training frequency on gains in muscular strength: a systematic review and meta-analysis. *Sports Medicine, 48*(5), 1207–1220.

Guzzoni, V., Selistre-de-Araújo, H., Marqueti, R., & de, C. (2018). Tendon remodeling in response to resistance training, anabolic androgenic steroids and aging. *Cells, 7*(12).

Haff, G., & Triplett, N. (2016). *Essentials of strength training and conditioning* (4th ed.). Human Kinetics.

Hammarström, D., Øfsteng, S., Koll, L., et al. (2020). Benefits of higher resistance-training volume are related to ribosome biogenesis. *The Journal of Physiology, 598*(3), 543–565.

Hartman, M., Clark, B., Bembens, D., et al. (2007). Comparisons between twice-daily and once-daily training sessions in male weight lifters. *International Journal of Sports Physiology and Performance, 2*(2), 159–169.

Haun, C., Vann, C., Mobley, C., et al. (2018). Effects of graded whey supplementation during extreme-volume resistance training. *Frontiers in Nutrition, 5.*

Heaselgrave, S., Blacker, J., Smeuninx, B., et al. (2019). Dose-response relationship of weekly resistance-training volume and frequency on muscular adaptations in trained men. *International Journal of Sports Physiology and Performance, 14*(3), 360–368.

Helms, E., Byrnes, R., Cooke, D., et al. (2018). RPE vs. Percentage 1RM loading in periodized programs matched for sets and repetitions. *Frontiers in Physiology, 9,* 247.

Henneman, E. (1957). Relation between size of neurons and their susceptibility to discharge. *Science, 126*(3287), 1345–1347.

Henselmans, M., & Schoenfeld, B. (2014). The effect of inter-set rest intervals on resistance exercise-induced muscle hypertrophy. *Sports Medicine, 44*(12), 1635–1643.

Hill-Haas, S., Bishop, D., Dawson, B., et al. (2007). Effects of rest interval during high-repetition resistance training on strength, aerobic fitness, and repeated-sprint ability. *Journal of Sports Sciences, 25*(6), 619–628.

Holloszy, J. (2005). Exercise-induced increase in muscle insulin sensitivity. *Journal of Applied Physiology, 99*(1), 338–343.

Hong, A., & Kim, S. (2018). Effects of resistance exercise on bone health. *Endocrinology and Metabolism, 33*(4), 435–444.

Hötting, K., & Röder, B. (2013). Beneficial effects of physical exercise on neuroplasticity and cognition. *Neuroscience and Biobehavioral Reviews, 37*(9), 2243–2257.

Hubal, M., Gordish-Dressman, H., Thompson, P., et al. (2005). Variability in muscle size and strength gain after unilateral resistance training. *Medicine and Science in Sports and Exercise, 37*(6), 964–972.

Humburg, H., Baars, H., Schröder, J., et al. (2007). 1-set vs. 3-set resistance training: a crossover study. *Journal of Strength and Conditioning Research, 21*(2), 578–582.

Hunter, G. (1985). Research: changes in body composition, body build and performance associated with different weight training frequencies in males and females. *Strength & Conditioning Journal, 7*(1), 26–28.

Ishii, T., Yamakita, T., Sato, T., et al. (1998). Resistance training improves insulin sensitivity in NIDDM subjects without altering maximal oxygen uptake. *Diabetes Care, 21*(8), 1353–1355.

Israetel, M., Feather, J., Faleiro, T., et al. (2019). Mesocycle progression in hypertrophy: volume versus intensity, *Strength and Conditioning Journal, 42*(5), 2–6.

Izquierdo-Gabarren, M., González De Txabarri Expósito, R., García-pallarés, J., et al. (2010). Concurrent endurance and strength training not to failure optimizes performance gains. *Medicine and Science in Sports and Exercise, 42*(6), 1191–1199.

Jones, D., Rutherford, O., & Parker, D. (1989). Physiological changes in skeletal muscle as a result of strength training. *Quarterly Journal of Experimental Physiology, 74*(3), 233–256.

Jones, D., & Rutherford, O. (1987). Human muscle strength training: The effects of three different regimens and the nature of the resultant changes. *The Journal of Physiology, 391*, 1–11.

Kidgell, D., Bonanno, D., Frazer, A., et al. (2017). Corticospinal responses following strength training: a systematic review and meta-analysis. *The European Journal of Neuroscience, 46*(11), 2648–2661.

Kraemer, W., & Ratamess, N. (2004). Fundamentals of resistance training: progression and exercise prescription. *Medicine and Science in Sports and Exercise, 36*(4), 674–688.

Krieger, J. (2009). Single versus multiple sets of resistance exercise: a meta-regression. *The Journal of Strength & Conditioning Research, 23*(6), 1890–1901.

Krieger J. (2010). Single vs. multiple sets of resistance exercise for muscle hypertrophy: a meta-analysis. *Journal of strength and conditioning research, 24*(4), 1150–1159.

Kubo, K., Kanehisa, H., & Fukunaga, T. (2002). Effects of resistance and stretching training programmes on the viscoelastic properties of human tendon structures in vivo. *The Journal of Physiology, 538*(1), 219–226.

Lagally, K., Robertson, R., Gallagher, K., et al. (2002). Perceived exertion, electromyography, and blood lactate during acute bouts of resistance exercise. *Medicine & Science in Sports & Exercise,* 34(3), 552–559.

Lamb, G. (2002). Excitation-contraction coupling and fatigue mechanisms in skeletal muscle: studies with mechanically skinned fibres. *Journal of Muscle Research and Cell Motility, 23*(1), 81–91.

Landrigan, J.-F., Bell, T., Crowe, M., et al. (2020). Lifting cognition: a meta-analysis of effects of resistance exercise on cognition. *Psychological Research, 84*(5), 1167–1183.

Lasevicius, T., Schoenfeld, B., Silva-Batista, C., et al. (2019). Muscle failure promotes greater muscle hypertrophy in low-load but not in high-load resistance training. *Journal of Strength and Conditioning Research.* Online publication.

Leal, L., Lopes, M., & Batista, M. (2018). Physical exercise-induced myokines and muscle-adipose tissue crosstalk: a review of current knowledge and the implications for health and metabolic diseases. *Frontiers in Physiology, 9.*

Lee, J., & Jun, H. (2019). Role of myokines in regulating skeletal muscle mass and function. *Frontiers in Physiology, 10.*

Leong, B., Kamen, G., Patten, C., et al. (1999). Maximal motor unit discharge rates in the quadriceps muscles of older weight lifters. *Medicine and Science in Sports and Exercise, 31*(11), 1638–1644.

Li, G., Wang, H., Wang, L., et al. (2014). Distinct pathways of ERK1/2 activation by hydroxy-carboxylic acid receptor-1. *PLoS ONE, 9*(3).

Lieber, R., & Fridén, J. (2000). Functional and clinical significance of skeletal muscle architecture. *Muscle & Nerve, 23*(11), 1647–1666.

Liu, Y., Ye, W., Chen, Q., et al. (2019). Resistance exercise intensity is correlated with attenuation of HbA1c and insulin in patients with type 2 diabetes: a systematic review and meta-analysis. *International Journal of Environmental Research and Public Health, 16*(1), 140.

Loenneke, J., Fahs, C., Wilson, J., et al. (2011). Blood flow restriction: the metabolite/volume threshold theory. *Medical Hypotheses, 77*(5), 748–752.

Loenneke, J., Wilson, J., Marín, P., et al. (2012). Low intensity blood flow restriction training: a meta-analysis. *European Journal of Applied Physiology, 112*(5), 1849–1859.

Looney, D., Kraemer, W., Joseph, M., et al. (2016). Electromyographical and perceptual responses to different resistance intensities in a squat protocol: does performing sets to failure with light loads produce the same activity? *Journal of Strength and Conditioning Research, 30*(3), 792–799.

MacDonald, H., Johnson, B., Huedo-Medina, T., et al. (2016). Dynamic resistance training as stand-alone antihypertensive lifestyle therapy: a meta-analysis. *Journal of the American Heart Association, 5*(10).

MacDougall, J., Sale, D., Alway, S., et al. (1984). Muscle fiber number in biceps brachii in bodybuilders and control subjects. *Journal of Applied Physiology, 57*(5), 1399–1403.

MacKenzie-Shalders, K., Kelly, J., So, D., et al. (2020). The effect of exercise interventions on resting metabolic rate: a systematic review and meta-analysis. *Journal of Sports Sciences, 38*(14), 1635–1649.

Maeo, S., Huang, M., Wu, Y., et al. (2021). Greater hamstrings muscle hypertrophy but similar damage protection after training at long versus short muscle lengths. *Medicine and Science in Sports and Exercise, 53*(4), 825–837.

Marcotte, G., West, D., & Baar, K. (2015). The molecular basis for load-induced skeletal muscle hypertrophy. *Calcified Tissue International, 96*(3), 196–210.

Martínez-Cava, A., Hernández-Belmonte, A., Courel-Ibáñez, J., et al. (2019). Bench press at full range of motion produces greater neuromuscular adaptations than partial executions after prolonged resistance training. *Journal of Strength and Conditioning Research.* Advance online publication.

Martorelli, S., Cadore, E., Izquierdo, M., et al. (2017). Strength training with repetitions to failure does not provide additional strength and muscle hypertrophy gains in young women. *European Journal of Translational Myology, 27*(2).

Mattocks, K., Jessee, M., Mouser, J., et al. (2018). The application of blood flow restriction: lessons from the laboratory. *Current Sports Medicine Reports, 17*(4), 129–134.

McKendry, J., Pérez-López, A., McLeod, M., et al. (2016). Short inter-set rest blunts resistance exercise-induced increases in myofibrillar protein synthesis and intracellular signalling in young males. *Experimental Physiology, 101*(7), 866–882.

Mclester, J., Bishop, P., Smith, J., et al. (2003). A series of studies- a practical protocol for testing muscular endurance recovery. *Journal of Strength & Conditioning Research, 17*(2), 259–273.

Methenitis, S., Mpampoulis, T., Spiliopoulou, P., et al. (2020). Muscle fiber composition, jumping performance and rate of force development adaptations induced by different power training volumes in females. *Applied Physiology, Nutrition, and Metabolism, 45*(9), 996–1006.

Millar, I., Barber, M., Lomax, M., et al. (1997). Mammary protein synthesis is acutely regulated by the cellular hydration state. *Biochemical and Biophysical Research Communications, 230*(2), 351–355.

Miranda, H., Maia, M., Paz, G., et al. (2018). Repetition performance and blood lactate responses adopting different recovery periods between training sessions in trained men. *Journal of Strength and Conditioning Research, 32*(12), 3340–3347.

Morán-Navarro, R., Pérez, C., Mora-Rodríguez, R., et al. (2017). Time course of recovery following resistance training leading or not to failure. *European Journal of Applied Physiology, 117*(12), 2387–2399.

Morton, R., Oikawa, S., & Wavell, C. (2016). Neither load nor systemic hormones determine resistance training-mediated hypertrophy or strength gains in resistance-trained young men. *Journal of Applied Physiology, 121*(1), 129–138.

Morton, R., Colenso-Semple, L., & Phillips, S. (2019). Training for strength and hypertrophy: an evidence-based approach. *Current Opinion in Physiology, 10*, 90–95.

Noorkõiv, M., Nosaka, K., & Blazevich, A. (2014). Neuromuscular adaptations associated with knee joint angle-specific force change. *Medicine and Science in Sports and Exercise, 46*(8), 1525–1537.

Nunes, J., Grgic, J., Cunha, P., et al. (2020). What influence does resistance exercise order have on muscular strength gains and muscle hypertrophy? A systematic review and meta-analysis. *European Journal of Sport Science*, 1–9.

Ogasawara, R., Akimoto, T., Umeno, T., et al. (2016). MicroRNA expression profiling in skeletal muscle reveals different regulatory patterns in high and low responders to resistance training. *Physiological Genomics, 48*(4), 320–324.

Oishi, Y., Tsukamoto, H., Yokokawa, T., et al. (2015). Mixed lactate and caffeine compound increases satellite cell activity and anabolic signals for muscle hypertrophy. *Journal of Applied Physiology*, 118(6), 742–749.

Orange, S., Metcalfe, J., Robinson, A., et al. (2019). Effects of in-season velocity-versus percentage-based training in academy rugby league players. *International Journal of Sports Physiology and Performance*, 1–8. Advance online publication.

Oranchuk, D., Storey, A., Nelson, A., et al., (2019). Isometric training and long-term adaptations: Effects of muscle length, intensity, and intent: A systematic review. *Scandinavian Journal of Medicine & Science in Sports, 29*(4), 484–503.

Paoli, A., Gentil, P., Moro, T., et al. (2017). Resistance training with single vs. Multijoint exercises at equal total load volume: effects on body composition, cardiorespiratory fitness, and muscle strength. *Frontiers in Physiology, 8*, 1105.

Pareja-Blanco, F., Rodríguez-Rosell, D., Aagaard, P., et al. (2020). Time course of recovery from resistance exercise with different set configurations. *Journal of Strength and Conditioning Research, 34*(10), 2867–2876.

Patterson, S., Hughes, L., Warmington, S., et al. (2019). Blood flow restriction exercise: considerations of methodology, application, and safety. *Frontiers in Physiology, 10*.

Pedersen, B., Akerström, T., Nielsen, A., et al. (2007). Role of myokines in exercise and metabolism. *Journal of Applied Physiology, 103*(3), 1093–1098.

Pedrosa, G., Lima, F., Schoenfeld, B., et al. (2021). Partial range of motion training elicits favorable improvements in muscular adaptations when carried out at long muscle lengths. *European Journal of Sport Science*, 1–11. Advance online publication.

Phillips, S. (2014). A brief review of critical processes in exercise-induced muscular hypertrophy. *Sports Medicine, 44*(S1), 71–77.

Radaelli, R., Fleck, S., Leite, T., et al. (2015). Dose-response of 1, 3, and 5 sets of resistance exercise on strength, local muscular endurance, and hypertrophy. *The Journal of Strength & Conditioning Research, 29*(5), 1349–1358.

Ralston, G., Kilgore, L., Wyatt, F., et al. (2017). The effect of weekly set volume on strength gain: a meta-analysis. *Sports Medicine, 47*(12), 2585–2601.

Raz, N., Ghisletta, P., Rodrigue, K., et al. (2010). Trajectories of brain aging in middle-aged and older adults: regional and individual differences. *NeuroImage, 51*(2), 501–511.

Roig, M., O'Brien, K., Kirk, G., et al. (2009). The effects of eccentric versus concentric resistance training on muscle strength and mass in healthy adults: a systematic review with meta-analysis. *British Journal of Sports Medicine, 43*(8), 556–568.

Roberts, M., Haun, C., Vann, C., et al. (2020). Sarcoplasmic hypertrophy in skeletal muscle: a scientific 'unicorn' or resistance training adaptation? *Frontiers in Physiology, 11.*

Rønnestad, B., Egeland, W., Kvamme, N., et al. (2007). Dissimilar effects of one- and three-set strength training on strength and muscle mass gains in upper and lower body in untrained subjects. *Journal of Strength and Conditioning Research, 21*(1), 157–163.

Saeidifard, F., Medina-Inojosa, J., West, C., et al. (2019). The association of resistance training with mortality: a systematic review and meta-analysis. *European Journal of Preventive Cardiology, 26*(15), 1647–1665.

Sánchez-Moreno, M., Cornejo-Daza, P., González-Badillo, J., et al. (2020). Effects of velocity loss during body mass prone-grip pull-up training on strength and endurance performance. *The Journal of Strength & Conditioning Research, 34*(4), 911–917.

Scarpelli, M., Nóbrega, S., Santanielo, N., et al. (2020). Muscle hypertrophy response is affected by previous resistance training volume in trained individuals. *Journal of Strength and Conditioning Research.* Online ahead of print.

Schoenfeld, B. (2012). Does exercise-induced muscle damage play a role in skeletal muscle hypertrophy? *Journal of Strength and Conditioning Research, 26*(5), 1441–1453.

Schoenfeld, B., Ogborn, D., & Krieger, J. (2015). Effect of repetition duration during resistance training on muscle hypertrophy: a systematic review and meta-analysis. *Sports Medicine, 45*(4), 577–585.

Schoenfeld, B., Contreras, B., Vigotsky, A., et al. (2016a). Effects of heavy versus moderate loads on measures of strength and hypertrophy in resistance-trained men. *Journal of Sports Science and Medicine, 15*(4), 715–722.

Schoenfeld, B., Ogborn, D., & Krieger, J. (2016b). Effects of resistance training frequency on measures of muscle hypertrophy: a systematic review and meta-analysis. *Sports Medicine, 46*(11), 1689–1697.

Schoenfeld, B., Pope, Z., Benik, F., et al. (2016c). Longer inter-set rest periods enhance muscle strength and hypertrophy in resistance-trained men. *Journal of Strength and Conditioning Research, 30*(7), 1805–1812.

Schoenfeld, B., Grgic, J., Ogborn, D., et al. (2017a). Strength and hypertrophy adaptations between low- vs. High-load resistance training: a systematic review and meta-analysis. *Journal of Strength and Conditioning Research, 31*(12), 3508–3523.

Schoenfeld, B., Ogborn, D., Vigotsky, A., et al. (2017b). Hypertrophic effects of concentric vs. Eccentric muscle actions: a systematic review and meta-analysis. *Journal of Strength and Conditioning Research, 31*(9), 2599–2608.

Schoenfeld, B., Contreras, B., Krieger, J., et al. (2019a). Resistance training volume enhances muscle hypertrophy but not strength in trained men. *Medicine and Science in Sports and Exercise, 51*(1), 94–103.

Schoenfeld, B., Grgic, J., & Krieger, J. (2019b). How many times per week should a muscle be trained to maximize muscle hypertrophy? A systematic review and meta-analysis of studies examining the effects of resistance training frequency. *Journal of Sports Sciences, 37*(11), 1286–1295.

Schoenfeld, B., & Grgic, J. (2020). Effects of range of motion on muscle development during resistance training interventions: a systematic review: *SAGE Open Medicine.*

Schuenke, M., Herman, J., Gliders, R., et al. (2012). Early-phase muscular adaptations in response to slow-speed versus traditional resistance-training regimens. *European Journal of Applied Physiology, 112*(10), 3585–3595.

Scott, W., Stevens, J., & Binder-Macleod, S. (2001). Human skeletal muscle fiber type classifications. *Physical Therapy, 81*(11), 1810–1816.

Senna, G., Willardson, J., Scudese, E., et al. (2016). Effect of different interest rest intervals on performance of single and multijoint exercises with near-maximal loads. *Journal of Strength and Conditioning Research, 30*(3), 710–716.

Seynnes, O., Boer, M., & Narici, M. (2007). Early skeletal muscle hypertrophy and architectural changes in response to high-intensity resistance training. *Journal of Applied Physiology, 102*(1), 368–373.

Shibata, K., Takizawa, K., Nosaka, K., et al. (2018). Effects of prolonging eccentric phase duration in parallel back-squat training to momentary failure on muscle cross-sectional area, squat one repetition maximum, and performance tests in university soccer players. *Journal of Strength and Conditioning Research, 35*(3), 668–674.

Siahkouhian, M., & Hedayatneja, M. (2010). Correlations of anthropometric and body composition variables with the performance of young elite weightlifters. *Journal of Human Kinetics, 25*(2010), 125–131.

Simpson, C., Kim, B., Bourcet, M., et al. (2017). Stretch training induces unequal adaptation in muscle fascicles and thickness in medial and lateral gastrocnemii. *Scandinavian Journal of Medicine & Science in Sports, 27*(12), 1597–1604.

Škarabot, J., Brownstein, C., Casolo, A., et al. (2021). The knowns and unknowns of neural adaptations to resistance training. *European Journal of Applied Physiology, 121*(3), 675–685.

Slater, L., & Hart, J. (2017). Muscle activation patterns during different squat techniques. *Journal of Strength and Conditioning Research, 31*(3), 667–676.

Stamatakis, E., Lee, I., Bennie, J., et al. (2018). Does strength-promoting exercise confer unique health benefits? A pooled analysis of data on 11 population cohorts with all-cause, cancer, and cardiovascular mortality endpoints. *American Journal of Epidemiology, 187*(5), 1102–1112.

Strasser, B., & Pesta, D. (2013). Resistance training for diabetes prevention and therapy: experimental findings and molecular mechanisms. *BioMed Research International, 2013*, 805217.

Suchomel, T., Nimphius, S., & Stone, M. (2016). The importance of muscular strength in athletic performance. *Sports Medicine, 46*(10), 1419–1449.

Sundstrup, E., Jakobsen, M., & Andersen, C. (2012). Muscle activation strategies during strength training with heavy loading vs. Repetitions to failure. *Journal of Strength and Conditioning Research, 26*(7), 1897–1903.

Tatsumi, R. (2010). Mechano-biology of skeletal muscle hypertrophy and regeneration: Possible mechanism of stretch-induced activation of resident myogenic stem cells. *Animal Science Journal, 81*, 11–20.

Tavares, L., Souza, E., Ugrinowitsch, C., et al. (2017). Effects of different strength training frequencies during reduced training period on strength and muscle cross-sectional area. *European Journal of Sport Science, 17*(6), 665–672.

Thyfault, J., & Bergouignan, A. (2020). Exercise and metabolic health: beyond skeletal muscle. *Diabetologia, 63*(8), 1464–1474.

Tresierras, M., & Balady, G. (2009). Resistance training in the treatment of diabetes and obesity: mechanisms and outcomes. *Journal of Cardiopulmonary Rehabilitation and Prevention, 29*(2), 67–75.

Trezise, J., & Blazevich, A. (2019). Anatomical and neuromuscular determinants of strength change in previously untrained men following heavy strength training. *Frontiers in Physiology, 10,* 1001.

Trezise, J., Collier, N., & Blazevich, A. (2016). Anatomical and neuromuscular variables strongly predict maximum knee extension torque in healthy men. *European Journal of Applied Physiology, 116*(6), 1159–1177.

Tsai, C., Wang, C., Pan, C., et al. (2015). The effects of long-term resistance exercise on the relationship between neurocognitive performance and GH, IGF-1, and homocysteine levels in the elderly. *Frontiers in Behavioral Neuroscience, 9,* 23.

Vigotsky, A., Contreras, B., & Beardsley, C. (2015). Biomechanical implications of skeletal muscle hypertrophy and atrophy: a musculoskeletal model. *PeerJ, 3,* e1462.

Vincent, K., & Braith, R. (2002). Resistance exercise and bone turnover in elderly men and women. *Medicine and Science in Sports and Exercise, 34*(1), 17–23.

Wackerhage, H., Schoenfeld, B., Hamilton, D., et al. (2019). Stimuli and sensors that initiate skeletal muscle hypertrophy following resistance exercise. *Journal of Applied Physiology, 126*(1), 30–43.

West, D., Kujbida, G., Moore, D., et al. (2009). Resistance exercise-induced increases in putative anabolic hormones do not enhance muscle protein synthesis or intracellular signalling in young men. *Journal of Physiology, 587*(21), 5239–5247.

Westcott, W., Winett, R., Anderson, E., et al. (2001). Effects of regular and slow speed resistance training on muscle strength. *The Journal of Sports Medicine and Physical Fitness, 41*(2), 154–158.

Wilke, J., Giesche, F., Klier, K., et al. (2019). Acute effects of resistance exercise on cognitive function in healthy adults: a systematic review with multilevel meta-analysis. *Sports Medicine, 49*(6), 905–916.

Willardson, J. (2007). The application of training to failure in periodized multiple-set resistance exercise programs. *Journal of Strength and Conditioning Research, 21*(2), 628–631.

Willardson, J., & Burkett, L. (2006). The effect of rest interval length on bench press performance with heavy vs. Light loads. *Journal of Strength and Conditioning Research, 20*(2), 396–399.

Willardson, J., & Burkett, L. (2008). The effect of different rest intervals between sets on volume components and strength gains. *Journal of Strength and Conditioning Research, 22*(1), 146–152.

Willoughby, D. (1993). The effects of mesocycle-length weight training programs involving periodization and partially equated volumes on upper and lower body strength. *Journal of Strength and Conditioning Research, 7*(1), 2–8.

Wilson, J., Loenneke, J., Jo, E., et al. (2012). The effects of endurance, strength, and power training on muscle fiber type shifting. *Journal of Strength and Conditioning Research, 26*(6), 1724–1729.

World Health Organization. (2020). *WHO guidelines on physical activity and sedentary behaviour.*

Yang, Y., Bay, P., Wang, Y., et al. (2018). Effects of consecutive versus non-consecutive days of resistance training on strength, body composition, and red blood cells. *Frontiers in Physiology, 9,* 725.

14 Training to improve body composition

Paul Hough

A common goal amongst personal training clients is to reduce body fat, more commonly known as 'losing weight'. Clients wishing to lose body fat intuitively focus on reducing body mass, using regular weigh-ins to monitor progress. Focusing on weight loss implies that all body mass is equal, and a reduction in body mass is a positive outcome, which is not the case. Instead, clients and trainers should focus on improving body composition (i.e., the proportion of fat and fat-free mass [FFM] in the body). A healthy body composition includes a lower proportion of body fat and a higher proportion of FFM, which consists of all bodily components other than fat tissue (e.g., muscle, bone, and organs). The preservation of muscle when reducing body fat is important as it has numerous essential functions and contributes to the resting metabolic rate (Bryner et al., 1999; Wolfe, 2006). Losing FFM, particularly protein from muscle and organs, is associated with increased appetite and weight regain, which is counterproductive to maintaining a lower body fat level (Turicchi et al., 2020). Furthermore, a loss of FFM could result in physiological changes that lead to hyperphagia (intense hunger) and excess fat gain to re-establish lean tissue homeostasis – this has been termed the 'fat overshooting' hypothesis (Dulloo et al., 2018). Therefore, fat loss programmes should focus on maintaining or increasing FFM while decreasing body fat.

Diet (energy in) is the principal determinant of body fat levels for most clients (Romieu et al., 2017), which can lead to the misguided assumption that exercise is unimportant for fat loss (Malhotra et al., 2015). Research indicates that a combined dietary *and* exercise approach is optimal for reducing body fat and, critically, maintaining fat-loss (Clark, 2015; Schwingshackl et al., 2013). Moreover, regular exercise improves numerous health aspects, which are independent of changes in body fat (e.g., cardiorespiratory fitness). Therefore, fat loss programmes should combine individualised dietary *and* exercise interventions to create an energy deficit (see Chapter 4). This chapter will explore how an exercise programme can be designed to improve body composition.

DOI: 10.4324/9781003204657-14

Endurance training for fat loss

Exercise recommendations for reducing body fat have historically focused on moderate-intensity continuous training (MICT), such as cycling and running (Donnelly et al., 2009; Haskell et al., 2007) because MICT or physical activity (PA) increases energy expenditure. Therefore, provided energy intake does not increase; performing MICT should create an energy deficit and reduce body fat. Research indicates that MICT can effectively reduce visceral fat, which is particularly detrimental to cardiometabolic health (Ismail et al., 2012). However, the evidence to support MICT for reducing total body fat (visceral and subcutaneous) mass is contentious, as several studies have reported either no change or only modest reductions in body fat following MICT (Donnelly et al., 2009; Swift et al., 2014). This discrepancy within the literature can be attributed to different dietary control levels, the volume of MICT performed between studies, and interindividual variation (discussed later).

What volume of physical activity or endurance exercise is required for fat loss?

Existing evidence indicates that 150–250 minutes/week of moderate-intensity PA is effective in preventing increases in body fat but only results in modest reductions in body fat (Donnelly et al., 2009; Thorogood et al., 2011). Higher volumes (>250 minutes/week) of PA or MICT are typically required to produce clinically significant reductions in body fat (Donnelly et al., 2009; Laskowski, 2012), but the exact volume of exercise required for fat loss is contentious. There is a dose-response relationship between exercise and positive health outcomes (see Chapter 10). However, a dose-response relationship between exercise volume and body fat is less clear, as increasing the volume of MICT does not always lead to further decreases in body fat (Friedenreich et al., 2019; Thomas et al., 2012). Indeed, several MICT programmes have not produced the magnitude of fat loss expected, based on the exercise's estimated energy expenditure (Church et al., 2009; Ross & Janssen, 2001; Slentz et al., 2004). For instance, similar reductions in body fat were reported between two groups during a 13-week exercise programme, despite one group performing double the volume of MICT than the other group (Rosenkilde et al., 2012).

A dose-response relationship between exercise and fat loss may exist (Friedenreich et al., 2015); however, programming more MICT is impractical for client's who are time-constrained (Sharifi et al., 2013). Therefore, increasing the intensity (and energy expenditure) of training sessions should be considered once a client consistently achieves up to 250 minutes/week of MICT or PA. Clients should be encouraged to maintain a minimum of 150 minutes/week of MICT or PA for health benefits and body composition maintenance (Catenacci & Wyatt, 2007).

What intensity of endurance exercise is optimal for fat loss?

The term 'the fat burning zone' is sometimes used to describe an intensity range where the body oxidises fat as a primary fuel. During low and moderate-intensity exercise, fat is oxidised (burned) at a high rate and gradually declines as exercise intensity (and carbohydrate oxidation) increases (Brooks & Mercier, 1994) (see Figure 14.1). The maximal rate of fat oxidation (FatMax) typically occurs at an intensity corresponding to 60–65% VO_{2max} (Achten & Jeukendrup, 2003; Achten et al., 2002). However, this varies (50–85% VO_{2max}) between individuals due to factors such as age, diet and training status (Achten & Jeukendrup, 2003; Carey, 2009).

A period of low to moderate-intensity endurance training can improve the muscle's capacity to oxidise fat, which is beneficial for metabolic health and potentially reducing body fat in the long-term (Barwell et al., 2009; Goodpaster & Sparks, 2017). However, fat loss requires creating an energy deficit, which means that dietary energy intake is lower than the body's energy requirements (Strasser et al., 2007). Exercise performed at FatMax (i.e., in the fat-burning zone) is not a time-efficient method for creating an energy deficit as the rate of energy expenditure is lower (i.e., kcal/minute) compared to higher intensity exercise (see Figure 14.2). Exercising above the FatMax intensity decreases the rate of fat oxidation, but the total energy expenditure will be higher during a time equated training session. Figure 14.2 shows fat oxidation and energy expenditure during a metabolic assessment of a runner. Fat oxidation decreased when the intensity was above FatMax (13 km), but energy expenditure increased. Consequently,

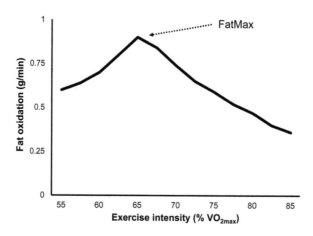

Figure 14.1 A typical pattern of fat oxidation during incremental endurance exercise.*

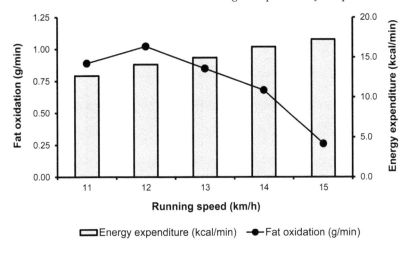

Figure 14.2 Fax oxidation and energy expenditure measured during exercise.

when a client has training time constraints, it is prudent to focus on endurance training that maximises total energy expenditure rather than the substrate used during exercise. A method that has become popular for maximising energy expenditure is high-intensity interval training (HIIT).

High-intensity interval training for fat loss

As MICT programmes performed without a dietary intervention often have a negligible effect on total body fat, researchers began studying the effect of HIIT on fat loss (Tremblay et al., 1994). Several theories have been proposed to explain why HIIT could be more effective than MICT for reducing body fat. The central theory is that HIIT provides a more time-efficient method to increase energy expenditure and create an energy deficit, as HIIT involves a higher degree of energy expenditure per unit of time (Skelly et al., 2014). Furthermore, after a HIIT session, there is an increase in energy expenditure due to an increase in oxygen uptake, known as excess post-exercise oxygen consumption or EPOC for short (LaForgia et al., 2006).

The EPOC is usually higher after HIIT compared to MICT due to an elevation in metabolic process, such as the removal of lactate/hydrogen ions and resynthesis of glycogen (Jung et al., 2019). These physiological processes can increase fat metabolism during and after exercise, which may positively affect metabolism and fat loss over time (Jung et al., 2019; Sevits et al., 2013; Williams et al., 2013). However, the EPOC following HIIT is relatively small compared to the energy expended during the session itself. For example, Tucker et al. (2016) reported that EPOC was higher after sprint interval training (SIT) than MICT. However, total net energy

272   *Paul Hough*

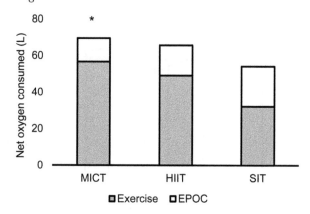

* indicates significantly greater overall net O$_2$ consumed in MICT compared with SIT

Figure 14.3 Net oxygen consumed during exercise and post-exercise for moderate-intensity continuous training (MICT), high-intensity interval training (HIIT), and sprint interval training (SIT). Reproduced with permission from Tucker et al. (2016).

expenditure (exercise + post-exercise) after SIT was less than MICT and HIIT (see Figure 14.3).

The magnitude of EPOC following HIIT is highly variable between individuals and appears to reduce as fitness improves (Børsheim & Bahr, 2003). Therefore, clients who are unaccustomed to HIIT may experience greater relative changes in energy expenditure and body fat when they perform regular HIIT (Børsheim & Bahr, 2003). However, the EPOC from HIIT is unlikely to be a significant contributor to energy expenditure and fat loss. A review of 22 studies reported that EPOC was higher following HIIT than MICT, but the difference in energy expenditure from the greater EPOC only equated to ~31 Calories (Panissa et al., 2020).

Does high-intensity exercise decrease appetite?

Exercise intensity can influence circulating levels of hormones that affect appetite. Therefore, another mechanism that may facilitate a negative energy balance following HIIT is a reduction in appetite and food intake. For example, ghrelin, a hunger-stimulating hormone, has been shown to decrease as exercise intensity increases (Broom et al., 2017). The mechanisms involved in suppressing appetite-stimulating hormones following high-intensity exercise are not fully understood, but research suggests increased lactate during/after exercise could be involved (Vanderheyden et al., 2020). Research examining the effect of HIIT on appetite and post-exercise energy intake has produced inconsistent results due to numerous confounding factors, such as genetic variation (Karra et al., 2013). Some individuals experience a large suppression in appetite following exercise, whereas others do not (Dorling et al., 2018). Nonetheless, individuals who perform regular PA seem to have improved appetite sensitivity, which may facilitate long-term energy balance and weight maintenance (Dorling et al., 2018).

Is HIIT more effective in practice for fat loss than MICT?

One of the first studies to investigate the effect of exercise intensity on fat loss compared MICT (cycling, 4–5 sessions/week for 30–45 minutes) to a mixed programme of MICT (25 sessions) and HIIT (35 sessions). The authors calculated that, when expressed relative to the exercise's energy cost, the reduction in body fat was nine times greater in the HIIT group (Tremblay et al., 1994). However, these seemingly impressive findings lack practical application, as the programme involved training five days per week and included MICT, which detracts from a primary advantage of HIIT (reduced training time). Consequently, other studies have adopted SIT protocols that are shorter and potentially more time efficient.

SIT studies have reported more significant reductions in body fat compared to MICT amongst sedentary women (Trapp et al., 2008) and recreationally active adults (Macpherson et al., 2011). However, other studies have not reported significant body fat changes after SIT (Astorino et al., 2013) or HIIT (Keating et al., 2014). The discrepancy between studies is due to methodological differences (e.g., level of dietary control, the HIIT protocol, and the population studied). For example, the amount of fat loss appears to be related to the individual's baseline (starting) body fat level. It is possible that HIIT can facilitate a decrease in body fat amongst relatively lean individuals (Shing et al., 2013); however, studies involving overweight/obese populations have typically reported larger reductions in total body fat compared to leaner participants (Gillen et al., 2013; Wewege et al., 2017). Another important consideration when comparing HIIT studies is the type of exercise performed. Running based HIIT is more likely to induce a higher energy expenditure than cycling and could, theoretically, induce a greater energy deficit and magnitude of fat loss (Wewege et al., 2017).

To address the conflicting findings between HIIT studies, researchers have analysed the results from multiple studies (meta-analysis) to establish if HIIT is superior to MICT for fat loss (see Table 14.1). Collectively, these meta-analyses indicate that HIIT or SIT are not superior methods for fat loss than MICT, as most HIIT will involve a similar or lower total energy expenditure than MICT. Indeed, a sub-analysis within one study indicated that HIIT protocols involving a lower energy expenditure than MICT tended to be less effective for reducing total body fat (Keating et al., 2017).

Table 14.1 The efficacy of HIIT versus MICT for reducing body fat

Study	Studies/participants	Key findings
Keating et al. (2017)	Meta-analysis (*n*=28)	No significant difference in fat mass (kg), body fat (%) or fat free mass (FFM) between HIIT and MICT.
	Participants (*n*=873)	HIIT and MICT achieved similar reductions in body fat (%) and total body fat mass (kg)
		Body fat %: HIIT −1.26% vs MICT −1.48% Fat mass (kg): HIIT −1.38 vs MICT −0.91
		Sub-group analysis
		Studies that employed HIIT protocols that were lower in time commitment than MICT tended to favour MICT for total body fat reduction.
Sultana et al. (2019)	Meta-analysis (*n*=47) Participants (*n*=1458)	No significant difference in fat mass (kg), body fat (%) or fat free mass (FFM) between HIIT and MICT.
Wewege et al. (2017)	Meta-analysis (*n*=13) Participants (*n*=424 overweight and obese adults)	No significant difference in fat mass (kg), body fat (%) or fat free mass (FFM) between HIIT and MICT.
		HIIT and MICT achieved reductions in whole-body fat mass and waist circumference.
		HIIT required ~40% less training time commitment

Why do some individuals lose more fat than others?

Regardless of the type of exercise (MICT or HIIT) adopted, a recurrent theme within the research is the large variability in fat loss between individuals following the same exercise programme (Barwell et al., 2009; King et al., 2008; Rosenkilde et al., 2012). This variability can be attributed to physiological and behavioural compensatory mechanisms that are activated during an energy deficit. Firstly, some individuals sub-consciously increase caloric intake when they exercise more, known as dietary compensation (Thomas et al., 2012). Additionally, when energy expenditure significantly increases (i.e., performing more exercise), total daily energy expenditure (TDEE) begins to plateau as the body adapts to maintain TDEE within a narrow range. This preservation of daily energy expenditure is the constrained total energy expenditure (CTEE) model conceptualised by Pontzer et al. (2016). Scientists have proposed that CTEE is an evolutionary mechanism where physiological compensatory mechanisms constrain TDEE when energy expenditure is significantly increased, thus ensuring TDEE remains relatively stable (Fernández-Verdejo et al., 2021; Pontzer et al., 2016). The CTEE model partly explains why exercise, without

---

BOX 14.1

Does training fasted promote fat loss?

Martin MacDonald

It has been suggested in the fitness industry and lay media that performing MICT before eating in the morning will lead to more significant body fat loss. The premise of this belief is that blood insulin levels will be low, cortisol will be high, glycogen stores will be lowered and, in the absence of food intake, the body will be forced to use stored fat as fuel (Spriet, 2014).

To obey the first law of thermodynamics, when it comes to longitudinal fat loss, fasted exercise would need to induce a negative energy balance either through increasing 24-hour energy expenditure or by reducing ad libitum energy intake. However, these effects have not been reported with fasted exercise (McIver et al., 2019). Exercising in the fasted state has been shown to increase fat oxidation during the exercise session itself; however, fat oxidation was shown to be greater in the fed group 12- and 24-hours post-exercise (Paoli et al., 2011). Another study where participants performed 100 minutes of fasted exercise (AM) vs exercise after lunch (PM) indicated that fasted training could lead to significant increases in 24-hour fat oxidation, while fed groups burned more carbohydrate (Iwayama et al., 2015). However, despite the greater fat oxidation in the fasted groups, the 24-hour energy balance was not different between groups (Iwayama et al., 2015). Furthermore, with limited carbohydrate stores in the body, the results of short-term studies cannot be extrapolated to the chronic effects of fasted exercise (Shimada et al., 2013).

Two interesting studies have investigated body composition changes when comparing exercise in the fed vs fasted state. The first looked at the effect of females performing 18 sessions of HIIT over six weeks in the fed vs fasted state. Both groups lost body fat and gained muscle; however, there was no difference between the two groups (Gillen et al., 2013). The second study by Schoenfeld et al. (2014) assigned females to a hypocaloric diet and then randomised them to one hour of aerobic exercise (three days per week) in either the fed or fasted state. Again, both groups showed significant weight and fat loss, but there were no significant differences between groups.

Based on the current research, it appears that exercising in the fasted state has no significant impact on long-term fat loss. Therefore, those undertaking MICT or HIIT to support the goal of fat loss can choose their preferred time of day to perform the exercise, whether in the fed or fasted state.

---

a dietary intervention, is not optimal for decreasing body fat. Examples of compensatory mechanisms that become activated following a significant increase in exercise/PA and subsequent energy deficit include:

- There is a change in the balance of hormones related to appetite, causing an increase in energy intake (Sumithran et al., 2011).

- Metabolic efficiency improves during exercise; burning fewer calories for the same volume/intensity of exercise (Amati et al., 2008).
- There is a decrease in resting energy expenditure (REE) as body mass decreases (Hopkins et al., 2014).
- There is a decrease in non-exercise activity thermogenesis (NEAT), which means doing less activity outside of planned exercise (Redman et al., 2009).

The physiological compensatory mechanisms (listed above) interact to varying degrees between individuals, which explains why some individuals experience more significant reductions in body fat than others, despite doing the same exercise programme (Riou et al., 2015).

Is endurance or high-intensity interval training necessary for fat loss?

Both MICT and HIIT improve cardiorespiratory fitness and are an important component of a holistic exercise programme, particularly for clients who are not achieving the PA guidelines (see Box 10.3). However, endurance training is not essential for fat loss as an energy deficit can be achieved without it. In some cases, extensive endurance training could be detrimental. For example, using endurance training to increase an already sizable energy deficit, coupled with insufficient protein intake, may produce the undesirable effect of reducing FFM and strength (Hammer et al., 1989; Villareal et al., 2011). Provided the fat loss programme is designed correctly (i.e., adequate-protein, induces a moderate energy deficit, and includes resistance training), judicious use of MICT and/or HIIT could increase the energy deficit without significantly reducing FFM or strength. HIIT should be prescribed carefully, as the high neuromuscular strain of some protocols (see Chapter 11) can increase residual fatigue and recovery time during periods of caloric restriction (Bishop et al., 2008; Helms et al., 2015; Stanley et al., 2013).

Practical application of MICT or HIIT within a fat loss programme

- MICT can be included for general health and maintaining a weight loss of 0.5–1% of body weight/week (Helms et al., 2014). The application of MICT depends on several factors, such as the client's personal preferences and time availability. Increasing daily PA is a practical method to increase energy expenditure when clients do not have time to perform structured MICT.
- When MICT is impractical or disliked, HIIT can be incorporated within a fat loss programme to increase energy expenditure with a lower time commitment to MICT. HIIT is also a time-efficient option to attain several health benefits.

- MICT does not include low-intensity PA, such as walking or everyday activities, which likely have little to no negative effect on recovery or RT adaptations (Schumann & Rønnestad, 2019). Several approaches can be used to increase daily PA and subsequent energy expenditure, such as setting daily step targets (see Chapter 10), using stairs instead of escalators and active commuting. The total duration of weekly endurance training should be limited to no more than half of the total duration of RT. For example, if a client does four hours of RT/week, he/she would limit MICT to two hours (Helms et al., 2019).
- In most cases, if fat loss has plateaued, energy intake should be reduced before increasing MICT or HIIT, unless further reducing energy intake would produce significant negative psychological and physiological symptoms (Helms et al., 2014).
- HIIT should be carefully programmed as it can increase recovery time between sessions.
- Although not necessary for fat loss, MICT and HIIT improve cardiorespiratory fitness and should not necessarily be excluded from a training programme.

Resistance training for fat loss
Paul Hough and Mike Matthews

As with MICT, research into the effects of resistance training (RT) on fat loss is conflicting. A period of RT has been demonstrated to decrease total body fat in some studies (Hunter et al., 2002; Prabhakaran et al., 1999), but not others (Bouchard et al., 2009; Ribeiro et al., 2016). Although the energy expenditure during RT is typically lower than MICT, it could increase the rate of fat loss over time through other mechanisms. For example, RT could increase daily PA, leading to increased TDEE (Hunter et al., 2015).

Resistance training to maximise energy expenditure

As fat loss is a function of energy expenditure exceeding energy intake, RT sessions can be designed to maximise energy expenditure and facilitate an energy deficit. For instance, one hour of RT can burn 200–500 ckcal, depending on the exercises used, the volume/intensity of the sets, and the individual's body mass (Brown et al., 1994; Morgan et al., 2003). High-intensity functional training (see Chapter 11) or circuit training approaches can be designed to maximise energy expenditure. However, RT sessions designed to maximise energy expenditure should be used sparingly. The main goal of RT within a fat loss programme is to preserve (or increase) FFM and minimise the compensatory effects (e.g., decreased RMR) associated with a chronic energy deficit (Bryner et al., 1999); these objectives can be achieved by training with sufficient volume and intensity (see page 279).

Does resistance training increase post-exercise energy expenditure?

Similar to HIIT, the anaerobic nature of RT increases oxygen uptake for a period after training (i.e., EPOC) to restore metabolic processes to their pre-exercise state. The magnitude of the EPOC response is variable between individuals and is dependent on the RT protocol. For example, resting metabolic rate (RMR) increased by 5%, three days after a RT session (one set of ten exercises) amongst untrained individuals (Heden et al., 2011). Conversely, RT sessions using load-volumes up to 20,000 kg did not significantly affect RMR in trained males (Abboud et al., 2013), which indicates the increase in RMR following RT decreases as fitness improves as part of the adaptive process (Børsheim & Bahr, 2003). The discrepancy in the EPOC responses between untrained and trained individuals can partly be attributed to untrained individuals experiencing more muscle damage and metabolic disruption after unaccustomed exercise. Trained individuals usually experience less muscle damage and metabolic disruption after training (Hyldahl et al., 2017). In summary, the increase in EPOC following RT is unlikely to be a fundamental mechanism that produces reductions in body fat.

The benefits of resistance training within a fat loss programme

As discussed in Chapter 13, RT can elicit numerous favourable metabolic adaptations and reduce cardiovascular and metabolic disease risk factors. For example, an improvement in insulin sensitivity could promote a favourable metabolic environment for fat burning (Nordby et al., 2015). Moreover, muscle tissue has a higher metabolic rate (i.e., expends more energy) than adipose tissue (Wolfe, 2006). Therefore, increasing muscle mass through RT can increase RMR (MacKenzie-Shalders et al., 2020). The magnitude of the increase in RMR depends on the amount of muscle gained and is usually modest. For example, a one kilogram increase in muscle tissue may only increase RMR by 20 kcal/day (Strasser & Schobersberger, 2011). Nevertheless, recent research indicates that regular RT could increase RMR by approximately 100 kcal/day (MacKenzie-Shalders et al., 2020), which could have a practically meaningful effect on weight management over time.

Regular RT is beneficial during an energy-restricted diet because it increases muscle protein synthesis, promoting muscle retention (see Chapter 13). Therefore, RT should be incorporated within a fat loss programme to increase the proportion of weight loss from fat while minimising/preventing muscle loss (Helms et al., 2015; Hunter et al., 2008; Willis et al., 2012). Furthermore, RT can also prevent a substantial decline in RMR (Bryner et al., 1999). Although an energy deficit can potentially restrict muscle hypertrophy, under the right conditions, RT could potentially increase muscle and decrease fat mass during caloric restriction – this is known as 'body recomposition' and will be discussed later.

Resistance training for fat loss guidelines

The RT guidelines for hypertrophy, presented in Chapter 13, can be applied within fat loss programmes. In general, each muscle group can be trained 2–3 times/week with a volume of ~40–70 repetitions/muscle group/session (Helms et al., 2015). However, performance during RT and recovery after RT sessions could be impaired during a prolonged energy-restricted diet (Huovinen et al., 2015; Ørtenblad et al., 2013). Therefore, training to failure (see Chapter 13) should be used sparingly and substantial increases in total training volume (hard sets) should be avoided. Indeed, to facilitate recovery between sessions, training volume could be reduced during a fat loss programme without compromising muscle size (Helms et al., 2015). Alternatively, training frequency can be increased to distribute volume. For example, performing the same total number of weekly sets over five instead of four sessions.

Combining endurance and resistance training (concurrent training)

Endurance training can interfere with adaptations to RT (see Chapter 10), reducing increases in strength and FFM (Baar, 2014). Running seems to be particularly detrimental in this regard. In contrast, other forms of low-impact endurance exercise, such as cycling, appear to have a less negative impact on strength and muscle hypertrophy (Wilson et al., 2012). Consequently, the following logistical considerations should be implemented within a fat loss programme:

- Limit the duration of MICT (<45 minutes). Low-intensity PA, such as walking or light cycling, do not need to be time-limited.
- Separate resistance and endurance training sessions by at least six hours, if possible
- Perform endurance and RT workouts that train the same muscle group on different days, if possible.
- Perform endurance training after RT (if the sessions cannot be separated) (Murach & Bagley, 2016).

Exercise for fat loss: Practical recommendations and summary

- While it is possible to reduce body fat by performing MICT without caloric restriction, this approach requires high volumes of exercise, which are impractical and unsustainable for most clients.
- An exercise programme without a dietary intervention does not usually produce a significant or permanent reduction in body fat. Therefore, all fat loss programmes should focus on a combination of diet and exercise.

- Along with appropriate dietary modifications (see Chapter 4), optimal and sustainable fat loss can be achieved using a combination of endurance and resistance exercise. Endurance training can facilitate an energy deficit and improve cardiorespiratory fitness. Alongside other health benefits, RT protects FFM.
- The magnitude of fat loss following any exercise programme is highly variable between individuals due to differences in total energy expenditure, compensatory dietary changes, and the complex effects of exercise on metabolism.
- RT should be included to preserve or increase FFM and minimise a reduction in RMR. Substantial increases in training volume should be avoided during a prolonged energy restricted diet.
- As total energy expenditure is an important determinant of fat loss over time, the use of higher intensity training methods, such as HIIT, can be included within a fat loss programme. Although HIIT is a time-efficient method for improving cardiorespiratory fitness, it is not a superior training method for reducing body fat.

Body recomposition
Mike Matthews

Body recomposition (BR) is the process of simultaneously decreasing fat mass and increasing the proportion of fat-free mass (FFM); it can be accomplished in three ways: (1) concurrently reducing fat mass and maintaining FFM; (2) maintaining fat mass and increasing FFM, and (3) reducing fat mass and increasing FFM. Typically, the term BR is used in the context of simultaneously reducing fat mass and increasing skeletal muscle mass; this form of BR will be the focus of this section. Some trainers may believe increasing muscle while concurrently decreasing fat mass can only occur in clients who are new to RT, whereas others may believe this form of BR is almost impossible. This section aims to clarify common misunderstandings clients might have regarding BR and provide evidence-based guidelines for concurrently reducing fat and increasing muscle.

Scientific evidence for body recomposition

Body recomposition in the form of simultaneous fat loss and muscle gain can occur to varying degrees between individuals under certain conditions. The most potent stimulus for BR is progressive resistance training (RT) which, when combined with a well-designed diet (energy deficit and adequate protein intake), can produce marked changes in body fat and FFM relative to total body mass. Individuals who have excess body fat (overweight/obesity) typically experience the largest BR effects, particularly if they are new to RT. For example, a study amongst sedentary, overweight police officers, with no RT background, reported significant BR effects in 12 weeks (Demling & DeSanti, 2000). Specifically, the participants followed a four-day/week progressive RT programme and an energy-restricted diet (1.4 g/kg of protein/day). After 12 weeks, the participants lost 4.2–7 kg of body fat and gained 2–4 kg of FFM, on average.

Research indicates BR can also occur in the elderly (Iglay et al., 2007), well-trained weightlifters (Paoli et al., 2012), women (Nindl et al., 2000), and very lean individuals (Garthe et al., 2011; MacKenzie-Shalders et al., 2016). However, the magnitude of the BR effect depends on several factors, and it does not always occur to the same extent (or at all) in all populations (Garthe et al., 2011; Hulmi et al., 2017; Josse & Phillips, 2012).

Body recomposition and training history

It is well-established that RT novices can gain muscle while losing significant body fat (Demling & DeSanti, 2000; di Palumbo et al., 2017; Josse et al., 2010; Nindl et al., 2000; Verreijen et al., 2017). However, individuals with a long RT history who are closer to their genetic potential for muscle gain are less likely to achieve BR, even if dietary and training conditions are optimal (Alway et al., 1992; Helms et al., 2014; Hulmi et al., 2017). While BR can occur in trained athletes, the magnitude tends to be much smaller and is often negligible or non-existent (Chappell et al., 2018; Hulmi et al., 2016; Robinson et al., 2015). For example, during a 12-week diet/RT exercise programme, athletes reduced body fat by ~5% but only increased FFM mass by ~1% (Garthe et al., 2011).

Body recomposition and body fat percentage

An energy deficit is required to lose body fat and achieve BR; however, as an individual becomes leaner, it becomes more difficult to preserve or increase muscle mass during an energy deficit (Hall, 2007; Helms et al., 2014). Thus, leaner individuals are less likely to experience BR than those with more body fat. People with significantly lower body fat levels than average (<10% for males and <20% for females) should not expect to gain much (if any) muscle mass while reducing their body fat but should endeavour to maintain muscle mass (Garthe et al., 2011).

Body recomposition and energy intake

Small to moderate energy deficits cause less muscle loss and facilitate BR in already lean individuals, whereas large energy deficits and rapid fat loss prevent gains in FFM and can even decrease FFM (Forbes, 2000; Hall, 2007; Huovinen et al., 2015). Even in obese individuals, larger energy deficits (i.e., extreme diets) tend to increase the percentage of weight loss from FFM (Redman et al., 2009), making more moderate energy deficits a better choice if the goal is BR. It is improbable that BR will occur in an energy surplus, regardless of training protocols adopted. Although muscle mass can increase, so will fat mass. Therefore, it is difficult, if not impossible, to build muscle and lose fat simultaneously while maintaining a net energy surplus (Aragon et al., 2017; Garthe et al., 2013).

Body recomposition and protein intake

Adequate protein intake is necessary to support gains in FFM, as insufficient protein intake can decrease the chances of achieving BR (Mettler et al., 2010). Higher protein intakes in conjunction with regular RT enhance FFM gains (or minimise losses) compared to lower protein intakes in relatively lean, female physique competitors (Campbell et al., 2018). Energy restriction, RT and low levels of body fat all increase protein requirements for building and maintaining muscle (Helms et al., 2014). Therefore, lean individuals (<10% body fat for males and <20% for females) should consider consuming 2.3–3.1 g of protein/kg of FFM per day to preserve and increase the likelihood of gaining muscle while losing fat (Helms et al., 2014).

Body recomposition practical recommendations and summary

* Resistance training should be prioritised within the training programme (see guidelines above and Chapter 13).
* The diet should be modified to produce a small to moderate energy deficit and elicit a gradual reduction in body fat.
* Individuals seeking BR should consume adequate protein (1.6-2 g/kg of body mass/day).
* Individuals with very low body fat levels (<10% for males; <20% for females) may benefit from increasing protein intake to >2–3.1 g/kg of FFM when dieting.

References

Abboud, G., Greer, B., & Campbell, S. (2013). Effects of load-volume on EPOC after acute bouts of resistance training in resistance-trained men. *The Journal of Strength & Conditioning Research*, 27(7), 1936–1941.

Achten, J., Gleeson, M., & Jeukendrup, A. (2002). Determination of the exercise intensity that elicits maximal fat oxidation. *Medicine and Science in Sports and Exercise*, 34(1), 92–97.

Achten, J., & Jeukendrup, A. (2003). The effect of pre-exercise carbohydrate feedings on the intensity that elicits maximal fat oxidation. *Journal of Sports Sciences*, 21(12), 1017–1024.

Alway, S., Grumbt, W., Stray-Gundersen, J., et al. (1992). Effects of resistance training on elbow flexors of highly competitive bodybuilders. *Journal of Applied Physiology*, 72(4), 1512–1521.

Amati, F., Dubé, J., Shay, C., et al. (2008). Separate and combined effects of exercise training and weight loss on exercise efficiency and substrate oxidation. *Journal of Applied Physiology, 105*(3), 825–831.

Aragon, A., Schoenfeld, B., Wildman, R., et al. (2017). International society of sports nutrition position stand: diets and body composition. *Journal of the International Society of Sports Nutrition, 14*, 16.

Astorino, T., Schubert, M., Palumbo, E., et al. (2013). Magnitude and time course of changes in maximal oxygen uptake in response to distinct regimens of chronic interval training in sedentary women. *European Journal of Applied Physiology, 113*(9), 2361–2369.

Baar, K. (2014). Using molecular biology to maximize concurrent training. *Sports Medicine, 44*(S2), 117–125.

Barwell, N., Malkova, D., Leggate, M., et al. (2009). Individual responsiveness to exercise-induced fat loss is associated with change in resting substrate utilization. *Metabolism: clinical and experimental, 58*(9), 1320–1328.

Bishop, P., Jones, E., & Woods, A. (2008). Recovery from training: a brief review. *Journal of Strength and Conditioning Research, 22*(3), 1015–1024.

Børsheim, E., & Bahr, R. (2003). Effect of exercise intensity, duration and mode on post-exercise oxygen consumption. *Sports Medicine, 33*(14), 1037–1060.

Bouchard, D., Soucy, L., Sénéchal, M., et al. (2009). Impact of resistance training with or without caloric restriction on physical capacity in obese older women. *Menopause, 16*(1), 66–72.

Brooks, G., & Mercier, J. (1994). Balance of carbohydrate and lipid utilization during exercise: the 'crossover' concept. *Journal of Applied Physiology, 76*(6), 2253–2261.

Broom, D., Miyashita, M., Wasse, L., et al. (2017). Acute effect of exercise intensity and duration on acylated ghrelin and hunger in men. *The Journal of Endocrinology, 232*(3), 411–422.

Brown, S., Clemons, J., He, Q., et al. (1994). Prediction of the oxygen cost of the deadlift exercise. *Journal of Sports Sciences, 12*(4), 371–375.

Bryner, R., Ullrich, I., Sauers, J., et al. (1999). Effects of resistance vs. aerobic training combined with an 800 calorie liquid diet on lean body mass and resting metabolic rate. *Journal of the American College of Nutrition, 18*(2), 115–121.

Campbell, B., Aguilar, D., Conlin, L., et al. (2018). Effects of high versus low protein intake on body composition and maximal strength in aspiring female physique athletes engaging in an 8-week resistance training program. *International Journal of Sport Nutrition and Exercise Metabolism, 28*(6), 580–585.

Carey, D. (2009). Quantifying differences in the "fat burning" zone and the aerobic zone: implications for training. *Journal of Strength and Conditioning Research, 23*(7), 2090–2095.

Catenacci, V., & Wyatt, H. (2007). The role of physical activity in producing and maintaining weight loss. *Nature Clinical Practice Endocrinology & Metabolism, 3*(7), 518–529.

Chappell, A., Simper, T., & Barker, M. (2018). Nutritional strategies of high level natural bodybuilders during competition preparation. *Journal of the International Society of Sports Nutrition, 15*, 4.

Church, T., Martin, C., Thompson, A., et al. (2009). Changes in weight, waist circumference and compensatory responses with different doses of exercise among sedentary, overweight postmenopausal women. *PLOS ONE, 4*(2), e4515.

Clark, J. (2015). Diet, exercise or diet with exercise: comparing the effectiveness of treatment options for weight-loss and changes in fitness for adults (18–65 years old) who are overfat, or obese: systematic review and meta-analysis. *Journal of Diabetes and Metabolic Disorders, 14*(1), 31.

Demling, R., & DeSanti, L. (2000). Effect of a hypocaloric diet, increased protein intake and resistance training on lean mass gains and fat mass loss in overweight police officers. *Annals of Nutrition & Metabolism, 44*(1), 21–29.

Donnelly, J., Blair, S., Jakicic, J., et al. (2009). American College of sports medicine position stand. Appropriate physical activity intervention strategies for weight loss and prevention of weight regain for adults. *Medicine and Science in Sports and Exercise, 41*(2), 459–471.

Dorling, J., Broom, D., Burns, S., et al. (2018). Acute and chronic effects of exercise on appetite, energy intake, and appetite-related hormones: the modulating effect of adiposity, sex, and habitual physical activity. *Nutrients, 10*(9), 1140.

Dulloo, A., Miles-Chan, J., & Schutz, Y. (2018). Collateral fattening in body composition autoregulation: its determinants and significance for obesity predisposition. *European Journal of Clinical Nutrition, 72*(5), 657–664.

Forbes, G. (2000). Body fat content influences the body composition response to nutrition and exercise. *Annals of the New York Academy of Sciences, 904*, 359–365.

Fernández-Verdejo, R., Alcantara, J., Galgani, J., et al. (2021). Deciphering the constrained total energy expenditure model in humans by associating accelerometer-measured physical activity from wrist and hip. *Scientific Reports, 11*(1), 12302.

Friedenreich, C., Neilson, H., O'Reilly, R., et al. (2015). Effects of a high vs moderate volume of aerobic exercise on adiposity outcomes in postmenopausal women: a randomized clinical trial. *JAMA Oncology, 1*(6), 766–776.

Friedenreich, C., Ruan, Y., Duha, A., et al. (2019). Exercise dose effects on body fat 12 months after an exercise intervention: follow-up from a randomized controlled trial. *Journal of Obesity, 2019*. ID 3916416

Garthe, I., Raastad, T., Refsnes, P., et al. (2011). Effect of two different weight-loss rates on body composition and strength and power-related performance in elite athletes. *International Journal of Sport Nutrition and Exercise Metabolism, 21*(2), 97–104.

Garthe, I., Raastad, T., Refsnes, P., et al. (2013). Effect of nutritional intervention on body composition and performance in elite athletes. *European Journal of Sport Science, 13*(3), 295–303.

Gillen, J., Percival, M., Ludzki, A., et al. (2013). Interval training in the fed or fasted state improves body composition and muscle oxidative capacity in overweight women. *Obesity, 21*(11), 2249–2255.

Goodpaster, B., & Sparks, L. (2017). Metabolic flexibility in health and disease. *Cell Metabolism, 25*(5), 1027–1036.

Hall, K. (2007). Body fat and fat-free mass inter-relationships: Forbes's theory revisited. *The British Journal of Nutrition, 97*(6), 1059–1063.

Hammer, R., Barrier, C., Roundy, E., et al. (1989). Calorie-restricted low-fat diet and exercise in obese women. *The American Journal of Clinical Nutrition, 49*(1), 77–85.

Haskell, W., Lee, I., Pate, R., et al. (2007). Physical activity and public health: updated recommendation for adults from the American College of sports medicine and the American heart association. *Medicine and Science in Sports and Exercise, 39*(8), 1423–1434.

Heden, T., Lox, C., Rose, P., et al. (2011). One-set resistance training elevates energy expenditure for 72 h similar to three sets. *European Journal of Applied Physiology, 111*(3), 477–484.

Helms, E., Fitschen, P., Aragon, A., et al. (2015). Recommendations for natural bodybuilding contest preparation: resistance and cardiovascular training. *The Journal of Sports Medicine and Physical Fitness, 55*(3), 164–178.

Helms, E., Zinn, C., Rowlands, D., et al. (2014). A systematic review of dietary protein during caloric restriction in resistance trained lean athletes: a case for higher intakes. *International Journal of Sport Nutrition and Exercise Metabolism, 24*(2), 127–138.

Helms, E., Morgan, A., & Valdez, A. (2019). *The muscle and strength pyramid: training.* 284.

Hopkins, M., Gibbons, C., Caudwell, P., et al. (2014). The adaptive metabolic response to exercise-induced weight loss influences both energy expenditure and energy intake. *European Journal of Clinical Nutrition, 68*(5), 581–586.

Hulmi, J., Isola, V., Suonpää, M., et al. (2017). The effects of intensive weight reduction on body composition and serum hormones in female fitness competitors. *Frontiers in Physiology, 7*, 689.

Hunter, G., Bryan, D., Wetzstein, C., et al. (2002). Resistance training and intra-abdominal adipose tissue in older men and women. *Medicine and Science in Sports and Exercise, 34*(6), 1023–1028.

Hunter, G., Byrne, N., Sirikul, B., et al. (2008). Resistance training conserves fat-free mass and resting energy expenditure following weight loss. *Obesity, 16*(5), 1045–1051.

Hunter, G., Fisher, G., Neumeier, W., et al. (2015). Exercise training and energy expenditure following weight loss. *Medicine and Science in Sports and Exercise, 47*(9), 1950–1957.

Huovinen, H., Hulmi, J., Isolehto, J., et al. (2015). Body composition and power performance improved after weight reduction in male athletes without hampering hormonal balance. *Journal of Strength and Conditioning Research, 29*(1), 29–36.

Hyldahl, R., Chen, T., & Nosaka, K. (2017). Mechanisms and mediators of the skeletal muscle repeated bout effect. *Exercise and Sport Sciences Reviews, 45*(1), 24–33.

Iglay, H., Thyfault, J., Apolzan, J., et al. (2007). Resistance training and dietary protein: effects on glucose tolerance and contents of skeletal muscle insulin signaling proteins in older persons. *The American Journal of Clinical Nutrition, 85*(4), 1005–1013.

Ismail, I., Keating, S., Baker, M., et al. (2012). A systematic review and meta-analysis of the effect of aerobic vs. Resistance exercise training on visceral fat. *Obesity Reviews, 13*(1), 68–91.

Iwayama, K., Kawabuchi, R., Park, I., et al. (2015). Transient energy deficit induced by exercise increases 24-h fat oxidation in young trained men. *Journal of Applied Physiology, 118*(1), 80–85.

Josse, A., & Phillips, S. (2010). Impact of milk consumption and resistance training on body composition of female athletes. *Medicine and Sport Science, 59*, 94–103.

Jung, W., Hwang, H., Kim, J., et al. (2019). Effect of interval exercise versus continuous exercise on excess post-exercise oxygen consumption during energy-homogenized exercise on a cycle ergometer. *Journal of Exercise Nutrition & Biochemistry, 23*(2), 45–50.

Karra, E., O'Daly, O., Choudhury, A., et al. (2013). A link between FTO, ghrelin, and impaired brain food-cue responsivity. *The Journal of Clinical Investigation, 123*(8), 3539–3551.

Keating, S., Johnson, N., Mielke, G., et al. (2017). A systematic review and meta-analysis of interval training versus moderate-intensity continuous training on body adiposity. *Obesity Reviews, 18*(8), 943–964.

Keating, S., Machan, E., O'Connor, H., et al. (2014). Continuous exercise but not high intensity interval training improves fat distribution in overweight adults. *Journal of Obesity, 2014*, 834865.

King, N., Hopkins, M., Caudwell, P., et al. (2008). Individual variability following 12 weeks of supervised exercise: identification and characterization of compensation for exercise-induced weight loss. *International Journal of Obesity, 32*(1), 177–184.

Laforgia, J., Withers, R., & Gore, C. (2006). Effects of exercise intensity and duration on the excess post-exercise oxygen consumption. *Journal of Sports Sciences, 24*(12), 1247–1264.

Lam, C., Chari, M., Wang, P., et al. (2008). Central lactate metabolism regulates food intake. *American Journal of Physiology – Endocrinology and Metabolism, 295*(2), 491–496.

Laskowski, E. (2012). The role of exercise in the treatment of obesity. *PM & R: The Journal of Injury, Function, and Rehabilitation, 4*(11), 840–844.

MacKenzie-Shalders, K., Kelly, J., So, D., et al. (2020). The effect of exercise interventions on resting metabolic rate: a systematic review and meta-analysis. *Journal of Sports Sciences, 38*(14), 1635–1649.

MacKenzie-Shalders, K., King, N., Byrne, N., et al. (2016). Increasing protein distribution has no effect on changes in lean mass during a rugby preseason. *International Journal of Sport Nutrition and Exercise Metabolism, 26*(1), 1–7.

Macpherson, R., Hazell, T., Olver, T., et al. (2011). Run sprint interval training improves aerobic performance but not maximal cardiac output. *Medicine and Science in Sports and Exercise, 43*(1), 115–122.

Malhotra, A., Noakes, T., & Phinney, S. (2015). It is time to bust the myth of physical inactivity and obesity: you cannot outrun a bad diet. *British Journal of Sports Medicine, 49*(15), 967–968.

Mettler, S., Mitchell, N., & Tipton, K. (2010). Increased protein intake reduces lean body mass loss during weight loss in athletes. *Medicine and Science in Sports and Exercise, 42*(2), 326–337.

McIver, V., Mattin, L., Evans, G., et al. (2019). The effect of brisk walking in the fasted versus fed state on metabolic responses, gastrointestinal function, and appetite in healthy men. *International Journal of Obesity, 43*(9), 1691–1700

Morgan, B., Woodruff, S., & Tiidus, P. (2003). Aerobic energy expenditure during recreational weight training in females and males. *Journal of Sports Science & Medicine, 2*(3), 117–122.

Murach, K., & Bagley, J. (2016). Skeletal muscle hypertrophy with concurrent exercise training: contrary evidence for an interference effect. *Sports Medicine, 46*(8), 1029–1039.

Nindl, B., Harman, E., Marx, J., et al. (2000). Regional body composition changes in women after 6 months of periodized physical training. *Journal of Applied Physiology, 88*(6), 2251–2259.

Nordby, P., Rosenkilde, M., Ploug, T., et al. (2015). Independent effects of endurance training and weight loss on peak fat oxidation in moderately overweight men: a randomized controlled trial. *Journal of Applied Physiology, 118*(7), 803–810.

Ørtenblad, N., Westerblad, H., & Nielsen, J. (2013). Muscle glycogen stores and fatigue. *The Journal of Physiology, 591*(18), 4405–4413.

di Palumbo, A., Guerra, E., Orlandi, C., et al. (2017). Effect of combined resistance and endurance exercise training on regional fat loss. *The Journal of Sports Medicine and Physical Fitness, 57*(6), 794–801.

Panissa, V., Fukuda, D., Staibano, V., et al. (2020). Magnitude and duration of excess of post-exercise oxygen consumption between high-intensity interval and moderate-intensity continuous exercise: a systematic review. *Obesity Reviews, 22*(1), e13099.

Paoli, A., Marcolin, G., Zonin, F., et al. (2011) Exercising fasting or fed to enhance fat loss? Influence of food intake on respiratory ratio and excess post-exercise oxygen consumption after a bout of endurance training. *International Journal of Sport Nutrition and Exercise Metabolism, 21,* 48–54

Paoli, A., Grimaldi, K., D'Agostino, D., et al. (2012). Ketogenic diet does not affect strength performance in elite artistic gymnasts. *Journal of the International Society of Sports Nutrition, 9*(1), 34.

Pontzer, H., Durazo-Arvizu, R., Dugas, L., et al. (2016). Constrained total energy expenditure and metabolic adaptation to physical activity in adult humans. *Current Biology, 26*(3), 410–417.

Prabhakaran, B., Dowling, E., Branch, J., et al. (1999). Effect of 14 weeks of resistance training on lipid profile and body fat percentage in premenopausal women. *British Journal of Sports Medicine, 33*(3), 190–195.

Redman, L., Heilbronn, L., Martin, C., et al. (2009). Metabolic and behavioral compensations in response to caloric restriction: implications for the maintenance of weight loss. *PLOS ONE, 4*(2), e4377.

Ribeiro, A., Schoenfeld, B., Souza, M., et al. (2016). Traditional and pyramidal resistance training systems improve muscle quality and metabolic biomarkers in older women: a randomized crossover study. *Experimental Gerontology, 79,* 8–15.

Richardson, C., Newton, T., Abraham, J., et al. (2008). A meta-analysis of pedometer-based walking interventions and weight loss. *Annals of Family Medicine, 6*(1), 69–77.

Riou, M., Jomphe-Tremblay, S., Lamothe, G., et al. (2015). Predictors of energy compensation during exercise interventions: a systematic review. *Nutrients, 7*(5), 3677–3704.

Robinson, S., Lambeth-Mansell, A., Gillibrand, G., et al. (2015). A nutrition and conditioning intervention for natural bodybuilding contest preparation: case study. *Journal of the International Society of Sports Nutrition, 12,* 20.

Romieu, I., Dossus, L., Barquera, S., et al. (2017). Energy balance and obesity: what are the main drivers? *Cancer Causes & Control, 28*(3), 247–258.

Rosenkilde, M., Auerbach, P., Reichkendler, M., et al. (2012). Body fat loss and compensatory mechanisms in response to different doses of aerobic exercise – a randomized controlled trial in overweight sedentary males. *American Journal of Physiology. Regulatory, Integrative and Comparative Physiology, 303*(6), 571.

Ross, R., & Janssen, I. (2001). Physical activity, total and regional obesity: dose-response considerations. *Medicine and Science in Sports and Exercise, 33*(6), S521–529.

Schoenfeld, B., Aragon, A., Wilborn, C., et al. (2014). Body composition changes associated with fasted versus non-fasted aerobic exercise. *Journal of the International Society of Sports Nutrition, 11*(1), 54

Schumann, B., & Rønnestad, B., (2019). *Concurrent aerobic and strength training: scientific basics and practical applications.* Springer International Publishing.

Schwingshackl,, L., Dias, S., Strasser, B., & Hoffmann, G. (2013). Impact of different training modalities on anthropometric and metabolic characteristics in overweight/obese subjects: a systematic review and network meta-analysis. *PLOS ONE, 8*(12), e82853.

Sevits, K., Melanson, E., Swibas, T., et al. (2013). Total daily energy expenditure is increased following a single bout of sprint interval training. *Physiological Reports, 1*(5), e00131.

Sharifi, N., Mahdavi, R., & Ebrahimi-Mameghani, M. (2013). Perceived barriers to weight loss programs for overweight or obese women. *Health Promotion Perspectives, 3*(1), 11–22.

Shing, C., Webb, J., Driller, M., et al. (2013). Circulating adiponectin concentration and body composition are altered in response to high-intensity interval training. *Journal of Strength and Conditioning Research, 27*(8), 2213–2218.

Shimada, K., Yamamoto, Y., Iwayama, K., et al. (2013) Effects of post-absorptive and postprandial exercise on 24 h fat oxidation. *Metabolism: Clinical and Experimental, 62*(6), 793–800.

Skelly, L., Andrews, P., Gillen, J., et al. (2014). High-intensity interval exercise induces 24-h energy expenditure similar to traditional endurance exercise despite reduced time commitment. *Applied Physiology, Nutrition, and Metabolism, 39*(7), 845–848.

Slentz, C., Duscha, B., Johnson, J., et al. (2004). Effects of the amount of exercise on body weight, body composition, and measures of central obesity: STRRIDE – a randomized controlled study. *Archives of Internal Medicine, 164*(1), 31–39.

Spriet, L. (2014). New insights into the interaction of carbohydrate and fat metabolism during exercise. *Sports Medicine, 44*(1), S87–96.

Stanley, J., Peake, J., & Buchheit, M. (2013). Cardiac parasympathetic reactivation following exercise: Implications for training prescription. *Sports Medicine, 43*(12), 1259–1277.

Strasser, B., Spreitzer, A., & Haber, P. (2007). Fat loss depends on energy deficit only, independently of the method for weight loss. *Annals of Nutrition & Metabolism, 51*(5), 428–432.

Strasser, B., & Schobersberger, W. (2011). Evidence for resistance training as a treatment therapy in obesity. *Journal of Obesity,* 2011.

Swift, D., Johannsen, N., Lavie, C., et al. (2014). The role of exercise and physical activity in weight loss and maintenance. *Progress in cardiovascular diseases, 56*(4), 441–447.

Sultana, R., Sabag, A., Keating, S., et al. (2019). The effect of low-volume high-intensity interval training on body composition and cardiorespiratory fitness: A systematic review and meta-analysis. *Sports Medicine, 49*(11), 1687–1721.

Sumithran, P., Prendergast, L., Delbridge, E., et al. (2011). Long-term persistence of hormonal adaptations to weight loss. *New England Journal of Medicine, 365*(17), 1597–1604.

Thomas, D., Bouchard, C., Church, T., et al. (2012). Why do individuals not lose more weight from an exercise intervention at a defined dose? An energy balance analysis. *Obesity Reviews, 13*(10), 835–847.

Thorogood, A., Mottillo, S., Shimony, A., et al. (2011). Isolated aerobic exercise and weight loss: a systematic review and meta-analysis of randomized controlled trials. *The American Journal of Medicine, 124*(8), 747–755.

Trapp, E., Chisholm, D., Freund, J., et al. (2008). The effects of high-intensity intermittent exercise training on fat loss and fasting insulin levels of young women. *International Journal of Obesity, 32*(4), 684–691.

Tremblay, A., Simoneau, J., & Bouchard, C. (1994). Impact of exercise intensity on body fatness and skeletal muscle metabolism. *Metabolism: Clinical and Experimental, 43*(7), 814–818.

Tucker, W., Angadi, S., & Gaesser, G. (2016). Excess post exercise oxygen consumption after high-intensity and sprint interval exercise, and continuous steady-state exercise. *Journal of Strength and Conditioning Research, 30*(11), 3090–3097.

Turicchi, J., O'Driscoll, R., Finlayson, G., et al. (2020). Associations between the proportion of fat-free mass loss during weight loss, changes in appetite, and subsequent weight change: results from a randomized 2-stage dietary intervention trial. *The American Journal of Clinical Nutrition, 111*(3), 536–544.

Vanderheyden, L., McKie, G., Howe, G., et al. (2020). Greater lactate accumulation following an acute bout of high-intensity exercise in males suppresses acylated ghrelin and appetite post exercise. *Journal of Applied Physiology, 128*(5), 1321–1328.

Verreijen, A., Engberink, M., Memelink, R., et al. (2017). Effect of a high protein diet and/or resistance exercise on the preservation of fat free mass during weight loss in overweight and obese older adults: a randomized controlled trial. *Nutrition Journal, 16*(1), 10.

Villareal, D., Chode, S., Parimi, N., et al. (2011). Weight loss, exercise, or both and physical function in obese older adults. *The New England Journal of Medicine, 364*(13), 1218–1229.

Wewege, M., van den Berg, R., Ward, R., et al. (2017). The effects of high-intensity interval training vs. moderate-intensity continuous training on body composition in overweight and obese adults: a systematic review and meta-analysis. *Obesity Reviews, 18*(6), 635–646.

Williams, C., Zelt, J., Castellani, L., et al. (2013). Changes in mechanisms proposed to mediate fat loss following an acute bout of high-intensity interval and endurance exercise. *Applied Physiology, Nutrition, and Metabolism, 38*(12), 1236–1244.

Willis, L., Slentz, C., Bateman, L., et al. (2012). Effects of aerobic and/or resistance training on body mass and fat mass in overweight or obese adults. *Journal of Applied Physiology, 113*(12), 1831–1837.

Wilson, J., Marin, P., Rhea, M., et al. (2012). Concurrent training: a meta-analysis examining interference of aerobic and resistance exercises. *Journal of Strength and Conditioning Research, 26*(8), 2293–2307.

Wolfe, R. (2006). Skeletal muscle protein metabolism and resistance exercise. *The Journal of Nutrition, 136*(2), 525S–528S.

15 Female clients

Jess Cunningham and Kay Robinson

Although the gender gap in exercise participation is decreasing worldwide, females remain under-represented throughout sport and exercise research (Bruinvels et al., 2017). While men's hormones remain relatively stable from day to day, the complexities of the menstrual cycle and its hormonal fluctuations have historically been thought to increase the complexity of sport and exercise studies. Therefore, most sport/exercise science research has involved male participants, meaning the findings of many studies may not be directly applicable to females.

Does the menstrual cycle affect exercise and performance?

In a global survey of active females, 74% of respondents reported their menstrual cycle negatively affected their performance, and >90% said it impacted training (Strava, 2019). Despite high rates of perceived negative effects on performance, most (82%) of the respondents had never discussed their menstrual cycle with their coach/trainer, and 72% had received no education regarding exercise and the menstrual cycle (Strava, 2019). Therefore, there is scope for trainers to optimise training programmes for female clients by adopting a cyclical approach to training based around the menstrual cycle, rather than traditional periodisation methods, which are usually based on research with males (see Chapter 8).

Trainers should be familiar with the hormonal fluctuations throughout the menstrual cycle, and how these can impact training and performance. Additionally, knowledge of the menstrual cycle enables trainers to optimise training programmes and facilitate open conversations with clients. It is also important for trainers to consider how changes in hormones and pelvic floor function are affected during pregnancy and menopause.

Overview of the menstrual cycle

The length of the menstrual cycle varies between women; however, the average cycle duration is considered to be 28 days, passing through high and low hormone phases, when hormonal contraception (HC) is not used

DOI: 10.4324/9781003204657-15

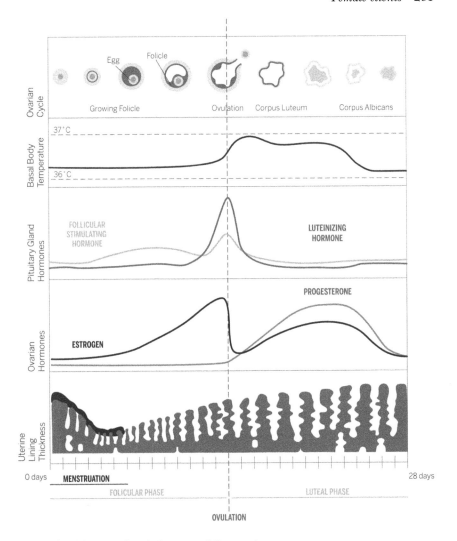

Figure 15.1 Menstrual cycle hormonal fluctuations.

(see Figure 15.1). During the *follicular phase*, that begins on the first day of menstruation, there is a gradual increase in oestrogen and luteinizing hormone, which stimulates the *ovulatory phase* and ovulation. In the ovulatory phase the uterus lining starts to thicken, preparing for the embryo. The *luteal phase* then uses the release of progesterone to support the uterus lining in preparation for fertilisation; if this does not occur progesterone secretion ceases, which results in menstrual bleeding (Constantini et al., 2005).

Menstrual cycle tracking

Before a cyclical approach to training can be considered, clients should be familiar with their menstrual cycle. Individual tracking for at least three months should be encouraged to obtain a clear understanding of the menstrual cycle and its effect on the client's mood, PMS (Premenstrual Syndrome), energy, etc. There are several menstrual cycle tracking apps that facilitate this process. The type and severity of symptoms experienced will be different for each client and may be impacted by HC use. Subsequently, a 'one size fits all' approach cannot be utilised when considering a cyclical approach to training. The exact methods and outcomes will be highly individual, with some clients experiencing significant benefits, while for others the benefits may be negligible.

Period tracking may assist trainers and their clients to identify how common menstrual symptoms (e.g., cramps, back pain, headaches, bloating, and fatigue) can affect their training and performance. Period tracking can also identify more severe symptoms that could indicate underlying menstrual dysfunctions (see Table 15.1). Trainers should advise clients who are unable to train due to pain or fatigue, and who report cycle irregularity to seek advice from their General Practitioner (GP) or Women's Health Physiotherapist to discuss any suspected dysfunctions or severe menstrual symptoms.

The effect of hormonal contraception on the menstrual cycle and exercise

The oral contraceptive pill (OCP) is the most commonly used HC (Martin et al., 2018) and is available as combined (estrogen and progesterone) or progesterone only. Progesterone only HC options, such as injections, implants and inter-uterine devices are also available. Since the introduction of the OCP, the use of HC has become more prevalent, with around 30% of the general population (Cea-Soriano et al., 2014; Daniels et al., 2014) and 50–70% of elite athletes (Martin et al., 2018) reporting using the OCP. Using HC lowers the levels of endogenous sex hormone concentrations and can be used to treat dysmenorrhea (painful periods) (Wong et al., 2009), which can subsequently increase exercise participation and performance (Schaumberg et al., 2018).

Athletic women who use HC are able to predict and/or manipulate the timing, frequency, and amount of menstrual bleeding (Martin et al., 2018). Indeed, 74% of OCP users have reported deliberately manipulating their menstrual cycle at least once during the previous year (Schaumberg et al., 2018). However, HC use can also have adverse effects, listed below. Trainers should be aware that a regular menstrual cycle is a barometer of female hormone health, and clients with long term HC use (particularly when OCP use started in teens) may have subsequent bone density issues

Table 15.1 Menstrual symptoms that may indicate potential underlying menstrual dysfunctions

---

Heavy Bleeding (Menorrhagia)

- Over 30% of exercising females are thought to suffer from heavy menstrual bleeding (Bruinvels et al., 2016), which could negatively impact training and performance due to the risk of anaemia/iron deficiency. Anaemia can lead to fatigue, weakness and decreased cognitive function.

Irregular Bleeding (Metrorrhagia) or Infrequent Periods (Oligomenorrhea)

- Cycle irregularities can be a symptom of Polycystic Ovarian Syndrome (PCOS), a complex hormonal condition where sufferers have increased levels of androgens (e.g., testosterone) (Hagmar et al, 2009).

Absent Periods (Amenorrhea)

- The absence of menstruation in athletic females, particularly endurance athletes, is not a natural side effect of training hard. Absent periods can be a sign of hormonal balance dysfunction, which indicates that training loads and nutrition should be addressed (Redman & Loucks, 2005).

Period Pain (Dysmenorrhea)

- Abdominal pains and cramping have been identified as the biggest performance limiters for females (Giacomoni et al., 2000).
- Severe and debilitating pain can be a sign of endometriosis.
- In the general population the incidence of endometriosis can be as high as 11% (AIHW, 2019), and 60% of females have reported missing training due to pain (Giacomoni et al., 2000). Therefore, trainers need to be aware that pain should not be considered a normal side effect of healthy menstruation.

Fatigue/Low Energy Availability (EA)

- Fatigue due to an imbalance of energy intake and expenditure (i.e., not eating enough).
- Relative Energy Deficiency in Sport (RED-S) is a disorder affecting a high proportion of female athletes. Symptoms of RED-S include periods ceasing, bone density loss, stress fractures, and eating disorders (Mountjoy et al., 2014; Williams et al., 2017).

---

or underlying undiagnosed menstrual dysfunction (endometriosis, PCOS) that has been masked (Gordon et al., 2017).

Potential negative effects of hormonal contraceptive use

- Cardiac and vascular arterial events
- DVT
- Prevention of achieving peak bone mass
- Impaired ovulatory cycle development
- Breast cancer, cervical cancer
- Interaction with gut flora
- Risk of inflammatory bowel disease

(Baillargeon et al., 2005; Khalili, 2016; Kemmeren et al., 2001; Prior et al., 2019)

The effect of HC use on performance is a complex area with much disagreement regarding how HC use affects the physiological factors related to performance and injury occurrence (Burrows & Peters, 2007; Rechichi et al., 2009). Although it has been suggested that a female's training programme can be designed to take advantage of hormonal fluctuations, further research is required to make definitive recommendations. Trainers should be aware of the emerging themes of research findings regarding training and performance at different stages of the menstrual cycle (see Table 15.2) and consider these when designing training programs.

Table 15.2 Menstrual cycle considerations to training and performance

Follicular Phase	• Starts on the first day of bleeding • Higher levels of testosterone – most 'like a man's' physiology at this phase • Favourable conditions for performance • Higher perceived energy levels • Likely to feel less pain and recover faster • Can make greater strength gains • Better suited to high-intensity training (Constantini et al., 2005; Sung et al., 2014)
Ovulatory Phase	• Increased ligament laxity and risk of ACL injury 'around the time of ovulation' (Balachandar et al., 2017; Herzberg et al., 2017).
Luteal Phase	• Reduced: reaction time, neuromuscular coordination and manual dexterity • Metabolism changes • Increasing insulin resistance and blood sugar levels – cravings, reduced energy levels • Increased ventilation and respiration – increased perceived exertion • Thermoregulation – increased body basal temperature • Fluid retention – bloating • Blood pressure – headaches • Harder to build muscle – less primed for high intensity training, progesterone increases the breakdown of muscle tissue • Inflammation • Prostaglandins released to help uterus contract and shed its lining • Cramping and GI issues • Reduced recovery capacity (Constantini et al., 2005; Gold et al., 2016)

Summary

Trainers should be aware of emerging themes regarding the training and performance of female clients.

- Discussion and education around the menstrual cycle and impact on performance should be encouraged.
- Trainers should urge clients to track periods and symptoms and seek further guidance from medical professionals when required.
- Trainers should be aware of HC options and their impact on the menstrual cycle.
- It is important for trainers to understand Relative Energy Deficiency Syndrome (RED-s) and how this may present.
- Training loads, nutrition/fluid balance, recovery, energy levels, body temperature, and injury risk/prevention should also be considered when programming for the female client.

References

Australian Institute of Health and Welfare. (2019). *Endometriosis in Australia: prevalence and hospitalisations.*

Baillargeon, J., McClish, D., Essah, P., et al. (2005). Association between the current use of low-dose oral contraceptives and cardiovascular arterial disease: a meta-analysis. *The Journal of Clinical Endocrinology and Metabolism, 90*(7), 3863–3870.

Balachandar, V., Marciniak, J. L., Wall, O., et al. (2017). Effects of the menstrual cycle on lower-limb biomechanics, neuromuscular control, and anterior cruciate ligament injury risk: a systematic review. *Muscles Ligaments Tendons Journal, 7*(1), 136–146.

Bruinvels, G., Burden, R., Brown, N., et al. (2016). The prevalence and impact of heavy menstrual bleeding (menorrhagia) in elite and Non-elite athletes. *PLOS One, 11*(2), e0149881.

Bruinvels, G., Burden, R., McGregor, A., et al. (2017). Sport, exercise and the menstrual cycle: where is the research? *British Journal of Sports Medicine, 51*(6), 487–488.

Burrows, M., & Peters, C. E. (2007). The influence of oral contraceptives on athletic performance in female athletes. *Sports Medicine, 37*(7), 557–574.

Cea-Soriano, L., Garcia Rodriguez, L., Machlitt, A., et al. (2014). Use of prescription contraceptive methods in the UK general population: a primary care study. *BJOG, 121*(1), 53–60; discussion 60–51.

Constantini, N., Dubnov, G., & Lebrun, C. (2005). The menstrual cycle and sport performance. *Clinical Sports Medicine, 24*(2), e51–82, xiii–xiv.

Daniels, K., Daugherty, J., & Jones, J. (2014). Current contraceptive status among women aged 15–44: United States, 2011–2013. *National Centre for Health Statistics Data Brief,* (173), 1–8.

Giacomoni, M., Bernard, T., Gavarry, O., et al. (2000). Influence of the menstrual cycle phase and menstrual symptoms on maximal anaerobic performance. *Medicine and Science in Sports and Exercise, 32*(2), 486–492.

Gold, E., Wells, C., & Rasor, M. (2016). The association of inflammation with pre-menstrual symptoms. *Journal of Women's Health, 25*(9), 865–874.

Gordon, C., Ackerman, K., Berga, S., et al. (2017). Functional hypothalamic amenorrhea: an endocrine society clinical practice guideline. *Journal Clinical Endocrinology and Metabolism, 102*(5), 1413–1439.

Hagmar, M., Berglund, B., Brismar, K., et al. (2009). Hyperandrogenism may explain reproductive dysfunction in Olympic athletes. *Medicine and Science in Sports and Exercise, 41*(6), 1241–1248.

Herzberg, S., Motu'apuaka, M., Lambert, W., et al. (2017). The effect of menstrual cycle and contraceptives on ACL injuries and laxity: a systematic review and meta-analysis. *Orthopaedic Journal of Sports Medicine, 5*(7), 2325967117718781.

Kemmeren, J., Algra, A., & Grobbee, D. (2001). Third generation oral contraceptives and risk of venous thrombosis: meta-analysis. *British Medical Journal, 323*(7305), 131–134.

Khalili, H. (2016). Risk of inflammatory bowel disease with Oral contraceptives and menopausal hormone therapy: current evidence and future directions. *Drug Safety, 39*(3), 193–197

Martin, D., Sale, C., Cooper, S., et al. (2018). Period prevalence and perceived side effects of hormonal contraceptive use and the menstrual cycle in elite athletes. *International Journal of Sports Physiology and Performance, 13*(7), 926–932.

Mountjoy, M., Sundgot-Borgen, J., Burke, L., et al. (2014). The IOC consensus statement: beyond the female athlete Triad—Relative energy deficiency in sport (RED-S). *British Journal of Sports Medicine, 48*(7), 491–497.

Prior, J., Whittaker, J., & Scott, A. (2019). Adolescent combined hormonal contraceptives and surgical repair of anterior cruciate tears: a risky recommendation based on an unproven causal relationship. *The Physician and Sports Medicine, 47*(3), 240–241.

Rechichi, C., Dawson, B., & Goodman, C. (2009). Athletic performance and the oral contraceptive. *International Journal of Sports Physiology and Performance, 4*(2), 151–162.

Redman, L., & Loucks, A. (2005). Menstrual disorders in athletes. *Sports Medicine, 35*(9), 747–755.

Schaumberg, M., Emmerton, L., Jenkins, D., et al. (2018). Use of oral contraceptives to manipulate menstruation in young, physically active women. *International Journal of Sports Physiology and Performance, 13*(1), 82–87.

Strava. (2019). *Press Release – Largest Global Study of Active Women.* https://www.fitrwoman.com/post/press-release-largest-global-studyof-active-women.

Wong, C., Farquhar, C., Roberts, H., et al. (2009). Oral contraceptive pill for primary dysmenorrhoea. *Cochrane Database Systematic Review,* (4), CD002120.

16 Older clients

Sean Wilson and Ben Kirk

Physical activity (PA) is an instrumental component of a healthy lifestyle and facilitates the maintenance of good physical function and quality of life (García-Hermoso et al., 2020; Raafs et al., 2020). The age-related rate of physiological deterioration is reduced by regular exercise (Neufer et al., 2015). Older adults that perform regular exercise can maintain significantly better physical function, muscle strength, muscle power (Carrick-Ranson et al., 2020; Zampieri et al., 2015), aerobic capacity (Westerståhl et al., 2018), bone density/strength (Leskinen & Kujala, 2015; Multanen et al., 2014), and balance (Bird et al., 2011; Sherrington et al., 2020). Therefore, older adults that possess excellent overall fitness and perform high levels of PA, particularly at moderate-to-vigorous intensities, demonstrate numerous health benefits including reduced incidence of chronic disease (Engelen et al., 2017; Ruiz et al., 2008), improved brain health (Vecchio et al., 2018), retention of cognitive functions (Noguera et al., 2019), decreased rates of falls, fractures, physical frailty (Elhakeem et al., 2019; Yeung et al., 2019), and substantially lowered risk of premature death (Kim et al., 2018; Lee et al., 2018).

Globally, the number of people aged over 60 years is predicted to more than double, exceeding two billion by 2050 (Thomson et al., 2016). To combat the growing prevalence of chronic disease and escalating expenditure on health (Harris & Sharma, 2018), primary care and public health initiatives that support and encourage the implementation of exercise into the daily lives of adults will be essential (Thornton et al., 2016). Less time spent sitting and more general PA should also be advocated, given that sedentarism increases with age (Hamer et al., 2012) and is independently associated with poor health outcomes, regardless of other exercise behaviours (Koster et al., 2012). Furthermore, exercise can produce robust and positive changes in quality of life (Raafs et al., 2020), improve mental health, and reduce the debilitating symptoms of mental illness (Stubbs & Rosenbaum, 2018). Thus, it is critically important for personal trainers working with older adults to provide ongoing education and encouragement to follow a physically active lifestyle. Based on the

DOI: 10.4324/9781003204657-16

current scientific evidence, the following activities are required for optimising improvements in health and fitness: (1) Cardiorespiratory activity; (2) Resistance training and high impact exercise; and (3) Balance and functional exercise. This section will briefly outline current PA and exercise guidelines for older adults.

Physical activity recommendations for older adults

Reduce sedentary activity and increase general daily PA

Older adults are strongly encouraged to sit less throughout the day and perform more general daily PA. Any PA, irrespective of intensity, is better than none as even small amounts of moderate-to-vigorous PA has been shown to elicit health benefits (Piercy et al., 2018).

Cardiorespiratory physical activity/exercise

Moderate-to-vigorous PA

PA guidelines (see Table 16.1) of health organisations recommend older adults 150–300 minutes/week of moderate-intensity, or 75–150 minutes/week of vigorous-intensity aerobic PA, or an equivalent combination of moderate and vigorous-intensity aerobic activity (Foster, 2019). Additional health benefits can be gained by performing more than 300 minutes (five hours) of moderate-intensity PA/week (Piercy et al., 2018), although this may not be feasible for many older adults. In addition to aerobic exercise, RT and high-impact loading are required to optimise musculoskeletal health (Hartley et al., 2020; Lambert et al., 2020).

High-intensity exercise

As discussed in Chapter 11, high-intensity interval training (HIIT) has been shown to result in marked improvements in both physical and mental health of older adults (Adamson et al., 2020; Martland et al., 2020). Moreover, compared to moderate-intensity activity, HIIT leads to similar and often better improvements in fitness, even when performed for shorter periods (Bouaziz et al., 2020; Boukabous et al., 2019).

Any PA is better than none

Older adults who are unable to achieve the recommended weekly levels of moderate-to-vigorous PA due to their social or personal circumstances should be assisted and encouraged to be as active as possible because every additional minute of PA will have a positive impact on health (Ekelund et al., 2019).

Table 16.1 Physical activity and exercise recommendations for older adults

Type of activity	Recommendation	Further details
General physical activity (PA)		
Sedentary activity (SA) & general PA	Reduce/minimise SA & increase general daily PA	Reducing SA and any increase in PA elicits health benefits. Long periods of sitting should be interspersed with 2–3 minutes of light PA.
Moderate-to-vigorous physical activity (MVPA)	150–300 minutes/week MPA or 75–150 minutes/week VPA, or equivalent combination of MVPA	RPE 12–13 (Borg scale 6–20), 55–69% maximum HR or 40–59% HRR is indicative of MPA. RPE 14–17, 70–89% maximum HR or 60–84% HRR is indicative of VPA.
High-intensity exercise (HIE)	1–2 sessions/week	HIE is safe for most older adults and may provide additional physiological benefits compared to MPA. Pre-screening and risk assessment should be conducted. A 4–6 week period of general strength and conditioning before commencing HIE is recommended.
Resistance training		
Modality	Free weight, machine-based, body weight, resistance bands and/or isometric exercises	Beginners or frail and deconditioned clients are advised to start RT using machines, resistance bands, body-weight and isometric exercises. Free-weight training can be included, provided it can be done safely.
Exercise selection	6–10 different exercises	Compound, multijoint exercises that target major muscle groups performed through different planes of motion.
Frequency	1–3 sessions/week	Two full body sessions/week optimises physiological and psychological benefits. One session/week may be sufficient for untrained older adults.
Intensity (load and effort)	50–85% of 1RM or OMNI 5–9	Improvements in muscle strength and hypertrophy can be achieved at most RT intensities. Lifting low ($\leq$50% 1RM) loads close to failure is associated with greater discomfort and displeasure.
Sets	1–2 sets per exercise per muscle group	Low volume RT is effective for older adults. High volume training may not be necessary.
Repetitions	6–30	Use higher repetitions ($\geq$12) for healthy beginners and frail/deconditioned older adults. Progression to lower repetitions ($\leq$8) is appropriate following a period (~6 weeks) of training. Performing sets to repetition failure is unnecessary.

(Continued)

Table 16.1 (Continued)

Type of activity	Recommendation	Further details
Rest periods	1–3 minutes	One-minute rests between sets is adequate for most older adults. Stronger and more experienced trainees benefit from 2 to 3 minutes rest periods.
Tempo	3–4 seconds eccentric 1–3 seconds concentric	A range of different RT movement speeds is effective (e.g., 3–4 seconds eccentric, 1–10 seconds concentric).
High-velocity RT	40–80% 1RM	High-velocity RT can be considered. Commence at light-to-moderate loads (40–60% 1RM). Training intensities (60–80% 1RM) may provide further benefits once familiarised. Avoid training to failure.
High-impact exercise and balance training		
High-impact exercise	As indicated	10–50 impacts/day, 3 times/week has shown benefit. Exercise modification may be required when musculoskeletal comorbidities exist. Progression from moderate (2–3 × body weight), multi-directional impact activities (e.g., heel drops) to higher (>4 × body weight) impact activities (e.g., jumping, hopping).
Balance/functional exercises	2–3 balance sessions/week	Significant challenges to balance should be safely provided and progressed by gradually decreasing the base of support, involving movements of centre of mass, and limiting the use of the upper limbs.
	Exercises that reflect activities of daily living	Incorporate exercises that reflect/mimic daily movement demands. Can be skill- or strength orientated (e.g., stair climbing or Farmer's walk).

RPE = Rating of perceived exertion, HR = heart rate, HRR = heart rate reserve, HIE = high intensity exercise, HIIT = high-intensity interval training, OMNI = OMNI-resistance exercise scale, RM = repetition maximum.

Resistance training and high-impact exercise

The age-related impairment of the neuromuscular and skeletal systems causes the atrophy (Nilwik et al., 2013) and loss of muscle fibres (McPhee et al., 2018), degeneration of neurological motor function (Beurskens & Dalecki, 2017), worsening muscle quality (Goodpaster et al., 2006), reduced bone and muscle strength (Havaldar et al., 2012; Zengin et al., 2016), and eventual reduction in overall functional capacity (Edholm et al., 2019). However, regular progressive RT counteracts these negative outcomes (Daly et al., 2020; Kemmler et al., 2020) and helps to maintain muscle function and morphology (Klitgaard et al., 1990; Papa et al., 2017).

Resistance training exercise selection

For most older adults, any type of RT will be beneficial and should be encouraged (Cunha et al., 2019; Izquierdo et al., 2004). Programmes should include compound, multiple-joint exercises that target major muscle groups performed through different planes of motion (Fragala et al., 2019). For example, exercises such as sit-to-stands, leg press, dead-lift, pulldowns, shoulder press, rows, bench press, and core exercises (see Chapter 12) are worthy inclusions within any RT programme. Isolation/single-joint movements should be utilised as supplementary exercises to address specific muscle groups that experience age-related deterioration, such as hip flexors (Ikezoe et al., 2011) or where there is inadequate stimulation from compound exercises (McKinnon et al., 2017).

It has been suggested that compound (multiple-joint) exercises should precede isolation (single-joint exercises) (Fragala et al., 2019); however, improvements in strength, muscle mass, and physical function can be achieved regardless of exercise order (Dib et al., 2020). There is limited evidence that free-weight exercises offer additional benefits compared to machine-based RT (Carpinelli, 2017), although there may be some advantages (Balachandran et al., 2016). For example, high functioning older adults may find free-weight RT more enjoyable and motivating (Schott et al., 2019).

Resistance training frequency

Twice-weekly RT involving 6–10 primarily compound exercises is recommended for older adults. However, healthy untrained older adults that perform one session/week can achieve significant improvements in muscle power, hypertrophy, neuromuscular function and cardiometabolic disease risk factors (Cunha et al., 2019; Foley et al., 2011; Izquierdo et al., 2004). The optimal frequency of RT sessions for older adults is unclear as superior physiological adaptations have been reported when more frequent sessions (2–3/week) were undertaken in some (Farinatti et al., 2013;

Fernández-Lezaun et al., 2017; Richardson et al., 2019) but not all studies (Grgic et al., 2018a). Increased RT volume may explain the discrepancies between studies as two sessions/week promoted similar improvements in muscular outcomes compared to three sessions, provided training volume was matched (Pina et al., 2020). Higher RT frequencies (2–3/week) may also be required when trying to maximise the effects on quality of life (Bampton et al., 2015; Hart & Buck, 2019), psychological functioning (Brunoni et al., 2015; Kekäläinen et al., 2018), and bone density/strength (Kemmler & Stengel, 2014; Nelson et al., 1994).

Most older trainees should not exceed three full body workouts/week that involve high-intensity training and/or multiple sets to muscle failure. Such training methods have been reported to induce muscle cell inflammation (Stec et al., 2017), which can delay recovery for several days (Orssatto et al., 2018) and may decrease overall safety and efficacy (Kamada et al., 2017; Kekäläinen et al., 2018; Pareja-Blanco et al., 2017). Therefore, the optimal RT frequency for older adults appears to be two sessions/week, although this may vary depending upon the client's training/health status and the goals of the programme.

Resistance training intensity

Low (<55% 1RM), moderate (55–75% 1RM) and high (>75% 1RM) intensity RT can all produce comparable changes in muscle strength, hypertrophy (Csapo & Alegre, 2016; Van Roie et al., 2013), muscle endurance (Rashidi et al., 2019), bone density/strength (Souza et al., 2020), and physical function (Nicholson et al., 2015; Shiotsu & Yanagita, 2018). However, progressive high-intensity RT (≥75% 1RM) is necessary to maximise gains in muscle strength (Borde et al., 2015; Raymond et al., 2013). Currently, there is no conclusive evidence that training to failure (see Chapter 13) provides additional benefits compared to submaximal efforts in older adults (Cadore et al., 2018; Davies et al., 2016). Training to failure using low loads can result in higher rates of perceived exertion, discomfort, and displeasure (Pritchett et al., 2009; Ribeiro et al., 2019). Therefore, trainers must consider how intensity and volume may impact levels of enjoyment, adherence, and effectiveness.

Resistance training volume

Performing one set/exercise may offer a time-efficient method to improve muscle strength, muscle quality, and functional performance for many older adults given that no further benefit has been shown versus higher (i.e., three sets per exercise) volume RT (Radaelli et al., 2013; Taaffe & Galvao, 2004). However, in the longer-term, higher volumes may be necessary to optimise neuromuscular adaptations, particularly in the lower limbs (Radaelli et al., 2014).

Resistance training inter-set rest periods

Longer (>2 minutes) rest periods are more effective for increasing muscle strength for individuals experienced in RT, whereas short-to-moderate (1–2 minutes) rest intervals are adequate for those without previous RT experience (Grgic et al., 2018b). Better inter-set recovery occurs in older versus younger adults (Bottaro et al., 2010; Theou et al., 2008), but optimal rest period duration during RT appears to be predominantly influenced by absolute muscle strength (Bottaro et al., 2010; Faigenbaum et al., 2008). Accordingly, short (~1 minute) inter-set rests appear adequate for older adults with limited RT experience and trained older women (Jambassi Filho et al., 2017; Villanueva et al., 2015). Stronger older adults may benefit from longer (≥2 minutes) rest periods to ensure that force production and the successful completion of the targeted repetitions is not compromised (Matos et al., 2020; Willardson et al., 2012).

Resistance training tempo

A range of movement velocities can be effective for increasing muscle strength, hypertrophy, and functional capacity (da Rosa Orssatto et al., 2019a; Westcott et al., 2001). Older adults unfamiliar with RT should focus on performing exercises correctly by conducting movements using a slow and controlled tempo (eccentric 3–4 seconds, concentric 2–3 seconds). When exercise technique is sound and improvements in overall strength and conditioning have been achieved (4–6 weeks minimum pre-training), alternative tempos, such as performing concentric muscle contractions 'as fast as possible' can be considered and gradually incorporated.

Explosive RT

Age-associated declines in muscle power occur at double the rate of muscle strength and is more strongly correlated to physical function (Byrne et al., 2016; McKinnon et al., 2017) and fall risk (Parsons et al., 2020). To evoke the greatest improvements in muscle power, RT conducted at faster movement speeds or with the intention to generate force rapidly, irrespective of movement speed, is required (Blazevich et al., 2020). Hence, explosive RT – where the concentric phase of an exercise is performed 'as fast as possible' – has been advocated as a safe and effective method for improving neuromuscular function in older adults (Cadore et al., 2018; Moran et al., 2018). When trying to maximise concurrent improvements in muscle strength, power and endurance, explosive RT performed at heavier loads may be more effective compared to low-to-moderate loads (De Vos et al., 2005). Explosive RT may provide additional benefits compared to conventional RT (Henwood et al., 2008; Miszko et al., 2003; Ramírez-Campillo et al., 2014), but more research is needed before any consensus is reached (da Rosa Orssatto et al., 2019b).

High-impact exercise

For older adults who are at risk of, or have developed osteopenia or osteoporosis, progressive, novel and multidirectional high-impact exercises (e.g., jumping, bounding, hopping) are recommended (Beck et al., 2017). Additionally, high-impact exercise improves balance, muscle strength and cardiorespiratory fitness which could enhance physical function and reduce fall-related risk factors (Allison et al., 2018; Multanen et al., 2014). However, optimal outcomes for musculoskeletal health are produced when high-impact exercise is combined with RT (Watson et al., 2018). An osteogenic response requires relatively few impacts (10–50/day, three times/week) and added benefit may be possible with more frequent (4–7 times/week) exposure (Beck et al., 2017). More frail individuals will require a phase of RT to build adequate strength before performing impact activities and further modification may be needed if there are other orthopaedic comorbidities (e.g., osteoarthritis).

Concurrent exercise

When conducting concurrent training sessions in older adults (i.e., endurance and resistance training), the order of exercises selected can influence the magnitude of improvement in neuromuscular performance, but more research is required to determine if there is an optimal sequence when attempting to maximise benefits (Moghadam et al., 2020; Cadore et al., 2013).

Balance and functional exercises

Older adults (>65 years) often experience falls, which can have disastrous consequences such as fractures, head injuries, and possible death (Downey et al., 2019; Sherrington et al., 2020). Balance and functional exercises can significantly reduce the rate of falls (Sherrington et al., 2020). For example, a high-level balance training and progressive moderate-intensity RT program resulted in a 55% fall rate reduction and significant improvement in physical performance of older adults (Hewitt et al., 2018). It is unclear whether programmes consisting primarily of RT, dance or walking are effective (Sherrington et al., 2020). While closed kinetic chain exercises are reportedly more effective than open kinetic chain for dynamic balance in young adults (Kwon et al., 2013), it is not clear if this applies to older adults for balance (Lee & Lee, 2019) or physical performance (Godin, 2003). Thus, it is recommended that balance and functional exercises be incorporated into the weekly physical activities of older adults (see

Table 16.1). Balance training programmes should safely attempt to provide significant challenges to balance and incorporate exercises that:

- *Progressively decrease the base of support*
  For example, standing with feet apart, standing with feet together, semi-tandem stance, tandem stance, standing on one leg. This principle can also be applied to balance exercises involving locomotion (e.g., semi-tandem walking to tandem walking)
- *Involve movements of centre of mass*
  For example, stepping up onto a step or over a hurdle or obstacle, moving forward, side-ways, backwards transferring body weight from one leg to another.
- *Restrict the use of the upper limbs*
  For example, when standing, decrease the dependency of the upper limbs for support, increasing the challenge by progressively moving from high to low levels of assistance (holding onto something with two hands to one hand to one finger to no hands).

Summary

Reductions in cardiorespiratory fitness, muscle size, quality, strength, balance and deterioration in bone density are hallmarks of the ageing process, which lead to worsening physical function and increased risk of chronic disease. Habitual sedentary behaviour exacerbates the physical and psychological changes that occur with ageing. However, regular PA and exercise can slow down the age-related degeneration in physiological and cognitive function. Indeed, adults with the highest levels of fitness and strength demonstrate the largest reductions in risk and rates of chronic disease, falls, fractures, frailty, and premature mortality. Consequently, regular PA and exercise are fundamental to improving the health, quality of life and physical function of older adults. Several factors (e.g., chronic disease, accessibility to services or equipment) may impact on the ability of some to meet the recommended PA guidelines. Thus, exercise should be tailored to the individual needs of each client. Any PA is better than none, although it is critical for personal trainers to acknowledge that clinical best practice requires the combination of several different activities and exercise modalities to optimise health and fitness (see Table 16.1).

References

Adamson, S., Kavaliauskas, M., Lorimer, R., et al. (2020). The impact of sprint interval training frequency on blood glucose control and physical function of older adults. *International Journal of Environmental Research and Public Health*, 17(2), 454.

Allison, S., Brooke-Wavell, K., & Folland, J. (2018). High and odd impact exercise training improved physical function and fall risk factors in community-dwelling older men. *Journal of Musculoskeletal & Neuronal Interactions*, 18(1), 100.

Balachandran, A., Martins, M., De Faveri, F., et al. (2016). Functional strength training: seated machine vs standing cable training to improve physical function in elderly. *Experimental Gerontology, 82*, 131–138.

Bampton, E., Johnson, S., & Vallance, J. (2015). Profiles of resistance training behavior and sedentary time among older adults: associations with health-related quality of life and psychosocial health. *Preventive Medicine Reports, 2*, 773–776.

Beck, B., Daly, R., Singh, M., & Taaffe, D. (2017). Exercise and Sports Science Australia (ESSA) position statement on exercise prescription for the prevention and management of osteoporosis. *Journal of Science and Medicine in Sport, 20*(5), 438–445.

Beurskens, R., & Dalecki, M. (2017). Physical activity: effects of exercise on neurological function. In *Physical activity and the aging brain* (pp. 185–198). Academic Press.

Bird, M., Hill, K., Ball, M., et al. (2011). The long-term benefits of a multi-component exercise intervention to balance and mobility in healthy older adults. *Archives of Gerontology and Geriatrics, 52*(2), 211–216.

Blazevich, A., Wilson, C., Alcaraz, P., et al. (2020). Effects of resistance training movement pattern and velocity on isometric muscular rate of force development: a systematic review with meta-analysis and meta-regression. *Sports Medicine*, 1–21.

Borde, R., Hortobágyi, T., & Granacher, U. (2015). Dose–response relationships of resistance training in healthy old adults: a systematic review and meta-analysis. *Sports Medicine, 45*(12), 1693–1720.

Bottaro, M., Ernesto, C., Celes, R., et al. (2010). Effects of age and rest interval on strength recovery. *International Journal of Sports Medicine, 31*(01), 22–25.

Bouaziz, W., Malgoyre, A., Schmitt, E., et al. (2020). Effect of high-intensity interval training and continuous endurance training on peak oxygen uptake among seniors aged 65 or older: a meta-analysis of randomized controlled trials. *International Journal of Clinical Practice*, e13490.

Boukabous, I., Marcotte-Chénard, A., Amamou, T., et al. (2019). Low-volume high-intensity interval training versus moderate-intensity continuous training on body composition, cardiometabolic profile, and physical capacity in older women. *Journal of Aging and Physical Activity, 27*(6), 879–889.

Brunoni, L., Schuch, F., Dias, C., et al. (2015). Strength training decreases the depressive symptoms and improves the health-related quality of life in older women. *Revista Brasileira de Educação Física e Esporte, 29*(2), 189–196.

Byrne, C., Faure, C., Keene, D., et al. (2016). Ageing, muscle power and physical function: a systematic review and implications for pragmatic training interventions. *Sports Medicine, 46*(9), 1311–1332.

Cadore, E., Pinto, R., Reischak-Oliveira, Á., et al. (2018). Explosive type of contractions should not be avoided during resistance training in elderly. *Experimental Gerontology, 102*, 81–83.

Cadore, E., Izquierdo, M., Pinto, S., et al. (2013). Neuromuscular adaptations to concurrent training in the elderly: effects of intrasession exercise sequence. *Age, 35*(3), 891–903.

Carpinelli, R. (2017). A critical analysis of the national strength and conditioning association's opinion that free weights are superior to machines for increasing muscular strength and power. *Medicina Sportiva Practica, 18*(2), 21–39.

Carrick-Ranson, G., Sloane, N., Howden, E., et al. (2020). The effect of lifelong endurance exercise on cardiovascular structure and exercise function in women. *The Journal of Physiology, 598*(13), 2589–2605.

Csapo, R., & Alegre, L. (2016). Effects of resistance training with moderate vs heavy loads on muscle mass and strength in the elderly: a meta-analysis. *Scandinavian Journal of Medicine & Science in Sports, 26*(9), 995–1006.

Cunha, P., Ribeiro, A., Nunes, J., et al. (2019). Resistance training performed with single-set is sufficient to reduce cardiovascular risk factors in untrained older women: the randomized clinical trial. Active aging longitudinal study. *Archives of Gerontology and Geriatrics, 81*, 171–175.

da Rosa Orssatto, L., Cadore, E., Andersen, L., et al. (2019a). Why fast velocity resistance training should be prioritized for elderly people. *Strength & Conditioning Journal, 41*(1), 105–114.

da Rosa Orssatto, L., de la Rocha Freitas, C., Shield, A., et al. (2019b). Effects of resistance training concentric velocity on older adults' functional capacity: a systematic review and meta-analysis of randomised trials. *Experimental Gerontology, 110731*, 1–14.

Daly, R., Gianoudis, J., Kersh, M., et al. (2020). Effects of a 12-month supervised, community-based, multimodal exercise program followed by a 6-month research-to-practice transition on bone mineral density, trabecular microarchitecture, and physical function in older adults: a randomized controlled trial. *Journal of Bone and Mineral Research, 35*(3), 419–429.

Davies, T., Orr, R., Halaki, M., et al. (2016). Effect of training leading to repetition failure on muscular strength: a systematic review and meta-analysis. *Sports Medicine, 46*(4), 487–502.

De Vos, N., Singh, N., Ross, D., et al. (2005). Optimal load for increasing muscle power during explosive resistance training in older adults. *The Journals of Gerontology Series A: Biological Sciences and Medical Sciences, 60*(5), 638–647.

Dib, M., Tomeleri, C., Nunes, J., et al. (2020). Effects of three resistance exercise orders on muscular function and body composition in older women. *International Journal of Sports Medicine, 41*(14), 1024–1031.

Downey, C., Kelly, M., & Quinlan, J. (2019). Changing trends in the mortality rate at 1-year post hip fracture-a systematic review. *World Journal of Orthopedics, 10*(3), 166.

Edholm, P., Nilsson, A., & Kadi, F. (2019). Physical function in older adults: impacts of past and present physical activity behaviors. *Scandinavian Journal of Medicine & Science in Sports, 29*(3), 415–421.

Ekelund, U., Tarp, J., Steene-Johannessen, J., et al. (2019). Dose-response associations between accelerometry measured physical activity and sedentary time and all-cause mortality: systematic review and harmonised meta-analysis. *British Medical Journal, 366*, 14570, 1–10.

Elhakeem, A., Hartley, A., Luo, Y., et al. (2019). Lean mass and lower limb muscle function in relation to hip strength, geometry and fracture risk indices in community-dwelling older women. *Osteoporosis International, 30*(1), 211–220.

Engelen, L., Gale, J., Chau, J., et al. (2017). Who is at risk of chronic disease? Associations between risk profiles of physical activity, sitting and cardio-metabolic disease in Australian adults. *Australian and New Zealand Journal of Public Health, 41*(2), 178–183.

Faigenbaum, A., Ratamess, N., McFarland, J., et al. (2008). Effect of rest interval length on bench press performance in boys, teens, and men. *Pediatric Exercise Science, 20*(4), 457–469.

Farinatti, P., Geraldes, A., Bottaro, M., et al. (2013). Effects of different resistance training frequencies on the muscle strength and functional performance of active women older than 60 years. *The Journal of Strength & Conditioning Research, 27*(8), 2225–2234.

Fernández-Lezaun, E., Schumann, M., Mäkinen, T., et al. (2017). Effects of resistance training frequency on cardiorespiratory fitness in older men and women during intervention and follow-up. *Experimental Gerontology, 95*, 44–53.

Foley, A., Hillier, S., & Barnard, R. (2011). Effectiveness of once-weekly gym-based exercise programmes for older adults post discharge from day rehabilitation: a randomised controlled trial. *British Journal of Sports Medicine, 45*(12), 978–986.

Foster, C. (2019). *UK chief medical officers' physical activity guidelines.* Department of Health and Social Care.

Fragala, M., Cadore, E., Dorgo, S., et al. (2019). Resistance training for older adults: position statement from the national strength and conditioning association. *The Journal of Strength & Conditioning Research, 33*(8).

García-Hermoso, A., Ramirez-Vélez, R., de Asteasu, M., et al. (2020). Safety and effectiveness of long-term exercise interventions in older adults: a systematic review and meta-analysis of randomized controlled trials. *Sports Medicine*, 1–12.

Godin, J. (2003). *Effect of closed-and open-kinetic chain resistance training on physical performance in older adults (PhD thesis).* The University of Connecticut.

Goodpaster, B., Park, S., Harris, T., et al. (2006). The loss of skeletal muscle strength, mass, and quality in older adults: the health, aging and body composition study. *The Journals of Gerontology Series A: Biological Sciences and Medical Sciences, 61*(10), 1059–1064.

Grgic, J., Schoenfeld, B., Davies, T., et al. (2018a). Effect of resistance training frequency on gains in muscular strength: a systematic review and meta-analysis. *Sports Medicine*, 1–14.

Grgic, J., Schoenfeld, B., Skrepnik, M., et al. (2018b). Effects of rest interval duration in resistance training on measures of muscular strength: a systematic review. *Sports Medicine, 48*(1), 137–151.

Hamer, M., Kivimaki, M., & Steptoe, A. (2012). Longitudinal patterns in physical activity and sedentary behaviour from mid-life to early old age: a substudy of the Whitehall II cohort. *Journal of Epidemiology and Community Health, 66*(12), 1110–1115.

Harris, A., & Sharma, A. (2018). Estimating the future health and aged care expenditure in Australia with changes in morbidity. *PLoS ONE, 13*(8), e0201697.

Hart, P., & Buck, D. (2019). The effect of resistance training on health-related quality of life in older adults: systematic review and meta-analysis. *Health Promotion Perspectives, 9*(1), 1.

Hartley, C., Folland, J., & Kerslake, R. (2020). High-impact exercise increased femoral neck bone density with no adverse effects on imaging markers of knee osteoarthritis in postmenopausal women. *Journal of Bone and Mineral Research, 35*(1), 53–63.

Havaldar, R., Pilli, S., & Putti, B. (2012). Effects of ageing on bone mineral composition and bone strength. *The International Organization of Scientific Research Journal of Dental and Medical Sciences, 1*(3), 12–16.

Henwood, T., Riek, S., & Taaffe, D. R. (2008). Strength versus muscle power-specific resistance training in community-dwelling older adults. *The Journals of Gerontology Series A: Biological Sciences and Medical Sciences, 63*(1), 83–91.

Hewitt, J., Goodall, S., Clemson, L., et al. (2018). Progressive resistance and balance training for falls prevention in long-term residential aged care: a cluster randomized trial of the sunbeam program. *Journal of the American Medical Directors Association, 19*(4), 361–369.

Ikezoe, T., Mori, N., Nakamura, M., et al. (2011). Age-related muscle atrophy in the lower extremities and daily physical activity in elderly women. *Archives of Gerontology and Geriatrics, 53*(2), e153–e157.

Izquierdo, M., Ibañez, J., Häkkinen, K., et al. (2004). Once weekly combined resistance and cardiovascular training in healthy older men. *Medicine & Science in Sports & Exercise, 36*(3), 435–443.

Jambassi Filho, J., Gurjão, A., Ceccato, M., et al. (2017). Chronic effects of different rest intervals between sets on dynamic and isometric muscle strength and muscle activity in trained older women. *American Journal of Physical Medicine & Rehabilitation, 96*(9), 627–633.

Kamada, M., Shiroma, E., Buring, J., et al. (2017). Strength training and all-cause, cardiovascular disease, and cancer mortality in older women: a cohort study. *Journal of the American Heart Association, 6*(11), e007677.

Kekäläinen, T., Kokko, K., Sipilä, S., et al. (2018). Effects of a 9-month resistance training intervention on quality of life, sense of coherence, and depressive symptoms in older adults: randomized controlled trial. *Quality of Life Research, 27*(2), 455–465.

Kemmler, W., & Stengel, V. (2014). Dose–response effect of exercise frequency on bone mineral density in post-menopausal, osteopenic women. *Scandinavian Journal of Medicine & Science in Sports, 24*(3), 526–534.

Kemmler, W., Weineck, M., Kohl, M., et al. (2020). High intensity resistance exercise training to improve body composition and strength in older men with osteosarcopenia. *Frontiers in Sports and Active Living, 2*(4), 1–12

Kim, Y., White, T., Wijndaele, K., et al. (2018). The combination of cardiorespiratory fitness and muscle strength, and mortality risk. *European Journal of Epidemiology, 33*(10), 953–964.

Klitgaard, H., Mantoni, M., Schiaffino, S., et al. (1990). Function, morphology and protein expression of ageing skeletal muscle: a cross-sectional study of elderly men with different training backgrounds. *Acta Physiologica Scandinavica, 140*(1), 41–54.

Koster, A., Caserotti, P., Patel, K., et al. (2012). Association of sedentary time with mortality independent of moderate to vigorous physical activity. *PLoS One, 7*(6), e37696.

Kwon, Y., Park, S., Jefferson, J., et al. (2013). The effect of open and closed kinetic chain exercises on dynamic balance ability of normal healthy adults. *Journal of Physical Therapy Science, 25*(6), 671–674.

Lambert, C., Beck, B., Harding, A., et al. (2020). Regional changes in indices of bone strength of upper and lower limbs in response to high-intensity impact loading or high-intensity resistance training. *Bone, 132*, 115192, 1–10.

Lee, I., Shiroma, E., Evenson, K., et al. (2018). Accelerometer-measured physical activity and sedentary behavior in relation to all-cause mortality: the women's health study. *Circulation, 137*(2), 203–205.

Lee, S., & Lee, D. Y. (2019). Effects of open and closed kinetic chain exercises on the balance using elastic bands for the health care of the elderly females. *Medico-Legal Update, 19*(2), 728–733.

Leskinen, T., & Kujala, U. M. (2015). Health-related findings among twin pairs discordant for leisure-time physical activity for 32 years: the TWINACTIVE study synopsis. *Twin Research and Human Genetics, 18*(3), 266–272.

Martland, R., Mondelli, V., Gaughran, F., et al. (2020). Can high-intensity interval training improve physical and mental health outcomes? A meta-review of 33 systematic reviews across the lifespan. *Journal of Sports Sciences*, 1–40.

Matos, F., Ferreira, B., Guedes, J., et al. (2020). Effect of rest interval between sets in the muscle function during a sequence of strength training exercises for the upper body. *The Journal of Strength & Conditioning Research*. Published Ahead of Print.

McKinnon, N., Connelly, D., Rice, C., et al. (2017). Neuromuscular contributions to the age-related reduction in muscle power: mechanisms and potential role of high velocity power training. *Ageing Research Reviews*, *35*, 147–154.

McPhee, J., Cameron, J., Maden-Wilkinson, T., et al. (2018). The contributions of fiber atrophy, fiber loss, in situ specific force, and voluntary activation to weakness in sarcopenia. *The Journals of Gerontology: Series A*, *73*(10), 1287–1294.

Miszko, T., Cress, M., Slade, J., et al. (2003). Effect of strength and power training on physical function in community-dwelling older adults. *The Journals of Gerontology Series A: Biological Sciences and Medical Sciences*, *58*(2), M171–M175.

Moghadam, B., Bagheri, R., Ashtary-Larky, D., et al. (2020). The effects of concurrent training order on satellite cell-related markers, body composition, muscular and cardiorespiratory fitness in older men with sarcopenia. *The Journal of Nutrition, Health & Aging*, 1–9.

Moran, J., Ramirez-Campillo, R., & Granacher, U. (2018). Effects of jumping exercise on muscular power in older adults: a meta-analysis. *Sports Medicine*, *48*(12), 2843–2857.

Multanen, J., Nieminen, M. T., Häkkinen, A., et al. (2014). Effects of high-impact training on bone and articular cartilage: 12-month randomized controlled quantitative MRI study. *Journal of Bone and Mineral Research*, *29*(1), 192–201.

Nelson, M., Fiatarone, M., Morganti, C., et al. (1994). Effects of high-intensity strength training on multiple risk factors for osteoporotic fractures: a randomized controlled trial. *The Journal of the American Medical Association*, *272*(24), 1909–1914.

Neufer, P., Bamman, M., Muoio, D., et al. (2015). Understanding the cellular and molecular mechanisms of physical activity-induced health benefits. *Cell Metabolism*, *22*(1), 4–11.

Nicholson, V., McKean, M., & Burkett, B. (2015). Low-load high-repetition resistance training improves strength and gait speed in middle-aged and older adults. *Journal of Science and Medicine in Sport*, *18*(5), 596–600.

Nilwik, R., Snijders, T., Leenders, M., et al. (2013). The decline in skeletal muscle mass with aging is mainly attributed to a reduction in type II muscle fiber size. *Experimental Gerontology*, *48*(5), 492–498.

Nóbrega, S., & Libardi, C. (2016). Is resistance training to muscular failure necessary? *Frontiers in Physiology*, *7*, Article 10, 1–4.

Noguera, C., Sánchez-Horcajo, R., Álvarez-Cazorla, D., et al. (2019). Ten years younger: practice of chronic aerobic exercise improves attention and spatial memory functions in ageing. *Experimental Gerontology*, *117*, 53–60.

Orssatto, L., Moura, B., Bezerra, E., et al. (2018). Influence of strength training intensity on subsequent recovery in elderly. *Experimental Gerontology*, *106*, 232–239.

Papa, E., Dong, X., & Hassan, M. (2017). Resistance training for activity limitations in older adults with skeletal muscle function deficits: a systematic review. *Clinical Interventions in Aging*, *12*, 955.

Pareja-Blanco, F., Rosell, D., Medina, L., et al. (2017). Effects of velocity loss during resistance training on athletic performance, strength gains and muscle adaptations. *Scandinavian Journal of Medicine & Science in Sports*, *27*(7), 724–735.

Parsons, C., Edwards, M., Cooper, C., et al. (2020). Are jumping mechanography assessed muscle force and power, and traditional physical capability measures associated with falls in older adults? Results from the Hertfordshire cohort study. *Journal of Musculoskeletal & Neuronal Interactions, 20*(2), 168.

Piercy, K., Troiano, R., Ballard, R., et al. (2018). The physical activity guidelines for Americans. *The Journal of the American Medical Association, 320*(19), 2020–2028.

Pina, F., Nunes, J., Schoenfeld, B., et al. (2020). Effects of different weekly sets-equated resistance training frequencies on muscular strength, muscle mass, and body fat in older women. *The Journal of Strength & Conditioning Research, 34*(10), 2990–2995.

Pritchett, R., Green, J., Wickwire, P., et al. (2009). Acute and session RPE responses during resistance training: bouts to failure at 60% and 90% of 1RM. *South African Journal of Sports Medicine, 21*(1), 23–26

Raafs, B., Karssemeijer, E., Van der Horst, L., et al. (2020). Physical exercise training improves quality of life in healthy older adults: a meta-analysis. *Journal of Aging and Physical Activity, 28*(1), 81–93.

Radaelli, R., Botton, C., Wilhelm, E., et al. (2014). Time course of low-and high-volume strength training on neuromuscular adaptations and muscle quality in older women. *Age, 36*(2), 881–892.

Radaelli, R., Botton, C., Wilhelm, E., et al. (2013). Low-and high-volume strength training induces similar neuromuscular improvements in muscle quality in elderly women. *Experimental Gerontology, 48*(8), 710–716.

Ramírez-Campillo, R., Castillo, A., Carlos, I., et al. (2014). High-speed resistance training is more effective than low-speed resistance training to increase functional capacity and muscle performance in older women. *Experimental Gerontology, 58*, 51–57.

Rashidi, E., Kakhak, H., Reza, S., et al. (2019). The effect of 8 weeks resistance training with low load and high load on testosterone, insulin-like growth factor-1, insulin-like growth factor binding protein-3 levels, and functional adaptations in older women. *Iranian Journal of Ageing, 14*(3), 356–367.

Raymond, M., Bramley-Tzerefos, R., Jeffs, K., et al. (2013). Systematic review of high-intensity progressive resistance strength training of the lower limb compared with other intensities of strength training in older adults. *Archives of Physical Medicine and Rehabilitation, 94*(8), 1458–1472.

Ribeiro, A., dos Santos, E., Nunes, J., et al. (2019). Acute effects of different training loads on affective responses in resistance-trained men. *International Journal of Sports Medicine, 40*(13), 850–855.

Richardson, D., Duncan, M., Jimenez, A., et al. (2019). Effects of movement velocity and training frequency of resistance exercise on functional performance in older adults: a randomised controlled trial. *European Journal of Sport Science, 19*(2), 234–246.

Ruiz, J., Sui, X., Lobelo, F., et al. (2008). Association between muscular strength and mortality in men: prospective cohort study. *British Medical Journal, 337*, a439, 1–9

Schott, N., Johnen, B., & Holfelder, B. (2019). Effects of free weights and machine training on muscular strength in high-functioning older adults. *Experimental Gerontology, 122*, 15–24.

Sherrington, C., Fairhall, N., Wallbank, G., et al. (2020). Exercise for preventing falls in older people living in the community: an abridged Cochrane systematic review. *British Journal of Sports Medicine, 54*(15), 885–891.

Shiotsu, Y., & Yanagita, M. (2018). Comparisons of low-intensity versus moderate-intensity combined aerobic and resistance training on body composition, muscle strength, and functional performance in older women. *Menopause, 25*(6), 668–675.

Souza, D., Barbalho, M., Ramirez-Campillo, R., et al. (2020). High and low-load resistance training produce similar effects on bone mineral density of middle-aged and older people: a systematic review with meta-analysis of randomized clinical trials. *Experimental Gerontology,* 110973.

Stec, M., Thalacker-Mercer, A., Mayhew, D., et al. (2017). Randomized, four-arm, dose-response clinical trial to optimize resistance exercise training for older adults with age-related muscle atrophy. *Experimental Gerontology, 99*, 98–109.

Stubbs, B., & Rosenbaum, S. (2018). *Exercise-based interventions for mental illness: physical activity as part of clinical treatment.* Academic Press.

Taaffe, D., & Galvao, D. (2004). High-and low-volume resistance training similarly enhances functional performance in older adults. *Medicine and Science in Sports and Exercise, 36*(5), S142–S142.

Theou, O., Gareth, J., & Brown, L. (2008). Effect of rest interval on strength recovery in young and old women. *The Journal of Strength & Conditioning Research, 22*(6), 1876–1881.

Thomson, R., Brinkworth, G., Noakes, M., et al. (2016). Muscle strength gains during resistance exercise training are attenuated with soy compared with dairy or usual protein intake in older adults: a randomized controlled trial. *Clinical Nutrition, 35*(1), 27–33.

Thornton, J., Frémont, P., Khan, K., et al. (2016). Physical activity prescription: a critical opportunity to address a modifiable risk factor for the prevention and management of chronic disease: a position statement by the Canadian academy of sport and exercise medicine. *British Journal of Sports Medicine, 50*(18), 1109–1114.

Van Roie, E., Delecluse, C., Coudyzer, W., et al. (2013). Strength training at high versus low external resistance in older adults: effects on muscle volume, muscle strength, and force–velocity characteristics. *Experimental Gerontology, 48*(11), 1351–1361.

Vecchio, L., Meng, Y., Xhima, K., et al. (2018). The neuroprotective effects of exercise: maintaining a healthy brain throughout aging. *Brain Plasticity, 4*(1), 17–52.

Villanueva, M., Lane, C., & Schroeder, E. (2015). Short rest interval lengths between sets optimally enhance body composition and performance with 8 weeks of strength resistance training in older men. *European Journal of Applied Physiology, 115*(2), 295–308.

Watson, S., Weeks, B., Weis, L., et al. (2018). High-intensity resistance and impact training improves bone mineral density and physical function in postmenopausal women with osteopenia and osteoporosis: the LIFTMOR randomized controlled trial. *Journal of Bone and Mineral Research, 33*(2), 211–220.

Westcott, W., Winett, R., Anderson, E., et al. (2001). Effects of regular and slow speed resistance training on muscle strength. *Journal of Sports Medicine and Physical Fitness, 41*(2), 154–158

Westerståhl, M., Jansson, E., Barnekow-Bergkvist, M., et al. (2018). Longitudinal changes in physical capacity from adolescence to middle age in men and women. *Scientific Reports, 8*(1), 1–10.

Willardson, J., Simão, R., & Fontana, F. (2012). The effect of load reductions on repetition performance for commonly performed multijoint resistance exercises. *The Journal of Strength & Conditioning Research, 26*(11), 2939–2945.

Yeung, S., Reijnierse, E., Pham, V., et al. (2019). Sarcopenia and its association with falls and fractures in older adults: a systematic review and meta-analysis. *Journal of Cachexia, Sarcopenia and Muscle, 10*(3), 485–500.

Zampieri, S., Pietrangelo, L., Loefler, S., et al. (2015). Lifelong physical exercise delays age-associated skeletal muscle decline. *Journals of Gerontology Series A: Biomedical Sciences and Medical Sciences, 70*(2), 163–173.

Zengin, A., Pye, S., Cook, M., et al. (2016). The relationship between muscle strength and bone outcomes in ageing UK men. In *43rd annual European calcified tissue society congress* (Vol. 5). BioScientifica.

17 Pregnant clients

Marlize De Vivo

Pregnancy is a unique life event characterised by significant anatomical, metabolic, cardiovascular, and pulmonary changes/adaptations (American College of Obstetricians and Gynaecologists [ACOG], 2020; Bø et al., 2018; Dipietro et al., 2019). Women with uncomplicated pregnancies are recommended to engage in 150 minutes of moderate-intensity physical activity (PA) per week and muscle-strengthening activities (e.g., resistance training) twice per week. However, the physiological and anatomical changes that occur during pregnancy mean that PA modifications may be required to ensure safe and effective participation.

The benefits of exercise during pregnancy

Alongside the benefits experienced by the general adult population, regular PA during pregnancy has specific benefits (see Figure 17.1). It is also important to recognise that there is no evidence of harm in relation to risk of preterm birth, small for gestational age, large for gestational age, or other complications for a new-born baby (Bø et al., 2016b; Department of Health and Social Care [DHSC], 2019a, 2019b). The evidence-based outcomes presented in Figure 17.1 are advocated by the United Kingdom's Chief Medical Officers' (DHSC, 2019a, 2019b).

Physiological changes that affect exercise capacity

According to the PA guidelines (see Figure 17.1), women with uncomplicated pregnancies can engage in activity, except for those with certain contraindications (see Table 17.1). Moderate-to-vigorous intensity PA (MVPA) is not recommended for women with absolute contraindications (see Table 17.1), as the risks outweigh the potential benefits and could result in adverse effects for the mother and/or foetus; however, activities of daily living may continue (Meah et al., 2020). Relative contraindications (see Table 17.1) refer to conditions where activity should be approached with caution and warrant further discussion with a healthcare professional.

DOI: 10.4324/9781003204657-17

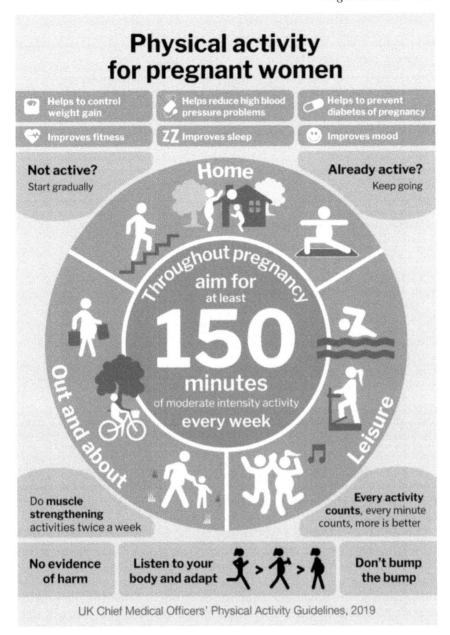

Figure 17.1 Physical activity guidelines for pregnant women.

Table 17.1 Absolute and relative contraindications to physical activity during pregnancy

---

Absolute Contraindications

- Severe respiratory diseases (e.g., chronic obstructive pulmonary disease, restrictive lung disease, cystic fibrosis, asthma, shortness of breath, chronic coughing, and chest tightness)
- Severe acquired or congenital heart disease with exercise intolerance
- Uncontrolled or severe arrhythmia
- Placental abruption
- Vasa previa
- Uncontrolled type 1 diabetes
- Intrauterine growth restriction (IUGR)
- Active preterm labour (i.e., regular and painful uterine contractions before 37 weeks of pregnancy
- Severe pre-eclampsia
- Cervical insufficiency

Relative Contraindications

- Mild respiratory disorders (see above)
- Mild congenital or acquired heart disease
- Well-controlled type 1 diabetes
- Mild pre-eclampsia
- Preterm premature rupture of membranes (PPROMs).
- Placenta previa after 28 weeks
- Untreated thyroid disease
- Symptomatic, severe eating disorders
- Multiple nutrient deficiencies and/or chronic undernutrition
- Moderate–heavy smoking (>20 cigarettes per day) in the presence of comorbidities

---

(Meah, Davies & Davenport, 2020)

The advantages and disadvantages of low-to-moderate intensity PA should be considered and may potentially proceed provided appropriate modifications are implemented and the training is supervised and monitored (Meah et al., 2020).

An initial assessment is required before continuing to train an existing client who has become pregnant or taking on a new client who is pregnant. In the absence of maternal or foetal contraindications, exercise programming during pregnancy is based on the same principles as those for the general adult population. However, as shown in Table 17.2, pregnancy is associated with significant anatomical and physiological changes that should be considered when designing a training programme (ACOG, 2020; Bø et al., 2018).

Endurance (cardiovascular) training recommendations

Regular cardiovascular training can produce measurable improvements in maternal cardiorespiratory fitness (ACOG, 2020; Mottola et al., 2006). Clients with uncomplicated pregnancies who are new to PA (i.e., sedentary

Table 17.2 Summary of anatomical and physiological adaptations to pregnancy

Musculoskeletal

- A shift in the centre of gravity occurs due to an expanding uterus, enlarged breasts and increased body mass.
- A displaced centre of gravity may result in progressive lumbar lordosis and anterior rotation of the pelvis on the femur.
- Increasing lumbar lordosis cause an increase in anterior flexion of the cervical spine and abduction of the shoulders.
- Significant decreases in both the length of the gait cycle and step length are observed as pregnancy progresses. This is associated with a significant increase in double support time whilst single support time is reduced, and step width is increased resulting in a wider stance.
- An increase in hormones, specifically relaxin, increase joint instability and the risk of injury.
- Postural balance is affected after the first trimester and increases the likelihood of falls and injury.

Cardiorespiratory

- Adaptations occur from the fifth week of gestation to ensure adequate blood supply to the foetus.
- Increases in oestrogen levels result in a primary reduction in afterload and an increase in venous capacitance. This is reflected in an increased resting cardiac output of approximately 50%.
- Remodelling of the heart increases the dimensions of the ventricular cavity without increasing wall thickness; increases aortic capacitance; and reduces peripheral vascular resistance.
- Resting heart rate increases by 15–20 bpm.
- By the end of the first trimester, before a significant improvement in maternal blood volume can be observed, stroke volume increases by approximately 10%. Blood volume may increase up to 50% above pre-pregnancy values by the end of the third trimester.
- An increase in respiratory sensitivity to carbon dioxide (CO_2) can be observed early in pregnancy. Because of the increase in tidal volume, minute ventilation increases up to 50%. These changes create a buffer that protects the foetus from any acute elevations in maternal CO_2 levels.
- During submaximal steady-state activities, perceptions of respiratory effort and dyspnoea appear reduced because maternal anatomical and mechanical respiratory adaptations reduce airway resistance, preserve breathing mechanics, minimise the effort of ventilation and thus increase minute ventilation.
- As a result of the physiologic decrease in the pulmonary reserve, ability to exercise anaerobically is reduced. During aerobic exercise, oxygen availability lags.

Metabolic

- Maternal metabolism adapts to ensure adequate glucose supply to support the growth of the fetoplacental unit.
- Several hormonal events lead to an increase in maternal blood glucose, decrease in liver glycogen storage, elevated liver glucose release, and an increase in maternal insulin levels.

(*Continued*)

Table 17.2 (Continued)

- The resulting increases in insulin resistance in skeletal muscle and decreased maternal utilisation of glucose in peripheral tissues, leaves more maternal glucose for foetal utilisation.
- The fetoplacental unit can use as much as 30–50% of the maternal glucose store in late stages of pregnancy.
- Due to the lipogenic action of higher maternal insulin concentrations, maternal body fat is stored early in pregnancy. These adipose stores may provide an alternative energy source for the mother later in pregnancy and preserve maternal blood glucose for foetal use.

Thermoregulatory

- Raising body core temperature above 39°C can increase the risk of foetal abnormalities during neural tube development which occurs 35–42 days from the last menstrual period.
- Exercising at 60–70% of VO_{2max} in a controlled environment for up to 60 minutes does not raise core temperature above 38°C.
- A higher body core temperature could be reached during strenuous exercise, such as marathon running, or being active outdoors in hot and humid weather.
- Whilst thermoregulation is dependent on hydration and environmental conditions, it steadily improves as pregnancy progresses. A lower body temperature threshold initiates sweating, resulting in evaporative heat loss starting at a lower body temperature.

(ACOG, 2020; Bø et al., 2016a)

or previously inactive) should start gradually and aim to accumulate 150 minutes of moderate intensity PA throughout the week (DHSC, 2019a, 2019b). Moderate intensity refers to activities performed whilst being able to hold a conversation (see Chapter 10).

Whilst it has been suggested that Borg's ratings of perceived exertion (RPE) scale may be an effective method to measure effort (ACOG, 2020), RPE ratings do not correlate strongly with heart rate (HR) during pregnancy, as women can potentially exercise at a higher HR than the RPE would suggest (Bø et al., 2016a). If HR zones (see Table 17.3) are to be used to guide training, HR should be measured using a HR monitor.

Pregnant clients with uncomplicated pregnancies who are already active should be encouraged to maintain their PA levels; however, adaptation of certain activities may be required as pregnancy progresses. For example, reducing training volume and replacing activities with suitable alternatives (DHSC, 2019a, 2019b).

Whilst research examining the safety and benefits of vigorous intensity PA are limited, women who regularly participate in such activities (e.g., running, cycling, rowing) before becoming pregnant may want to continue doing so (Dipietro et al., 2019). These women can continue with vigorous intensity activities but adaption of the activity and/or nutritional uptake may be required if they start to lose weight (ACOG, 2019) and consultation with a healthcare professional is advised (Mottola et al., 2018). In

Table 17.3 Heart rate ranges for women with uncomplicated pregnancies

Maternal age	Intensity	HR range (B/min)
<29	Light	102–124
	Moderate*	125–146
	Vigorous**	147–169***
30+	Light	101–120
	Moderate*	121–141
	Vigorous**	142–162***

(Mottola et al., 2018)

* Moderate intensity physical activity (40%–59% heart rate reserve (HRR))

** Vigorous intensity physical activity (60%–80% HRR).

*** Limited evidence regarding the impact of physical activity at the upper end of the vigorous-intensity HR ranges; pregnant clients wishing to be active at this intensity (or beyond) should consult their healthcare professional.

general, however, it is recommended that women consider how they might adjust their activity to what is comfortable and suitable. Pregnant clients who are new to PA should avoid engaging in vigorous intensity activities (see Figure 17.1).

Strength training recommendations

Women with uncomplicated pregnancies should engage in muscle strengthening activities (e.g., resistance training) involving the major muscle groups of the upper and lower body twice per week (DHSC, 2019a, 2019b; Department of Health [DOH], 2017). Resistance training using free weights or machines at a low-to-moderate intensity, has no adverse health effects during pregnancy (Bø et al., 2016a). Indeed, large improvements in strength have been reported in healthy untrained women who performed resistance training twice per week for 12 weeks during pregnancy (O'Connor et al., 2011).

Overall, there is limited research on strenuous strength training in the pregnant population (Bø et al., 2016a). However, trained women who continue to engage in strenuous resistance training during their pregnancies should pay attention to technique and safety (Bø et al., 2018). Specifically, the Valsalva manoeuvre causes a rapid increase in blood pressure and intra-abdominal pressure, which may temporarily decrease blood flow to the foetus (Bø et al., 2016a). The effects of temporary increases in blood and intra-abdominal pressure on the foetus remain unknown. However, women should be aware that large increases in intra-abdominal pressure may damage the pelvic floor and increase the risk of complications, such as urinary or anal incontinence and pelvic organ prolapse (Bø et al., 2016a).

To prevent blood from pooling in a specific area of the body, splitting a full-body routine and performing a single exercise for each of the major muscle groups is recommended (Schoenfeld, 2011). Whist beginners should start with one set of 10–15 repetitions per exercise, trained women can perform up to three sets. A two-minute rest period between sets should allow for sufficient recovery of maternal HR, although this will be based on the client's fitness level.

Exercises to avoid during pregnancy

Activities such as walking, swimming, dancing, stationary cycling, yoga/ Pilates (modified for pregnancy), low impact aerobics and resistance training are safe to initiate or continue for women with uncomplicated pregnancies (ACOG, 2019, 2020). However, pregnant women who are not already active should avoid high intensity activities (e.g., running, racquet sports, plyometrics) and strenuous resistance training (DOH, 2017; Schoenfeld, 2011).

Whilst various types of exercises can be recommended to pregnant clients, it is important to be aware of the risks of certain activities. For example, activities with an increased risk of trauma where there is a higher risk of falling or sustaining high impact or contact injuries (e.g., skiing, gymnastics, horse riding) should be avoided (DOH, 2017; Mottola et al., 2018). Activities associated with physiological risk factors (e.g., scuba diving, sky diving, high altitude training) are not advised (DOH, 2017; Mottola et al., 2018).

Due to progressive weight gain, a shift in the centre gravity, and increase in the hormone relaxin, postural balance can be affected, which increases the risk of falls and injury (ACOG, 2020; Bø et al., 2018). Therefore, it is advisable that pregnant clients have support available when performing stretches and balance type activities (DOH, 2017). Exercises that require forward flexion at the hips and/or waist should be avoided after the first trimester and alternate positions such as all-fours or seated exercises should be considered (Schoenfeld, 2011). Overhead lifting movements that exacerbate lumbar stress should be substituted with alternative movements targeting the same muscle groups (Schoenfeld, 2011).

Exercises performed in the supine position after the first trimester are not recommended because there is an increased risk of reduced cardiac output and orthostatic hypotension that can occur as the uterus enlarges (ACOG, 2020; DOH, 2017). Yoga or Pilates classes that have been modified for pregnancy should not include these exercises and can be encouraged (DOH. 2017).

Additional considerations

Pregnant women should stay hydrated, wear loose clothing and avoid excessive exposure to heat during exercise (DOH, 2017). Exercising for long durations (over one hour), especially in hot humid conditions, is not advised. In

Table 17.4 Warning signs to stop exercise whilst pregnant

Vaginal bleeding
Abdominal pain
Regular and painful contractions
Amniotic fluid leakage indicating rupture of the membranes
Difficulty breathing before exertion
Persistent excessive shortness of breath that does not resolve with rest
Persistent dizziness or faintness that does not resolve on rest
Headache
Chest pain
Muscle weakness affecting balance
Calf pain or swelling

(ACOG, 2020; Mottola et al., 2018)

general, pregnant clients should be encouraged to continue if the PA feels pleasant but should stop and seek advice from a healthcare professional if anything feels uncomfortable or if they experience any warning signs (see Table 17.4).

Summary of exercise recommendations

Women with uncomplicated pregnancies are recommended to accumulate 150 minutes of aerobic activity throughout the week and engage in muscle strengthening activities twice per week. Already active clients are advised to maintain their PA levels, although the training programme may need to be adapted as pregnancy progresses. Pregnant women who are new to activity should start gradually and avoid vigorous-intensity activities. Whilst a variety of activities can be recommended, it is important for trainers to be aware of the risks of certain activities and the modifications that may be required. Finally, trainers should be able to recognise the signs and symptoms that necessitate a pregnant client to stop exercising and seek advice.

References

American College of Obstetricians and Gynaecologists (ACOG). (2019). *Frequently asked questions No. 119: exercise during pregnancy*. Retrieved from www.acog.org.

American College of Obstetricians and Gynaecologists (ACOG) (2020). Committee opinion No. 804: physical activity and exercise during pregnancy and the postpartum period. *Obstetrics & Gynecology, 135*(4), e178–e188.

Bø, K., Artal, R., Barakat, R., et al. (2016a). Exercise and pregnancy in recreational and elite athletes: 2016 evidence summary from the IOC expert group meeting, Lausanne. Part 1—exercise in women planning pregnancy and those who are pregnant. *British Journal of Sports Medicine, 50*(10), 571–589.

Bø, K., Artal, R., Barakat, R., et al. (2016b). Exercise and pregnancy in recreational and elite athletes: 2016 evidence summary from the IOC expert group meeting, Lausanne. Part 2—the effect of exercise on the fetus, labour and birth. *British Journal of Sports Medicine, 50*(21), 1297–1305.

Bø, K., Artal, R., Barakat, R., et al. (2018). Exercise and pregnancy in recreational and elite athletes: 2016/2017 evidence summary from the IOC expert group meeting, Lausanne. Part 5. Recommendations for health professionals and active women. *British Journal of Sports Medicine*, *52*(17), 1080–1085.

Department of Health (DOH). (2017). Physical activity in pregnancy infographic guidance. Retrieved from: https://assets.publishing.service.gov.uk/government/uploads/system/uploads/attachment_data/file/831430/Withdrawn_Physical_activity_pregnancy_infographic_guidance.pdf

Department of Health and Social Care (DHSC). (2019a). *UK Chief Medical Officers' Physical Activity Guidelines*. Retrieved from https://www.gov.uk/government/publications/physical-activity-guidelines-uk-chief-medical-officers-report

Department of Health and Social Care (DHSC). (2019b). *Physical activity in pregnancy infographic: guidance*. Retrieved from https://assets.publishing.service.gov.uk/government/uploads/system/uploads/attachment_data/file/829894/5-physical-activity-for-pregnant-women.pdf

Dipietro, L., Evenson, K. R., Bloodgood, B., et al. (2019). Benefits of physical activity during pregnancy and postpartum: an umbrella review. *Medicine and Science in Sports and Exercise*, *51*(6), 1292–1302.

Meah, V., Davies, G., & Davenport, M. (2020). Why can't I exercise during pregnancy? Time to revisit medical 'absolute' and 'relative' contraindications: systematic review of evidence of harm and a call to action. *British Journal of Sports Medicine*, 1–12.

Mottola, M., Davenport, M., Brun, C., et al. (2006). VO_{2peak} prediction and exercise prescription for pregnant women. *Medicine and Science in Sports and Exercise*, *38*(8), 1389–1395.

Mottola, M., Davenport, M., Ruchat, S., et al. (2018). 2019 Canadian guideline for physical activity throughout pregnancy. *British Journal of Sports Medicine*, *52*(21), 1339–1346.

O'Connor, P., Poudevigne, M., Cress, M., et al. (2011). Safety and efficacy of supervised strength training adopted in pregnancy. *Journal of Physical Activity and Health*, *8*(3), 309–320.

Schoenfeld, B. (2011). Resistance training during pregnancy: safe and effective program design. *Strength & Conditioning Journal*, *33*(5), 67–75.

18 Recovery from training

Paul Hough and Shona Halson

When a progressive overload is applied during exercise, both fitness and fatigue effects occur concurrently. The fatigue from training causes a short-term reduction in fitness; however, during the post-exercise recovery period there is a restoration of homeostasis and fitness levels return to, or exceed, previous levels (see Chapter 6). Therefore, the recovery period following exercise is a vital component of the training process. Inadequate recovery (aka under-recovery) results in sub-optimal performance in the next training session or during competition for athletes. Inadequate recovery can lead to negative physiological and psychological consequences; therefore, it is important for trainers and clients to recognise common symptoms of inadequate recovery (see Figure 18.1). This chapter will focus on the role of sleep in recovery and common post-exercise strategies that are used to promote muscle recovery between bouts of exercise.

Sleep

Sleep is often described as the best recovery strategy available to athletes and individuals who are involved in physically demanding occupations. This is due to the important physiological and psychological functions that occur during sleep. Disturbed sleep has been shown to result in decreases in performance, impaired cognitive function, mood disturbance, altered metabolism and increased risk of injury (Halson, 2014). Interestingly, research in athletes has shown that sleep quality and/or quantity is impaired compared to the general population (Leeder et al., 2012) and is often outside the recommended range of 7–8 hours (Lastella et al., 2015, 2020)

Sleep restriction can reduce maximal and sub-maximal strength and sport-specific performance (Walsh et al., 2020). Further, sleep restriction is more likely to affect performance in sports that involve higher-level cognitive and mental tasks rather than gross-motor execution (Reilly & Deykin, 1983). It is likely that reduced motivation and higher ratings of perceived exertion explain part of the reason why sleep restriction impairs performance (Thun et al., 2015).

DOI: 10.4324/9781003204657-18

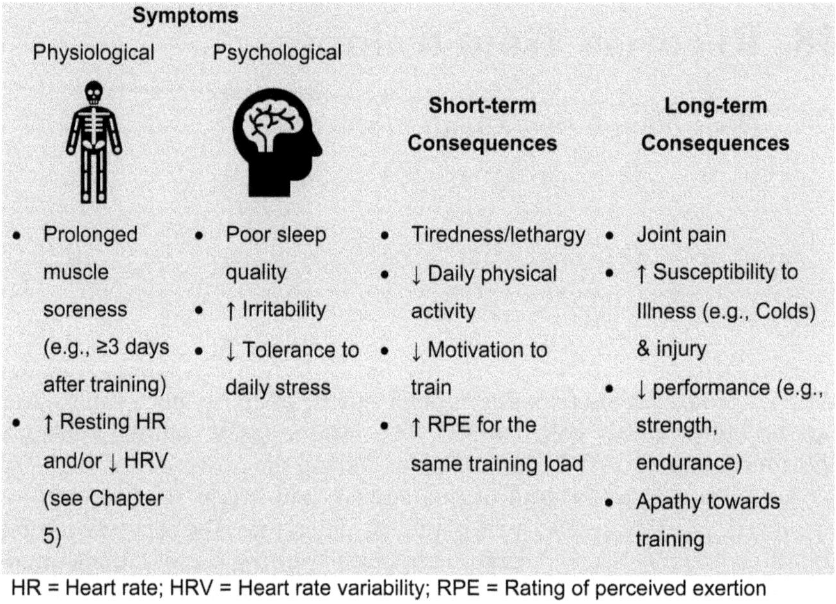

Figure 18.1 Common symptoms and consequences of inadequate recovery after training.

There are several reasons why athletes may have difficulty obtaining an appropriate duration of sleep or may have disturbed sleep resulting in poor quality sleep. Although some factors affecting athletes sleep are unique to high-level athletes (e.g., competition schedules), many factors are also experienced by the general population of a similar age. These include early morning or late evening training sessions, afternoon or evening caffeine ingestion, psychological and emotional stressors (e.g., occupational workloads), social media and video gaming, extensive travelling, and jetlag (van Rensburg et al., 2020; Walsh et al., 2020).

Measuring sleep has become popular in both high-level athletes and the general population (see Chapter 5). Good sleep is generally considered when an individual falls asleep within 30 minutes, sleeps for 7–8 hours, and wakes feeling refreshed most mornings of the week.

Some recommendations for good sleep include:

- Establish a consistent sleep-wake pattern (i.e., go to bed and wake at the same time)
- Create a non-stimulating before bed routine
- Avoid napping in the late afternoon
- Limit caffeine in the afternoon

- Maintain a cool (19–21°C), dark, and quiet bedroom
- Avoid electronic device use 30 minutes before bed.

Reducing post-exercise fatigue

Athletes often perform specific recovery protocols following training and competition to accelerate recovery and reduce fatigue. However, there are numerous types and causes of fatigue; for example, muscular fatigue from physical activity and cognitive fatigue due to sleep loss. Furthermore, the type of training influences the time-course and nature of post-exercise fatigue (Nuuttila et al., 2020). Before selecting a recovery strategy, it is important to identify the nature of the client's fatigue (i.e., what is the client recovering from?). Exercise can induce different types of fatigue (e.g., metabolic, and central nervous system); the most common type of fatigue clients will experience and wish to recover from is muscle fatigue.

Timing of recovery strategies

It is important to consider the timing and long-term implications of the recovery strategy. Most of the recovery strategies discussed below originated from elite sport when athletes have limited time to recover between competition periods (Thomas et al., 2017); in these scenarios, the athletes' priority is to recover as quickly as possible. However, rapid recovery is not always essential for clients who are training to improve health and fitness. A well-designed programme (see Chapter 8) should allow sufficient recovery time between training sessions, and the fatiguing aftereffects from the previous sessions will have dissipated. Thus, specialist recovery strategies, such as cryotherapy (discussed later), are not usually required. Furthermore, some post-exercise recovery strategies could be counterproductive in some instances. For example, cold water immersion (CWI) can diminish acute molecular responses that regulate muscle hypertrophy, which could impede muscle hypertrophy in the long-term (Fyfe et al., 2019; Roberts et al., 2015). Therefore, trainers should have a thorough knowledge of the relevant research before recommending novel recovery strategies.

Strategies to promote muscle recovery after exercise

The production of muscle force depends on complex contractile mechanisms within the muscle fibres. Failure at any site within the motor pathway (brain to muscle) reduces muscle force production (i.e., muscle fatigue). During exercise, repeated muscle actions and tissue vibrations can cause muscle fatigue due to central (nervous system) and peripheral (within the muscle) factors. Both the type and intensity of exercise affect where muscle fatigue originates within the motor pathway; however, a discussion of the complex aetiology of muscle fatigue is beyond this chapter's scope.

Prolonged exercise can also lead to dehydration, muscle damage and the depletion of muscle glycogen, all of which reduce muscle force capacity. Thus, post-exercise nutritional considerations, such as carbohydrate and protein intake, and rehydration, are also an important part of the recovery process (see Chapter 4).

Unaccustomed or strenuous exercise often causes exercise-induced muscle damage (EIMD) and associated muscle soreness. Several physiological mechanisms interact to cause acute or delayed muscle soreness following exercise (Cleak & Eston, 1992). Damaged connective tissue stimulates mechanically sensitive receptors and nociceptors, which causes soreness and pain when the tissue is stretched or pressed. The tissue damage also initiates an inflammatory response, which can cause swelling. Consequently, EIMD causes site-specific muscle pain, decreased range of movement (ROM), reduced force production and contributes to the delayed onset of muscle soreness (DOMS), which occurs approximately 12 hours following strenuous exercise. DOMS usually lasts for 48–72 hours, although it can last longer if the exercise is particularly intensive or novel (Law & Herbert, 2007).

The following sections will focus on strategies to accelerate recovery from EIMD and reduce DOMS: active cool-down, static stretching (SS), massage, foam rolling (FR), compression and water immersion. Most of the post-exercise recovery strategies presented aim to decrease EIMD and inflammation through several mechanisms, such as reducing the available space for swelling and oedema formation, and increasing blood and lymph flow to facilitate the transport of metabolites and damaged proteins (Barnett, 2006; Kovacs & Baker, 2014).

Active cool-down

An active cool-down (also known as a warm-down) describes the period at the end of a training session where low to moderate-intensity exercise is performed to restore homeostasis more quickly than passive rest (Popp et al., 2017). The cool-down aims to reduce sympathetic nervous system activity and gradually reduce cardiorespiratory parameters (e.g., heart rate, blood pressure, respiration). In clients with suspected or diagnosed clinical conditions, a cool-down is performed to minimise the risk of cardiovascular complications following exercise, such as syncope and postural hypotension (MacDonald, 2002). An active cool-down is also thought to enhance muscle recovery via increasing blood flow to muscles, thus facilitating the transport of nutrients and removal of metabolic by-products (e.g., lactate and hydrogen ions), and possibly reducing muscle tension (Cheung et al., 2003).

A moderate intensity (50–75% VO_{2max}) cool-down can facilitate the recovery of cardiorespiratory variables, such as heart rate and respiration (Takahashi et al., 2002). A cool-down may also elicit a temporary reduction in blood pressure (BP), below resting values, known as post-exercise

Table 18.1 Cool-down guidelines

Exercise type	Intensity	Volume	Considerations
Active cool-down: dynamic, rhythmic exercises (e.g., cycling, jogging)	• Low-Moderate (~50–75% $VO_{2\,max}$) • RPE 8–12	• 5–30 minutes	Avoid high impact exercises to prevent exacerbating muscle damage.
Static stretching	• Low (40–70% of maximum perceived stretch)	• 2–3 sets/ stretch • 30–60 seconds/ stretch	Avoid stretching to the point of pain or discomfort. Practise deep breathing during each stretch.
Foam rolling	• Light-moderate pressure (≤6 on a 0–10 pain scale)	• 30–60 seconds/ muscle group	Volume should be modified based on individual needs. Self-experimentation is required. Practise deep breathing when rolling.

RPE = Rating of perceived exertion (Borg Scale 6–20).

hypotension (PEH), for minutes or hours after exercise (MacDonald et al., 1999). The exact duration and mechanisms responsible for PEH are variable between individuals (MacDonald, 2002). However, a significant drop in BP after exercise can cause a loss of consciousness (syncope) (Krediet et al., 2004). A cool-down may decrease the likelihood of post-exercise syncope and cardiovascular complications by increasing blood flow to the heart and brain and reducing blood pooling in the lower extremities (Romero et al., 2017). Therefore, trainers should be aware of PEH and consider monitoring BP during a cool-down in clients who have borderline or diagnosed hypertension. Cool-down guidelines to facilitate the recovery of cardiorespiratory variables are presented in Table 18.1.

Does a cool-down enhance next-day performance and reduce the delayed onset of muscle soreness?

The scientific evidence for the efficacy of a cool-down on next-day performance and recovery of neuromuscular function is equivocal. Some studies indicate moderate performance benefits after performing a cool-down compared with passive rest (Takahashi et al., 2006); conversely, other studies have reported no performance or neuromuscular benefits (Raeder et al., 2017; Rey et al., 2012; Wiewelhove et al., 2016). Research is also equivocal regarding the effect of a cool-down on DOMS, musculotendinous stiffness and indirect markers of muscle damage in the days following exercise (Law & Herbert, 2007; Rey et al., 2012; Takahashi et al., 2006).

The mixed findings on the effectiveness of a cool-down on next-day performance, DOMS and musculotendinous stiffness is due to differences between studies in the exercise protocols used to induce fatigue and the type of exercise performed in the cool-down. For instance, some studies have implemented protocols, such as 300 countermovement jumps, that would likely cause more DOMS than a regular training session (Wahl et al., 2017). Although unconfirmed in the literature, the type of exercise performed during the cool-down could also influence DOMS. For example, weight-bearing activities, such as running, could conceivably worsen DOMS compared to cycling or swimming.

According to current research, a cool-down does not significantly accelerate the recovery of neuromuscular function or reduce DOMS; however, a cool-down is not detrimental to recovery, provided the intensity is moderate. A cool-down could offer some psychological benefits as it provides an opportunity for clients to relax, socialise and reflect on the training session. Furthermore, a cool-down could enhance perceived recovery compared to a passive cool-down (Cortis et al., 2010; Tavares et al., 2017).

Cool-down summary

A moderate-intensity cool-down can accelerate the recovery of cardiorespiratory measures after exercise, and potentially reduce post-exercise syncope. However, performing a cool-down does not significantly accelerate the recovery of physiological function or performance the following day. The effect of a cool-down on DOMS, indirect markers of muscle damage and musculotendinous stiffness is also negligible. However, an active cool-down may offer some psychological benefits.

Static stretching

Stretching involves the application of force to increase flexibility and joint range of motion (ROM) (Weerapong et al., 2004). SS involves slowly stretching a musculotendinous unit (MTU) and holding the stretched position for a specific period, usually 15–60 seconds. Historically, SS was recommended before exercise to reduce injury risk and improve subsequent performance, although both theories are contentious (see Chapter 9). SS is often performed after exercise as it is thought to facilitate recovery by reducing DOMS and musculotendinous stiffness after exercise (Torres et al., 2012). However, standardising the intensity of stretches is difficult, which makes comparisons between studies problematic. Most research indicates that SS does not significantly reduce DOMS (Dupuy et al., 2018; Herbert et al., 2011; Henschke & Lin, 2011), although low intensity stretching (30–40% of maximum perceived stretch) could provide moderate improvements in perceived muscle soreness (Apostolopoulos et al., 2018). Overall, the current empirical evidence suggests that post-exercise SS has a minimal effect on reducing EIMD and DOMS, but it may have other beneficial effects, discussed below.

Benefits of post-exercise static stretching

Several studies suggest that regular SS can alter the length and stiffness of the MTU and improve ROM (Davis et al., 2005; LaRoche & Connolly, 2006). Improving ROM could be beneficial for certain clients; for instance, a lack of ROM may restrict movement and compromise exercise technique or result in sub-optimal performance in activities requiring a high level of flexibility (e.g., gymnastics).

During SS, blood flow and muscle oxygenation decrease (Poole et al., 1997). However, a hyperemic response has been observed when the stretch is released, meaning blood flow significantly increases above the pre-stretching levels (Kruse et al., 2016). The hyperemic response after SS may quicken the delivery of nutrients and removal of metabolites to the muscle; however, it is unclear if this has a meaningful impact on muscle recovery.

In general, the nervous system's parasympathetic branch is more active during periods of recovery than the sympathetic branch, which is more active during exercise (see Chapter 5). Several studies have reported an increase in parasympathetic nervous system activity following SS, suggesting SS could promote relaxation following exercise (Eda et al., 2020; Farinatti et al., 2011). However, stretches must be performed carefully, as stretching too quickly or intensely (to the point of pain) could increase hemodynamic (e.g., BP and heart rate) responses (Lima et al., 2015). Therefore, SS should be performed at a moderate intensity (below 70% of maximum perceived stretch) as stretching too intensely could increase sympathetic nervous system activity and possibly worsen DOMS (Smith et al., 1993).

Massage

Effects on delayed onset of muscle soreness

Massage is a widely used therapy to reduce DOMS and promote relaxation. Research indicates that massage effectively reduces *perceived* muscle soreness and pain in the hours and days after exercise (Mancinelli et al., 2006; Smith et al., 1993; Zainuddin et al., 2005). Although the mechanisms by which massage might reduce DOMS are uncertain, it has been speculated that massage can decrease the inflammatory response to strenuous exercise by enhancing blood and lymph flow, which decreases the accumulation of fluid in the affected area (Mancinelli et al., 2006; Zainuddin et al., 2005). However, debate persists whether massage enhances muscle blood flow; indeed, some authors have suggested that massage increases skin blood flow and potentially diverts blood away from muscle (Hinds et al., 2004).

Although there are inconsistencies in protocols and findings between massage studies (Weerapong et al., 2005), massage could potentially mediate molecular process linked to inflammation and reduce tissue damage and accelerate recovery (Best & Crawford, 2017). For example, massage can decrease inflammation via stimulating an increase in neutrophils (Smith et al., 1993) whilst reducing cytokines and cortisol (Field et al., 2005; Rapaport et al., 2010). The current body of evidence suggests that post-exercise massage can help alleviate DOMS after intensive exercise (Guo et al., 2017). However, the reduction in DOMS could be brief, with one study suggesting the positive effects diminish within an hour (Andersen et al., 2013).

Effects on pain and performance

The mechanical action of massage could have pain-relieving effects due to a combination of neurological, biochemical and mechanical effects. A popular theory is that massage stimulates large nerve fibres and 'blocks' the smaller fibres that detect pain – this is known as the Gate-Control Theory (Mendell, 2014; Weerapong et al., 2005). Massage has also been shown to elicit similar effects to SS (see above) in increasing the parasympathetic response alongside reducing cortisol, which in turn leads to reduced pain and enhanced immune function (Field, 2014). Although post-exercise massage can reduce the soreness and pain associated with DOMS, there is insufficient evidence that it promotes quicker recovery of performance outcomes, such as strength and speed (Hemmings et al., 2000; Torres et al., 2012).

Psychological effects

Most post-exercise massage research has focussed on physiological and performance outcomes; however, post-exercise massage can also induce psychological benefits, such as improving perceptions of recovery after exercise (Hemmings et al., 2000). Massage likely elicits psychophysiological effects whereby the proposed mechanisms for reducing perceived DOMS and pain (see above) perhaps play a role in enhancing mood and perceptions of recovery after the massage. For instance, increases in the neurotransmitters serotonin and dopamine (Field et al., 2005) and augmented heart rate variability (see Chapter 5) could contribute to subjective improvements in relaxation and wellbeing (Meier et al., 2020).

Massage summary

Post-exercise massage can reduce ratings of muscle soreness and pain. However, these positive effects might be brief and do not seem to accelerate the recovery of performance outcomes. Massage likely exerts positive psychophysiological effects, which could promote feelings of perceived recovery and wellbeing. Massage does not appear to be detrimental to recovery outcomes. However, it is financially and practically unfeasible for most clients to have a massage after every training session. Therefore, more practical and financially viable strategies that mimic the effects of a post-exercise massage, such as foam rolling, have become established.

Foam rolling

Foam rolling (FR) is a form of self-manual therapy where the user compresses targeted muscles using a tool, such as a foam roller, massage ball or stick. With a foam roller, the individual uses his/her body weight to apply pressure to the soft tissues during a rolling motion. The pressure applied from FR can be used to mimic the pressure applied by a massage therapist; thus, FR is also known as self-massage. FR is performed as part of a warm-up and cool-down to increase mobility and reduce DOMS, respectively. As with massage, improvements in mobility and perceptions of muscle soreness/pain following FR have been attributed to hemodynamic (e.g., increased blood flow), mechanical (e.g., reduced tissue stiffness), neurological, and psychophysiological mechanisms (Aboodarda et al., 2015; Kelly & Beardsley, 2016; Phillips et al., 2018).

FR has been proposed to reduce or 'release' myofascial constrictions caused by scar tissue, muscle spasms and other pathologies; thus, the term self-myofascial release (SMR) is often used to describe FR. Although FR can influence tissue stiffness by changing blood flow, fascial hydration and thixotropic (gel-like) tissue properties, it is unlikely that FR provides enough pressure to significantly affect the mechanical properties of the fascia (Schleip, 2003). Accordingly, using the term SMR to describe FR is inaccurate (Behm & Wilke, 2019).

Effects of FR on the recovery of performance and delayed onset of muscle soreness

Numerous mechanisms have been proposed to explain how FR might reduce exercise-induced decreases in performance, reduce soreness and pain, and promote muscle relaxation (Behm & Wilke, 2019). The positive effects of FR are likely due to a combination of peripheral (e.g., increased blood flow and fascial hydration) and neurological effects. A recent meta-analysis reported that post-exercise FR appears to restore exercise-induced decreases in sprint and strength performance faster than passive recovery (Wiewelhove et al., 2019). Faster recovery of strength and speed after FR could be due to a quicker restoration of soft-tissue function, the restoration of central factors, or a combination of both responses (Wiewelhove et al., 2019).

Post-exercise FR has been consistently demonstrated to reduce perceived muscle pain and soreness following strenuous exercise (Cheatham & Baker, 2017; Wiewelhove et al., 2019). Various physiological, mechanical, neurological, and psychophysiological mechanisms (similar to massage) have been presented to explain how FR could decrease perceived muscle pain and soreness (Behm & Wilke, 2019). The central nervous system influences muscle tone, and some research indicates that FR could induce temporary neurological effects. For example, FR can induce a non-localised effect where the pressure applied from rolling the left leg can induce ROM improvements and decreased pain in the right leg (Cheatham & Baker, 2017). The pressure exerted on tissue from FR could also activate sensory receptors within the skin and muscle that could induce muscle relaxation by inhibiting sympathetic activity (Behm & Wilke, 2019). For instance, applying pressure to sensitive, tender spots (aka trigger points) within muscles could cause a brief and non-localised analgesic effect through the ascending pain inhibitory system – see Gate Control Theory, discussed above (Aboodarda et al., 2015; Cheatham & Baker, 2017).

In summary, FR can reduce the sensation of muscle soreness and pain, which could improve the user's comfort, readiness to exercise and subsequent physical performance. The physiological effects of FR are still being studied, and there is no consensus regarding the optimal method of rolling to enhance post-exercise recovery.

Foam rolling protocol

An optimal FR protocol has not been identified due to dissimilarities between studies (e.g., small sample sizes, participant characteristics, and methods). The intensity (pressure applied) of the rolling action should be individualised based on the roller's density and the client's tissue morphology and pain threshold. The optimal volume (number of rolls/duration) and intensity will be different for each client, and self-experimentation is required.

In general, users should begin rolling large muscle groups with slow motions to identify tender areas. Applying extreme or maximal pressure to a specific region should be avoided. Applying a high pressure is unlikely to disrupt fascial adhesions or scar tissue and could initiate counterproductive responses, such as increased heart rate and muscle tension (Behm & Wilke, 2019). When a tender area (a rating of ≥6 on a 0–10 pain scale) is identified, the user can maintain light pressure on the area for 30 seconds while concentrating on taking long and deep breathes to promote a parasympathetic response (Weerapong et al., 2005). When the perceived tenderness dissipates, active movements can be performed against the roller to target the tissues dynamically; for example, flexing the knee when applying pressure to the quadriceps. Most studies have implemented FR protocols that last 10–20 minutes, and it is possible that FR for three consecutive days (20 minutes/day) could provide a temporary decrease in muscle soreness and pain (Cheatham et al., 2015).

Compression

Compression garments and pneumatic compression devices are popular with athletes as a means of enhancing recovery. The general aim of compression garments is to increase blood flow and venous return, resulting in reduced inflammation and soreness (Brown et al., 2017). Recent evidence also suggests compression garments may decrease muscle oscillation during exercise (Broatch et al., 2020a) and enhance proprioception in individuals with poor proprioception (Broatch et al., 2020b). Pressure applied from compression garments generally increases from the distal to proximal portions of an arm or leg. This pressure increases venous blood flow resulting in enhanced removal of muscle metabolites, and reduced muscle damage and swelling. These effects on muscle damage are thought to increase repeat performance and reduce fatigue and soreness. From a performance recovery perspective, more research has been conducted on compression garments in comparison to pneumatic compression, with garments being shown to increase recovery of strength, power and cycling performance (Brown et al., 2017).

Pneumatic compression commonly involves compression applied to the legs or arms using sleeves that are inflated mechanically. The amount of compression applied by pneumatic devices is greater than compression garments. For example, mechanical, pneumatic boots apply up to 110 mmHg compared to ˜30 mmHg for compression garments (Winke & Williamson, 2018). Anecdotally, many athletes report enhanced recovery and reduced soreness when using pneumatic compression, but there is limited research to support increased recovery from these devices.

In general, compression garments should have a pressure of >20 mmHg to influence blood flow adequately, and they should be worn for at least 30 minutes after exercise. Recommendations for pneumatic compression are limited, so users should follow the manufacturers' guidelines.

Water immersion

Water immersion strategies such as cold-water immersion (CWI), contrast water therapy (CWT), and hot water immersion (HWI) are another popular recovery strategy for athletes. Each water immersion strategy elicits different physiological responses due to the differences in water temperature. Consequently, the aim of each strategy is slightly different.

Cold water immersion

CWI is typically performed in water ranging from 5 to 20°C, for 3–20 minutes, with immersions being performed either continuously or intermittently (Versey et al., 2013). CWI aims to reduce body temperature and blood flow leading to a reduction in swelling, inflammation and pain (Stephens et al., 2018).

Contrast water immersion

CWT involves alternating between CWI (5–20°C) and HWI (≥36°C) 3–7 times for 1–2 minutes per immersion (Versey et al., 2013). CWT aims to enhance blood flow, clear metabolic waste and reduce inflammation (Dupuy et al., 2018).

Hot water immersion

HWI involves immersion in hot (≥ 36°C) water for 10–24 minutes (Versey et al., 2013). HWI is believed to reduce muscle tension and increase blood flow to assist in the removal of metabolic waste and increase nutrient delivery to the cells (Versey et al., 2013).

Water immersion research

Research has generally demonstrated improvements in acute recovery (<72 hours) when using CWI and CWT, with less research examining HWI for recovery (Stephens et al., 2017; Versey et al., 2013). The question of the potential blunting of adaptation from long-term CWI usage has recently been examined (Poppendieck et al., 2020). The available evidence amongst recreational athletes suggests the chronic use of CWI may have small negative effects on strength training adaptations, such as strength and muscle hypertrophy (Poppendieck et al., 2020). Therefore, CWI should be carefully planned and periodised based on the client's short versus long term goals. For a review of the periodisation of recovery, refer to Mujika et al. (2018).

Placebo and belief effects

Several definitions exist for the term 'placebo' and 'the placebo effect'. All the definitions have limitations due to the placebo phenomenon's complexity (Shahar & Shahar, 2013). In this discussion, a placebo describes 'a treatment that has no direct physical effect, but may have a psychological effect' (Shahar & Shahar, 2013, p. 824). A 'placebo effect' is any beneficial effect attributable to the brain-mind responses to the context in which the treatment is delivered, rather than to the treatment's specific actions (Wager & Atlas, 2015).

A placebo is used in scientific studies to test an intervention's effectiveness and minimise the placebo effect. For example, in clinical drug trials, the participants' responses are compared against others taking a placebo (e.g., a sugar pill). Using a placebo enables researchers to understand if the treatment's effect was due to factors outside of the drug's medicinal properties (e.g., the participants' expectations). Historically, treatments that produced similar outcomes to placebo were thought to be ineffective (i.e., the placebo effect was not valued). However, research indicates that a placebo exerts several complex neurobiological effects that have real therapeutic benefits, such as increasing certain neurotransmitters and upregulating activity in specific brain regions (Halson & Martin, 2013; Wager & Atlas, 2015).

Studies that have investigated FR, water immersion and sleep extension have faced the difficulty of blinding (concealing) the participants to the treatment using a placebo, which increases the possibility of an (unmeasurable) placebo effect. Although the psychological effects of recovery strategies are challenging to measure, all the interventions discussed above could induce a meaningful placebo effect. In other words, the client's perception of the recovery method could influence its efficacy. For example, clients who believe or feel the recovery method has reduced their DOMS and musculotendinous stiffness (even if it has not physiologically) are likely to perform better in subsequent training (Cook & Beaven, 2013). Therefore, even without substantial scientific support, recovery methods may have positive effects if three criteria are met: (1) the client believes the method is beneficial; (2) the method does not have harmful effects; and (3) the method is practically viable (e.g., not too time-consuming or expensive).

Summary

Recovery is an essential component of the training and adaptation process. Several important physiological and psychological functions occur during sleep that facilitates recovery; therefore, all clients should be encouraged to achieve adequate sleep on a daily basis. Clients will vary in their ability to recover from exercise. The use of post-exercise recovery strategies can provide benefits to clients seeking to accelerate aspects of recovery, such as reducing perceived muscle soreness and pain. The regular use of some recovery methods, such as cold-water immersion, are more applicable to advanced level athletes and are typically unnecessarily for clients training to improve health and fitness. The mechanisms by which recovery strategies facilitate recovery are complex, but it is likely that all methods can improve perceived recovery, which could have a positive effect on clients' wellbeing and subsequent performance.

References

Aboodarda, S., Spence, A., & Button, D. (2015). Pain pressure threshold of a muscle tender spot increases following local and non-local rolling massage. *BMC Musculoskeletal Disorders, 16,* 265.

Andersen, L., Jay, K., Andersen, C., et al. (2013). Acute effects of massage or active exercise in relieving muscle soreness: randomized controlled trial. *Journal of Strength and Conditioning Research, 27*(12), 3352–3359.

Apostolopoulos, N., Lahart, I., Plyley, M., et al. (2018). The effects of different passive static stretching intensities on recovery from unaccustomed eccentric exercise—A randomised controlled trial. *Applied Physiology, Nutrition, and Metabolism, 43*(8), 806–815.

Barnett, A. (2006). Using recovery modalities between training sessions in elite athletes: does it help? *Sports Medicine, 36*(9), 781–796.

Behm, D., & Wilke, J. (2019). Do self-myofascial release devices release myofascia? Rolling mechanisms: a narrative review. *Sports Medicine, 49*(8), 1173–1181.

Best, T., & Crawford, S. (2017). Massage and post exercise recovery: the science is emerging. *British Journal of Sports Medicine, 51*(19), 1386–1387.

Broatch, J., Brophy-Williams, N., Phillips, E., et al. (2020a). Compression garments reduce muscle movement and activation during submaximal running. *Medicine and Science in Sports and Exercise, 52*(3), 685–695.

Broatch, J., Halson, S., Panchuk, D., et al. (2020b). Compression enhances lower-limb somatosensation in individuals with poor somatosensation, but impairs performance in individuals with good somatosensation. *Translational Sports Medicine.* Published online ahead of print.

Brown, F., Gissane, C., Howatson, G., et al. (2017). Compression garments and recovery from exercise: a meta-analysis. *Sports Medicine, 47*(11), 2245–2267.

Cheatham, S., & Baker, R. (2017). Differences in pressure pain threshold among men and women after foam rolling. *Journal of Bodywork and Movement Therapies, 21*(4), 978–982.

Cheatham, S., Kolber, M., Cain, M., et al. (2015). The effects of self-myofacial release using a foam roll or roller massager on joint range of motion, muscle recovery, and performance: a systematic review. *International Journal of Sports Physical Therapy, 10*(6), 827–838.

Cheung, K., Hume, P., & Maxwell, L. (2003). Delayed onset muscle soreness: treatment strategies and performance factors. *Sports Medicine, 33*(2), 145–164.

Cleak, M., & Eston, R. (1992). Delayed onset muscle soreness: mechanisms and management. *Journal of Sports Sciences, 10*(4), 325–341.

Cook, C., & Beaven, C. (2013). Individual perception of recovery is related to subsequent sprint performance. *British Journal of Sports Medicine, 47*(11), 705–709.

Cortis, C., Tessitore, A., D'Artibale, E., et al. (2010). Effects of post-exercise recovery interventions on physiological, psychological, and performance parameters. *International Journal of Sports Medicine, 31*(5), 327–335.

Davis, D., Ashby, P., McCale, K., et al. (2005). The effectiveness of 3 stretching techniques on hamstring flexibility using consistent stretching parameters. *Journal of Strength and Conditioning Research, 19*(1), 27–32.

Dupuy, O., Douzi, W., Theurot, D., et al. (2018). An evidence-based approach for choosing post-exercise recovery techniques to reduce markers of muscle damage, soreness, fatigue, and inflammation. *Frontiers in Physiology, 9*, 403.

Eda, N., Ito, H., & Akama, T. (2020). Beneficial effects of yoga stretching on salivary stress hormones and parasympathetic nerve activity. *Journal of Sports Science & Medicine, 19*(4), 695–702.

Farinatti, P., Brandão, C., Soares, P., et al. (2011). Acute effects of stretching exercise on the heart rate variability in subjects with low flexibility levels. *Journal of Strength and Conditioning Research, 25*(6), 1579–1585.

Field, T. (2014). Massage therapy research review. *Complementary Therapies in Clinical Practice, 20*(4), 224–229.

Field, T., Hernandez-Reif, M., Diego, M., et al. (2005). Cortisol decreases and serotonin and dopamine increase following massage therapy. *The International Journal of Neuroscience, 115*(10), 1397–1413.

Fyfe, J., Broatch, J., Trewin, A., et al. (2019). Cold water immersion attenuates anabolic signaling and skeletal muscle fiber hypertrophy, but not strength gain, following whole-body resistance training. *Journal of Applied Physiology, 127*(5), 1403–1418.

Guo, J., Li, L., Gong, Y., et al. (2017). Massage alleviates delayed onset muscle soreness after strenuous exercise: a systematic review and meta-analysis. *Frontiers in Physiology, 8,* 747.

Halson, S. (2014). Sleep in elite athletes and nutritional interventions to enhance sleep. *Sports Medicine, 44*(1), 13–23.

Halson, S., & Martin, D. (2013). Lying to win-placebos and sport science. *International Journal of Sports Physiology and Performance, 8*(6), 597–599.

Hemmings, B., Smith, M., Graydon, J., et al. (2000). Effects of massage on physiological restoration, perceived recovery, and repeated sports performance. *British Journal of Sports Medicine, 34*(2), 109–114.

Herbert, R., Noronha, M. de, & Kamper, S. (2011). Stretching to prevent or reduce muscle soreness after exercise. *Cochrane Database of Systematic Reviews, 7.*

Henschke, N., & Lin, C. (2011). Stretching before or after exercise does not reduce delayed-onset muscle soreness. *British Journal of Sports Medicine, 45*(15), 1249–1250.

Hinds, T., McEwan, I., Perkes, J., et al. (2004). Effects of massage on limb and skin blood flow after quadriceps exercise. *Medicine and Science in Sports and Exercise, 36*(8), 1308–1313.

Kelly, S., & Beardsley, C. (2016). Specific and cross-over effects of foam rolling on ankle dorsiflexion range of motion. *International Journal of Sports Physical Therapy, 11*(4), 544–551.

Kovacs, M., & Baker, L. (2014). Recovery interventions and strategies for improved tennis performance. *British Journal of Sports Medicine, 48,* i18–i21.

Krediet, C., Wilde, A., Wieling, W., et al. (2004). Exercise related syncope, when it's not the heart. *Clinical Autonomic Research, 14*(1), i25–i36.

Kruse, N., Silette, C., & Scheuermann, B. (2016). Influence of passive stretch on muscle blood flow, oxygenation and central cardiovascular responses in healthy young males. *American Journal of Physiology. Heart and Circulatory Physiology, 310*(9), H1210–1221.

LaRoche, D., & Connolly, D. (2006). Effects of stretching on passive muscle tension and response to eccentric exercise. *The American Journal of Sports Medicine, 34*(6), 1000–1007.

Lastella, M., Roach, G., Halson, S., et al. (2015). Sleep/wake behaviours of elite athletes from individual and team sports. *European Journal of Sport Science, 15*(2), 94–100.

Lastella, M., Roach, G., Vincent, G., et al. (2020). The impact of training load on sleep during a 14-day training camp in elite, adolescent, female basketball players. *International Journal of Sports Physiology and Performance, 15*(5), 724–730.

Law, R., & Herbert, R. (2007). Warm-up reduces delayed-onset muscle soreness but cool-down does not: a randomised controlled trial. *Australian Journal of Physiotherapy, 53*(2), 91–95.

Leeder, J., Glaister, M., Pizzoferro, K., et al. (2012). Sleep duration and quality in elite athletes measured using wristwatch actigraphy. *Journal of Sports Sciences, 30*(6), 541–545.

Lima, T., Farinatti, P., Rubini, E., et al. (2015). Hemodynamic responses during and after multiple sets of stretching exercises performed with and without the Valsalva maneuver. *Clinics (Sao Paulo, Brazil), 70*(5), 333–338.

MacDonald, J., MacDougall, J., & Hogben, C. (1999). The effects of exercise intensity on post exercise hypotension. *Journal of Human Hypertension, 13*(8), 527–531.

MacDonald, J. (2002). Potential causes, mechanisms, and implications of post exercise hypotension. *Journal of Human Hypertension, 16*(4), 225–236.

Mancinelli, C., Davis, D., Aboulhosn, L., et al. (2006). The effects of massage on delayed onset muscle soreness and physical performance in female collegiate athletes. *Physical Therapy in Sport, 7*(1), 5–13.

Meier, M., Unternaehrer, E., Dimitroff, S., et al. (2020). Standardised massage interventions as protocols for the induction of psychophysiological relaxation in the laboratory: a block randomised, controlled trial. *Scientific Reports, 10*(1), 14774.

Mendell, L. (2014). Constructing and deconstructing the gate theory of pain. *Pain, 155*(2), 210–216.

Mujika, I., Halson, S., Burke, L., et al. (2018). An integrated, multifactorial approach to periodisation for optimal performance in individual and team sports. *International Journal of Sports Physiology and Performance, 13*(5), 538–561.

Nuuttila, O, Kyröläinen, H., Häkkinen, K., et al. (2020). Acute physiological responses to four running sessions performed at different intensity zones. *International Journal of Sports Medicine, 42*(6), 513-522

Phillips, J., Diggin, D., King, D., et al. (2018). Effect of varying self-myofascial release duration on subsequent athletic performance. *Journal of Strength and Conditioning Research, 35*(3), 746–753.

Poole, D., Musch, T., & Kindig, C. (1997). In vivo microvascular structural and functional consequences of muscle length changes. *The American Journal of Physiology, 272*(2), H2107– H2114.

Popp, J., Bellar, D., Hoover, D., et al. (2017). Pre- and post-activity stretching practices of collegiate athletic trainers in the United States. *Journal of Strength and Conditioning Research, 31*(9), 2347–2354.

Poppendieck, W., Wegmann, M., Hecksteden, A., et al. (2020). Does cold-water immersion after strength training attenuate training adaptation? *International Journal of Sports Physiology and Performance,* 1–7.

Raeder, C., Wiewelhove, T., Schneider, C., et al. (2017). Effects of active recovery on muscle function following high-intensity training sessions in elite Olympic weightlifters. *Advances in Skeletal Muscle Function Assessment, 1*, 3–12.

Rapaport, M., Schettler, P., & Breese, C. (2010). A preliminary study of the effects of a single session of Swedish massage on hypothalamic-pituitary-adrenal and immune function in normal individuals. *Journal of Alternative and Complementary Medicine, 16*(10), 1079–1088.

Reilly, T., & Deykin, T. (1983). Effects of partial sleep loss on subjective states, psychomotor and physical performance tests. *Journal of Human Movement Studies, 9*, 157–170.

van Rensburg, D., van Rensburg, A., Fowler, P., et al. (2020). How to manage travel fatigue and jet lag in athletes? A systematic review of interventions. *British Journal of Sports Medicine, 54*(16), 960–968.

Rey, E., Lago-Peñas, C., Lago-Ballesteros, J., et al. (2012). The effect of recovery strategies on contractile properties using tensiomyography and perceived muscle soreness in professional soccer players. *Journal of Strength and Conditioning Research, 26*(11), 3081–3088.

Roberts, L., Raastad, T., Markworth, J., et al. (2015). Post-exercise cold water immersion attenuates acute anabolic signalling and long-term adaptations in muscle to strength training. *The Journal of Physiology, 593*(18), 4285–4301.

Romero, S., Minson, C., & Halliwill, J. (2017). The cardiovascular system after exercise. *Journal of Applied Physiology, 122*(4), 925–932.

Schleip, R. (2003). Fascial plasticity – a new neurobiological explanation: part 1. *Journal of Bodywork and Movement Therapies, 7*(1), 11–19.

Shahar, E., & Shahar, D. (2013). Causal diagrams, the placebo effect, and the expectation effect. *International Journal of General Medicine, 6*, 821–828.

Smith, L., Brunetz, M., Chenier, T., et al. (1993). The effects of static and ballistic stretching on delayed onset muscle soreness and creatine kinase. *Research Quarterly for Exercise and Sport, 64*(1), 103–107.

Stephens, J., Halson, S., Miller, J., et al. (2017). Cold-water immersion for athletic recovery: one size does not fit all. *International Journal of Sports Physiology and Performance, 12*(1), 2–9.

Stephens, J., Halson, S., Miller, J., et al. (2018). Effect of body composition on physiological responses to cold-water immersion and the recovery of exercise performance. *International Journal of Sports Physiology and Performance, 13*(3), 382–389.

Takahashi, T., & Miyamoto, Y. (1998). Influence of light physical activity on cardiac responses during recovery from exercise in humans. *European Journal of Applied Physiology and Occupational Physiology, 77*(4), 305–311.

Takahashi, J., Ishihara, K., & Aoki, J. (2006). Effect of aqua exercise on recovery of lower limb muscles after downhill running. *Journal of Sports Sciences, 24*(8), 835–842.

Tavares, F., Healey, P., Smith, T., et al. (2017). The usage and perceived effectiveness of different recovery modalities in amateur and elite Rugby athletes. *Performance Enhancement & Health, 5*(4), 142–146.

Thomas, K., Dent, J., Howatson, G., et al. (2017). Etiology and recovery of neuromuscular fatigue after simulated soccer match play. *Medicine and Science in Sports and Exercise, 49*(5), 955–964.

Thun, E., Bjorvatn, B., Flo, E., et al. (2015). Sleep, circadian rhythms, and athletic performance. *Sleep Medicine Reviews, 23*, 1–9.

Torres, R., Ribeiro, F., Alberto Duarte, J., et al. (2012). Evidence of the physiotherapeutic interventions used currently after exercise-induced muscle damage: systematic review and meta-analysis. *Physical Therapy in Sport, 13*(2), 101–114.

Versey, N., Halson, S., & Dawson, B. (2013). Water immersion recovery for athletes: effect on exercise performance and practical recommendations. *Sports Medicine, 43*(11), 1101–1130.

Wager, T., & Atlas, L. (2015). The neuroscience of placebo effects: connecting context, learning and health. *Nature Reviews. Neuroscience, 16*(7), 403–418.

Walsh, N., Halson, S., Sargent, C., et al. (2020). Sleep and the athlete: narrative review and 2021 expert consensus recommendations. *British Journal of Sports Medicine.*

Weerapong, P., Hume, P., & Kolt, G. (2004). Stretching: mechanisms and benefits for sport performance and injury prevention. *Physical Therapy Reviews, 9*(4), 189–206.

Weerapong, P., Hume, P., & Kolt, G. (2005). The mechanisms of massage and effects on performance, muscle recovery and injury prevention. *Sports Medicine, 35*(3), 235–256.

Wahl, P., Sanno, M., Ellenberg, K., et al. (2017). Aqua cycling does not affect recovery of performance, damage markers, and sensation of pain. *Journal of Strength and Conditioning Research, 31*(1), 162–170.

Wiewelhove, T., Döweling, A., Schneider, C., et al. (2019). A meta-analysis of the effects of foam rolling on performance and recovery. *Frontiers in Physiology, 10,* 376.

Wiewelhove, T., Raeder, C., Meyer, T., et al. (2016). Effect of repeated active recovery during a high-intensity interval-training shock microcycle on markers of fatigue. *International Journal of Sports Physiology and Performance, 11*(8), 1060–1066.

Winke, M., & Williamson, S. (2018). Comparison of a pneumatic compression device to a compression garment during recovery from DOMS. *International Journal of Exercise Science, 11*(3), 375–383.

Zainuddin, Z., Newton, M., Sacco, P., et al. (2005). Effects of massage on delayed-onset muscle soreness, swelling, and recovery of muscle function. *Journal of Athletic Training, 40*(3), 174–180.

Index